# Medical Photography

## Study Guide

Illustrated throughout by

**Mike Duffy**

Formerly Senior Medical Artist
Charing Cross Hospital Medical School

# Medical Photography Study Guide

Edited by

**Robin Williams**

A Publication of the London School of Medical Photography

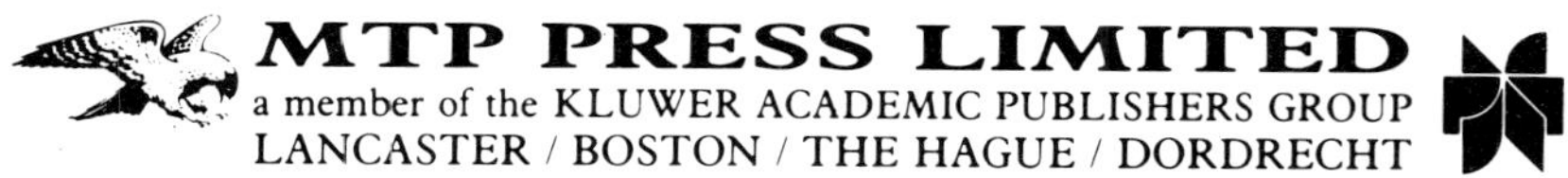
MTP PRESS LIMITED
a member of the KLUWER ACADEMIC PUBLISHERS GROUP
LANCASTER / BOSTON / THE HAGUE / DORDRECHT

Published in the UK and Europe by
MTP Press Limited
Falcon House
Lancaster, England

**British Library Cataloguing in Publication Data**

Medical photography study guide.–4th ed.
1. photography, Medical
I. Williams, Robin
610′.28 TR708

ISBN 0–85200–742–6

Published in the USA by
MTP Press
A division of Kluwer Boston Inc
190 Old Derby Street
Hingham, MA 02043, USA

**Library of Congress Cataloging in Publication Data**

Main entry under title:

Medical photography study guide.

"A publication of the London School of Medical Photography."
Bibliography: p.
Includes index.
1. Photography, Medical. I. Williams, Robin, 1952 Oct. 5– . II. London School of Medical Photography.
TR708.M43 1984 610′.28 84–7891
ISBN 0–85200–742–6



Printed in Great Britain by
Butler & Tanner Ltd, Frome and London

# Contents

# Contributors to the 4th edition

**Dr A.C. Branfoot**, MA, BM, FRCS, FRCPath.
Senior Lecturer in Histopathology
Westminster Medical School.

**Dr P.N. Cardew**, MRCS, LRCP, FRPS, FBPA, AIMBI.
Director of Audio-visual Communications
St Mary's Hospital and Medical School.

**K.P. Duguid**, FBIPP, FRPS, AIMBI.
Head of Medical Illustration
Westminster Hospital and Medical School.

**R.T. Fletcher**, AIMBI.
Formerly Head of Medical Photography
Institute of Ophthalmology and
Moorfields Eye Hospital.

**M.K. Johns**, FIMBI, ARPS.
Deputy Director of Medical Illustration
Institute of Child Health and Hospitals
for Sick Children.

**R.J. Lunnon**, MPhil, FBIPP, FRPS, AIMBI, SBStj.
Director of Medical Illustration
Institute of Child Health and Hospitals
for Sick Children.

**R.R. Phillips**, FBIPP, FRPS.
Head of Medical Illustration
Middlesex Hospital and Medical School.

**Carole Reeves**, FIMBI, ABIPP.
Senior Photographer
Institute of Child Health and Hospitals
for Sick Children.

**S.J. Robertson**, BA, ABIPP, ARPS, AIMBI.
Director of Medical Illustration
Institute of Dermatology and
St John's Hospital for Diseases of the Skin.

**D. Tredinnick**, FRPS, AIMBI.
Head of Medical Illustration
St Bartholomew's Hospital and Medical College.

**A.R. Williams**, MPhil, FBIPP, FBPA, FRPS, AIMBI.
Head of Medical Illustration and Teaching Services
Charing Cross Hospital and Medical School.

# Contributors to previous editions

**Dr W.F. Berg**
Kodak Research Laboratories
Harrow.

**Dr T.B. Boulton**
Department of Anaesthetics
St. Bartholomew's Hospital.

**Dr. R.J. Cureton**
Department of Morbid Anatomy
St. Bartholomew's Hospital.

**C.E. Engel**
Department of Medical Illustration
Guy's Hospital Medical School.

**Dr P. Hansell**
Department of Medical Illustration
Westminster Medical School.

**N. Jeffreys**
Department of Medical Illustration,
Institute of Ophthalomology.

**B. Jones**
Photographic Department
Guy's Hospital Dental School.

**Wanda Kimpton**
Department of Medical Illustration
Institute of Ophthalmology.

**D. Martin**
Department of Medical Photography
Hospital for Sick Children.

**Patricia Turnbull**
Department of Medical Photography
Charing Cross Hospital.

**R.J. Whitley**
Department of Medical Photography
Royal National Orthopaedic Hospital.

**E.V. Willmott**
Department of Medical Photography
London Postgraduate Hospital.

# Preface

The study of medical photography is fraught with difficulties. The small number of people involved professionally inevitably means that formal courses of instruction are both few and widely dispersed geographically. The student is, therefore, frequently faced with the prospect of a 'self learning' course of study. The few texts which exist are either hopelessly out-of-date or inadequate in depth or breadth of coverage. The knowledge required of a medical photographer in terms of medical conditions, their visual appearance and nomenclature is vast. Finding this information is difficult in conventional texts on medicine, which for obvious reasons, devote a large proportion of their content to such aspects as aetiology, differential diagnosis, treatment and prognosis. Much of the work on the specialized application of medical photography has been confined to publication in specialist journals. The serious student of medical photography, therefore, faces some difficulty.

This book was never intended to be an exhaustive treatise on the subject – its origins lie in the set of course notes issued to students of the London School of Medical Photography – and its present format is essentially the same, being a 'source book' and a 'guide to study'. The intention is that it should provide the student with a baseline of essential information and steer him in the right direction to further reading, as well as setting written and practical assignments. It is designed to assist students working for the qualifications of the British Institute of Professional Photography, the Institute of Medical and Biological Illustration and the Biological Photographic Association of America, but is equally suited to students studying for university or higher degrees in the subject. Unfortunately in order to keep the price of the book within easy reach of the student it has not been possible to include colour and tone illustrations but many excellent examples of these can be found in its sister volume '*A Guide to Medical Photography*', edited by Peter Hansell and also published by MTP Press.

Ample space has been left around the text for the student to make his own notes. The practical assignments and examination questions to be found at the end of each section are more than testing assignments – they are actually part of the learning process and once completed add to the body of knowledge presented in the text. Some of them are straightforward self-learning exercises, but some will require assessment and students are recommended to ask their Head of Department or senior colleagues in the profession for assistance.

This edition of the study guide contains over 600 references designed to cater both for the basic student and for the advanced worker needing a source for further information. No apology is made for some of the references being old – the information they contain is relevant to the contemporary student. Similarly 'well-known' sources have occasionally been omitted either because they are no longer available or simply because they are out of date. For the convenience of students on both sides of the Atlantic wherever possible references have been quoted from both *Medical and Biological Illustration* (or *Journal of Audio-Visual Media in Medicine*) and from the *Journal of the Biological Photographic Association*, even if they duplicate one another in content. The advanced student is strongly advised to consult these references for more specialized knowledge.

*Robin Williams*
*London, 1984*

# Acknowledgements

A work of this type is not possible without the help and cooperation of a large number of people and it would be remiss not to record special thanks to some of them here.

Firstly to fellow authors and contributors whose expertise made my work as editor easy; and to Mike Duffy my artist whose skilled interpretations have added immeasurably to the text. Secondly to the examinations boards of the Biological Photographic Association, The British Institute of Professional Photography and the Institute of Medical and Biological Illustration, whose examination questions acted as models for those set in this edition.

The onerous task of typing and preparing the manuscripts was diligently undertaken by Susanne Stevens, whose capable assistance and friendship I value immensely. I am deeply indebted to Dr Peter Hansell, FRCP, HonFRPS, HonFIMBI, FBPA, formerly Director of Medical Audiovisual Services, Westminster Medical School and Institute of Ophthalmology for his constant guidance, advice and constructive criticism. This project, and many others, would not have been possible were it not for his generosity as guide, mentor and friend.

Finally the greatest thanks of all must go to my wife Angela whose understanding and forbearance allowed me to concentrate on the book.

*Robin Williams*

# Foreword

There are very few texts on medical photography in the world. This is one which has survived through constant demand to enjoy four editions since the year 1960.

It has never been supplanted as an intensely practical and provocative *guide* to teachers and students alike. It is unique in giving direction in all sorts of ways – posing questions, but not giving answers; suggesting further reading without quoting from the literature; and setting practical tasks which provide their own particular challenge to the student. In this edition specimen examination questions have also been included.

To go back some way in time, the London School of Medical Photography was at first loosely formed in 1952 as a philanthropic association between the medical photographic or illustration departments of eight London teaching hospitals, largely as a self-protective measure, having the aim of ultimately generating a continuing flow of well-trained staff through the interchange of students; a foresighted policy as witnessed by the number of heads of present-day departments who have passed through the School at some time in the past.

Order soon prevailed and sections of the syllabus for the new Final Examination of the Institute of British Photographers in Medical Photography were duly apportioned to member departments of the School, which mounted a fifteen-month full-time course on a rotational basis for a limited number of students.

Rationalization was the next necessary step and the 'LSMP Study Guide', as it ultimately came to be called, began to take shape. At first it comprised no more than a series of telegraphic data sheets, issued at random as and when prepared by individual teaching units and handed out to students in attendance. These sheets were, however, prepared to a master pattern, but took over 3 years to complete in loose leaf form. Sections A–Z having been exhausted. Sections AA, BB, etc. were included as new topics were added to the curriculum and a whole new chunk on anatomy, physiology and terminology was soon in place to form the basis of the second edition.

Wider circulation and the notion of commercial publication forced the teachers of the school into the persuasion that the third edition should necessarily be made more readable – a dubious decision. However, this edition too survived to meet the demand of change.

The present editor's decision to return to an aggressive text, albeit expanded and more freely illustrated, is probably a wise one, thus producing a more detached work of universal usefulness and potential following.

Having been associated with this venture in one way or another since its inception and having cobbled together the first slender edition, it naturally affords me the greatest pleasure and pride to be invited to pen a few words of introduction to this virtually new work which will undoubtedly find favour wherever medical photography is taught or practised, and which will surely form the basis of several editions to come.

*Peter Hansell*
*Bath*

# Section 1
# The practice of medical photography

**A.R. Williams,** MPhil, FBIPP, FRPS, FBPA, AIMBI
Head of Medical Illustration and Teaching Services
Charing Cross Hospital and Medical School

## 1.1 THE USES OF MEDICAL PHOTOGRAPHY

All teaching hospitals and many non-teaching hospitals have medical photographic units. The work they do assists four main categories of hospital work: (1) Clinical, (2) Research, (3) Publication, (4) Teaching.

***(1) Clinical:***
The clinical work of a photographer is essentially the photography of patients, recording stages in the history of disease. In most cases, the object is to assist in assessing progress but occasionally the work may be diagnostic, as for example, in fluorescein angiography. These routine clinical photographs often provide material for medical research, publication and teaching.

***(2) Research:***
The features of photography which make it particularly useful in research are its ability:

- –to provide an objective record from which measurements can be made
- –to change magnification or time scale
- –to visualize events occurring outside the normal visual spectrum.

The photographs may be either an invaluable objective record or part of the research method itself.

***(3) Publication:***
Much of the photographer's work will involve preparing illustrations for books or journals. In order to provide good originals, an understanding of the graphic reproduction processes is essential. The importance of this is increasing because of the demands for domestic printing (for example by photo-offset lithography from typed originals).

***(4) Teaching:***
Prints, transparencies, tape/slide programmes, films and television tapes are the standard means of illustration in teaching. They must be prepared so as to reveal the specific points the teacher wishes to illustrate. In some cases, drawings are preferable to photographs and sometimes a combination of both is more effective.

In a busy teaching hospital the work may be difficult to classify in this way. For example, a photograph might be taken of a patient's leg as part of a research project on the healing rate of ulcers. The same photograph would be of immense value for assessing the patient's own progress, and may be used as part of a lecture to students on leg ulcers or indeed appear in a publication on the treatment of such conditions.

## 1.2 THE MEDICAL PHOTOGRAPHER

The photographer who works in a hospital community must develop or acquire a personality which fits him for the job. To be a responsible medical photographer demands qualities other than mere competence in photography. Within a hospital community the photographer has an important responsibility towards the medical staff whom he serves and more especially to patients who come under his complete charge for clinical photography. The following points are essential to the work of a hospital photographer.

***(a) Attitude to patients.***
Tact, understanding, infinite patience, and the avoidance of embarrassment are qualities required. It is essential that the photographer presents a professional image to the patient. This entails various factors such as personal appearance and dress, a firm precise manner of speech, kindliness without being condescending and above all an obvious efficiency which will inspire confidence.

***(b) Work in the operating theatre.***
There is a definite ritual attached to work in the operating room and the photographer must acquaint himself with the special clothing involved, sterile and unsterile areas and viewpoints which are accessible to him without risk. Explosion hazards should also be understood. Hyperefficiency is called for, as is the ability to work as part of the theatre team.

***(c) Morbid specimens.***
The handling of specimens, culture plates and potentially infectious material invariably forms part of the daily work. Precautions as laid down by your own institution must be observed. Various statutory regulations, such as the Health and Safety at Work Act and the Howie Code in the UK, affect the way this kind of photography is undertaken and they must be studied carefully.

***(d) Relations with medical staff.***
At all times the medical photographer must remember that he is primarily providing a service akin to radiology or pathology for the benefit of the medical staff and the patients under their care. He has therefore, to develop a sense of duty to the community in general and the service which he provides must be efficient, rapid and reliable, and at all times linked to the needs of the client. Never forget that were it not for the patients and doctors there would be no medical photography department. Always remember that the consultant has absolute jurisdiction over his patients and that even to ask a patient to stand, or give him a drink, could on occasions endanger his life.

***(e) Handling of equipment.***
Much of the material, either living or dead, which passes through the photographer's hands is likely to be irreplaceable, delicate, or valuable, and this factor must be borne in mind at all times. For this reason, the necessity for re-takes should be avoided wherever possible.

## 1.3 THE RANGE OF WORK

A study of the contents of this guide indicates the wide range of disease entities which a medical photographer may encounter. The recording of each of these may require the use of a particular approach and specialized photographic techniques. The more important of these techniques, such as infrared, ultraviolet, endoscopic photography etc. are also covered.

Patients may need to be photographed in the delivery room, studio, ward, clinic, operating room or autopsy room; all involve their own special problems. A medical photographer may take pictures of patients from before they are born until after they die, in all states of health and disease.

Anatomical and morbid specimens are frequently recorded by photography both to show their gross appearance and also their structure under the microscope. Bacterial and viral cultures as well as immunological and biochemical methods are ephemeral and require permanent records of their appearances.

Apparatus and instruments may need to be demonstrated. Radiographic reproduction and flat copy work, particularly of graphs and tables, are of great importance. As the numbers involved can be very great, standardization and semi-automated techniques may need to be adopted.

Photography is frequently involved in recording instruments. In many instances, particularly with modern automated equipment, this will be operated by non-photographic staff, but the medical photographer will be expected to give expert advice on the photographic design of such equipment and on the photographic aspects of its operation.

The medical photographer can usefully extend the range of visualization that can be encompassed by the doctor. The physical scale can be altered for example, by enlarging microscopically small subjects with photomacrography or photomicrography or by reducing large – scale artwork to microscopically small dimensions by microphotography for the custom-made manufacture of electronic microchips. The timescale of events can be changed for example, by high-speed photography which can slow down the vibration of the vocal cords, or by time-lapse photography which can speed up the growth of a bacterial culture. Photography can extend the spectral sensitivity of the eye into for example, the ultraviolet region where melanin pigmentation is clearly delineated or into the infrared region where venous patterns beneath the skin are revealed. Small changes in refractive index hidden to the medical researcher can be revealed for example, by schlieren photography which is able to show the flow of heat around the body or by photo-elastic stress analysis which is able to show stress patterns in diseased joints. Photography can be used to measure patients as for example, in photogrammetry where tumour volume can be measured, or in reflection densitometry where skin surface roughness can be quantified.

In addition to his specialist skills the medical photographer will be expected to be a proficient general photographer taking portraits of VIPs, architectural shots of buildings and advertising pictures for promotional brochures.

Apart from pure photography, the medical illustration department frequently organizes projection and other lecture theatre services and now extends its influence into the wider aspects of audio-visual aids and automated self-teaching, including computer assisted learning with interactive videotape. Frequently the medical photographer will be working in conjunction with the medical artist, audio-visual technician and television engineer to produce a wide range of instructional material.

Finally, a medical photographer should be capable of not only designing his own department, but also should be able to give advice on the design of lecture theatres and teaching areas.

## 1.4 BASIC CLINICAL PHOTOGRAPHY

As stated previously the object of photographing patients is either to assist in assessing progress or to provide material for medical research, publication and teaching. These primary aims of clinical photography demand that the photographs are of the highest standard as regards technical qualities; sharpness of detail, clarity of image, use of lighting, perspective and the accuracy of reproduction of both colour and form.

The general technical photographic skills common to the production of good photography are essential to the establishment of a basic technique. In addition, specific details and modifications are necessary due to the subject being a sick person. In order to fulfil its purpose the photograph must:

(1) Provide an accurate record
(2) Be comparable with others taken over a period of time
(3) Be obtained with the least inconvenience to the patient
(4) Meet the intention of the request
(5) Be in accord with current methods of presenting medical data.

Arrangements in the studio or on the wards; the choice of camera and lenses; choice of backgrounds and of film and lighting and positioning of the patient are all parts of the basic technique and are considered here together with some aspects of printing and presentation.

### 1.4.1 The Studio

For clinical photography the studio should be large enough to allow for adequate camera–subject distances. For example, it must permit the use of the correct focal length lens when photographing the standing patient full length. In the absence of a separate film/TV studio, the general studio must have sufficient length for filming the walking or standing figure.

To allow for such filming and to provide enough clear space for clinical photography including, if desired, space for backlighting an illuminated background, a studio should have minimum dimensions of:

Length: 9 metres, Width: 5 metres, Height: 4 metres.

The standard room height of around 3 metres is severely limiting, preventing the use of a full range of lighting technique and precluding the use of ceiling mounted equipment such as background rolls.

There is no doubt that in an ideal situation many special forms of photography carried out in a department would have their own particular space and equipment. Photography of the teeth and photography of the eyes are examples. The nearer one can get to this ideal the better, as constant changing over of equipment and rearrangements of the studio space is very time wasting. The use of portable screening for temporary divisions in the studio can enable more than one photographer to work at the same time. Thus one large studio may be divided into two and then opened out again when required.

It is essential that accommodation for lighting equipment, background rolls, camera stands and so forth should be as convenient as possible for both the photographer and the patient. If headspace allows, the overhead suspended lighting system should be considered as offering both convenience and safety. It is essential that the studio can be blacked out totally when necessary.

### 1.4.2 Cameras

Camera equipment available on the market changes with the times, and choice of any particular model will be determined largely by financial considerations. It is not the object of this guide to suggest individual cameras or manufacturers but whatever equipment is chosen it must be capable of producing photographs which meet the requirements given in the introduction to this section. Thus, particular care must be given to:

(1) Image quality
(2) Suitability for making records to definite and repeatable scales
(3) Ease of operation
(4) Portability
(5) Ability over a wide range of image magnification
(6) The range of film stock available
(7) Accuracy of the screen image and the ease of viewing.

For many years the most popular choice of format for clinical photography was the 5″ × 4″ view camera complete with a full range of camera movements. The choice was made to give the highest possible quality while yet not being too unwieldy. At the same time, however, all departments use 35 mm cameras for the production of transparancies. The increased quality of equipment and film now obtainable in the smaller formats, together with the financial constraints and greater quantity of work required, has led many departments to adopt the 35 mm format for all clinical photography.

The amount of close-up work required in clinical photography and the need for really accurate viewing at short distances dictates that the single lens reflex camera is the apparatus of choice. It has the following advantages:

(1) Extremely portable, ideal for working on wards and in operating rooms
(2) Ease of handling, especially when working to scale or with children
(3) Has a large range of lenses, extensions and other accessories
(4) Economy of film costs and a wide range of available emulsions.

Loss of quality when using 35 mm equipment has often been put forward as an argument against its use but most workers are now agreed that good technique and careful quality control will give results indistinguishable from large format negatives, when prints not larger than 30 × 20 cm are required.

### 1.4.3 Choice of lenses

In basic photography of the patient the size of the subject field extends from the maximum height of the full length figure down to, for example, the area of a single eye, to be photographed at a magnification of 1:1. This range will need to be covered both in the studio and in the ward. In the operating theatre the range will be rather less, though even here it is possible to have to photograph the whole body, as for example in the case of extensive burns. Whatever camera system is used it is essential to have available lenses to cover the above. This will usually mean:

For 35 mm format – 35 mm, 50 mm, 100 mm
For 6 × 6 cm format – 65 mm, 85 mm, 120 mm
For 9 × 12 cm (5″ × 4″) format – 90 mm, 150 mm, 200 mm.

The high proportion of close-up pictures required, coupled with the need to maintain working distances sufficient to avoid exaggerated perspective, make the lens of longer than standard focal length extremely useful. When using a 35 mm system, for example, a 100 mm lens can be mounted on a suitable bellows extension to give focussing from 1:1 to full length. Such a combination will cover the subject areas likely to be required in the theatre without the need to change lenses. Almost the same range is available from some manufacturers in the form of 'Macro' lenses which have an extension sufficient to give a magnification of 1:1 at the closest working distance. These lenses have the useful additional feature of being marked with magnification ratios, which is most useful in achieving standardized results.

Several manufacturers supply what they call 'medical' lenses which are essentially macro lenses with a built-in ringflash facility. Whilst these are valuable for cavity, intra-oral and operative photography the

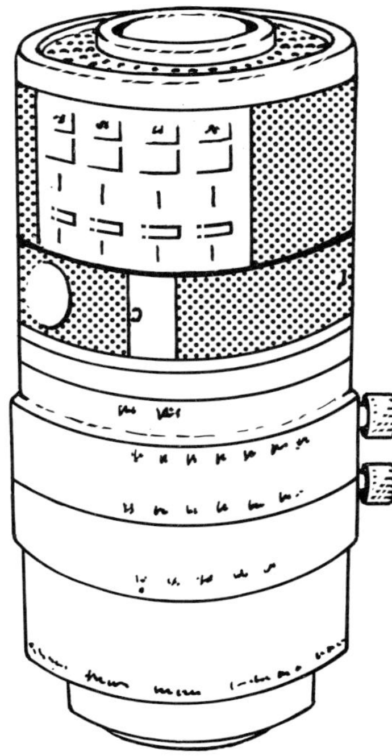

***Figure 1.1*** *The Nikon medical Nikkor lens is especially designed for medical photography in that it has a long focal length, built-in ringflash and a range of supplementary lenses to give fixed reproduction ratios down to very close ranges*

flat lighting and low output of the ringflash makes them unsuitable for the majority of clinical photographs.

Wide angle lenses are necessary to deal with the occasions when full length pictures are required in restricted conditions, as for example when photographing the patient confined to bed.

For speed of working all lenses must have fully automatic diaphragm control and the smaller the minimum aperture the better. The maximum aperture is not of prime importance here since adequate lighting will be available for focussing except in rare and special cases. For use in the operating theatre the zoom lens may have some merit but in studio work possible distortion and problems of scaling may arise. It is preferable to use fixed focal length lenses.

### 1.4.4 Lighting

Attainment of good photographic quality depends more on lighting technique than any other part of the photographic procedure. It is the key to excellence in medical photography just as in other branches of photography although the principles of photographic lighting may have to be modified to suit the medical subject.

Lighting must achieve several aims in its 'natural' portrayal of the medical subject. It must clearly demonstrate the contour, shape and outline of the lesion and surrounding anatomy. The basic component of photographic lighting is the modelling or 'key' light. This is usually a directional source which is positioned to cast shadows to show contour and shape. Shadows should always be cast downwards to preserve a natural appearance. The keylight alone will produce a lighting contrast ratio which is too high. Therefore the shadows cast are 'filled-in' with a soft 'flood' type lamp which is positioned at a point close to the lens axis, and at a distance which will lower the lighting ratio by the appropriate amount for the film in use.

After key – and fill-in lighting are positioned, effects lights may then be placed in position. These are used to stop the subject being lost against a dark background. Effects lights include back light and side light. These principles may be followed irrespective of the type of lamp used, although electronic flash lamps with proportional modelling lights are of great value in assessing how the light is cast. Directionality or softness is usually achieved by changing the type of reflector used on the electronic flash head.

The shape of the human body dictates that certain departures from the above technique are necessary. Cavity lighting,

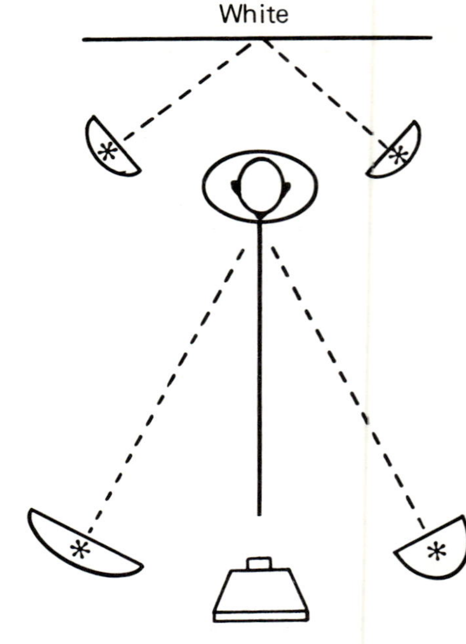


***Figure 1.2*** *White backgrounds must be illuminated evenly without flare. Simple clinical photography can be accomplished with a single key light and a single fill-in floodlight*

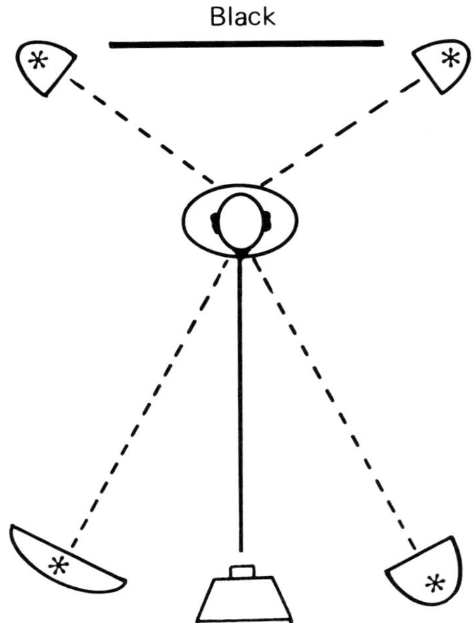


***Figure 1.3*** *Black backgrounds demand that the subject has some back-light or rim-light to lift it from the background. Otherwise key and fill are the same as for a white background*

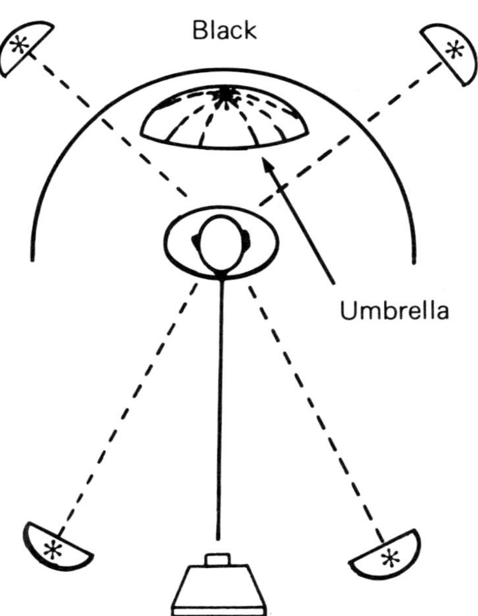


***Figure 1.4*** *A 'pool' of front– and back-light can be used with a curved black background to give a very flexible arrangement. The lights remain fixed while the subject/photographer move around to obtain the desired viewpoint. This is especially useful for children*

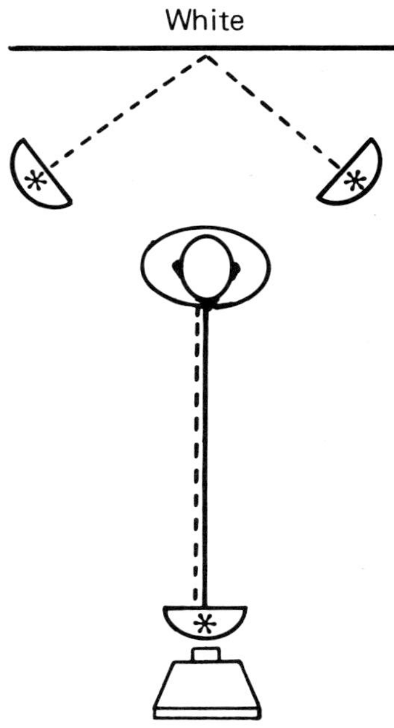


***Figure 1.5*** *A single axially placed front light can be used with advantage. It is highly standardized, gives reasonable modelling and darker edges to the subject which are ideal for an illuminated white or coloured background*

infrared lighting and endoscopy are cases which illustrate this point. In straightforward clinical photography deviations from the basic lighting technique are usual in order to demonstrate a lesion or limb against backgrounds which differ in tone, e.g. black backgrounds demand effects lights which rim-light any part of the limb, whereas the outline of the body will be lost by rim-lighting against a white background. White backgrounds need a lighting set-up which provides a darker outline of the patient than the white background.

Complex lighting set-ups are difficult to repeat, therefore the simplest arrangements should be used whenever possible. Many departments advocate a single flash head with a white background separately illuminated as being the most suitable and easily repeated lighting.

For cine and television it is still necessary to use tungsten lamps of the photoflood or tungsten-halogen type, which are hot, of comparatively low intensity and are unstable for colour balance. Remember when filming patients that the heat can at times become unbearable. Metal objects in the field view, e.g. instruments in the operating field, have been known to get so hot they inflicted serious burns.

Remember also that flash may alarm children or the elderly but usually no problems occur if the patient is warned and shown what is about to happen. Constant intensity enables exposure charts to be calibrated for each lens/film combination.

Special lamps include ringflash and texture lights, both of which are dealt with in the sections on cavity photography and photomacrography.

Wherever possible trailing leads to lights should be avoided – the risk of elderly patients tripping over them is too great. This can be done by using ceiling mounted lights which are attached to a gantry to allow positioning and by using only one synchronization cable to the camera and firing all the other sources by remote slave cells.

### 1.4.5 Backgrounds

The choice of background needs careful consideration. Its purpose is to exclude other subjects, or parts of the subject, so as to focus the attention on the object in question, and to provide adequate contrast with the subject. Choice of background, therefore, is inextricably linked with lighting technique.

A plain white background will flare if over illuminated and show shadows if under illuminated, whilst a black background rarely reproduces well and requires rim-lighting to prevent the loss of subject edges in shadow. Coloured backgrounds may induce colour casts and are very difficult to standardize. Generally a background suitable for monochrome work is unsuitable for colour; therefore some compromise has usually to be effected.

A slightly off-white background is ideal for all subjects and can be illuminated independently of the subject to reproduce as white regardless of subject size or emulsion choice. Meticulous care needs to be exercised, however, to avoid flare. Some departments advocate mid-grey as the all purpose background being equally suitable for colour or black-and-white and for light or dark subjects.

For colour photography either pale blue or green are often recommended. Green reflects 50–75% of the incident light and therefore affords a light background and the persistence of vision from red (which most medical subjects are) is green, so it is particularly restful on the eye. (Hence the choice of green for operating room gowns and towels.)

Various specialist backgrounds can be devised, such as large transilluminated ones, or ones with grids etched on them for patient measurement. The further the patient is from the background the easier it is to independently control the lighting and obtain a harmonious and uniform background.

Where different backgrounds are used for monochrome or colour work the change from one to the other should be easy (e.g. pull-down background stored on ceiling mounted rolls). Ideally backgrounds should also be disposable – or at the very least easily cleaned and disinfected. If a continuous paper roll is used for background and floor make certain it cannot slide on a slippery floor surface and endanger the unstable or elderly patient.

### 1.4.6 Choice of film

Like other branches of photography, medical photography utilizes a wide range of film emulsions so that the widely differing subjects may be reproduced satisfactorily as prints or transparencies. Unlike many other branches of photography however, black-and-white emulsions still play an active part in medical photography where a monochrome print for the patient's notes can be just as useful as a colour print and much more economic.

Panchromatic emulsions are now the routine for all monochrome clinical photography and may be used to show detail in dark-red or red tissues respectively, e.g. 'varicose' ulcers. Conversely pale skin lesions such as erythema or contact dermatitis may not show up well against the surrounding normal skin. Detail in human tissue photographed on panchromatic film will be less sharp than with film of non-red sensitivity because of diffusion of the deeply penetrating red light. The use of a deep cyan filter, however, overcomes this problem and often gives a much enhanced result – very similar to that which used to be obtained by using orthochromatic emulsions.

Colour films vary considerably in their rendering of individual colours and each person interprets colour differently. For these reasons selection of a colour film for medical subjects is bound to be subjective. However, selection of film is generally based on the rendering of red and also the skin tone. An added factor influencing choice is film speed. Certain colour films may be suitable for specific purposes. An example of this is a medium speed film which has exceptionally good rendition of red which would be very suitable for photography of surgery. Inherent colour contrast may also influence choice of a film.

Modern colour films are increasingly reliable and consistent, especially in regard to manufacturing and processing standards, but perhaps the greatest inconsistency lies in batch-to-batch colour matching. Often, medical photographers will not have a sufficient quantity of film to make accurate colour processing in the department a viable proposition. A reliable laboratory is therefore essential and it must also provide an 'urgent' service. In sending any clinical photographic material out for processing confidentiality of the records becomes a problem. Discretion must be used and some laboratories make special arrangements in this respect for dealing with medical photographs. The most satisfactory method of controlling colour balance is to bulk-buy the film stock, test for the necessary filtration for the camera lenses, then store the stock of film in a domestic fridge. It is also necessary to include a control colour wedge on the first frame of every film used to assess the colour balance of the processing or any shift in colour temperature of the lighting.

Some hospitals resort to placing specially mounted colour transparencies in the case notes but in most cases a colour print will be preferred. Colour fidelity and permanence are, however, serious worries with colour prints. The choice of emulsions is vast and every individual has his own preferences, but in medical photography, where insufficient light is rarely a problem, it is usual to choose a slower, higher resolution film with good tone and colour rendition.

There are, of course, several specialist films for such applications as photomicrography or infrared photography but these are dealt with in the appropriate sections.

### 1.4.7 Development

Due to the considerable contrast variations in medical subjects some variation of development contrast must be achieved. This can be done by using two, or more, developers with different inherent contrast characteristics, or less drastic variation gained by alteration of either dilution or period of development. Skin is low in contrast – especially in the young child – and will require a considerable contrast boost in a developer of high contrast characteristics. Morbid specimens, radiographs and apparatus are typical of subjects which require lower development contrast as the subject contrast may be high.

Standardization of processing is, however, the key factor – time, temperature, agitation, etc. must all be fixed for any one type of subject so that the doctor is furnished with a consistently accurate record.

### 1.4.8 Printing and presentation

Quality of printing and presentation is an important factor, because not only does the quality of the finished print affect the interpretation and usefulness of the result but also the way in which the print is presented is important. In so far as the mechanics of printing is concerned, medical photography has few requirements which do not occur in general photography.

Attention must be given to accurate scaling and positioning of the image within the format so that, for example, in three photographs of the face (AP, L. Lat., R.Lat.) the features of the face such as the eyes and tip of the nose are at the same level in each print. To be able to do this, attention must be given at the camera stage to frame the image so that sufficient background is available. Maintaining scale in a set of prints may demand attention before commencing to print. For example, in a set of three prints of the full head (AP, L. Lat., R.Lat.) the lateral must be framed before the AP shot, due to the difference in width accommodated by the lateral head as opposed to that taken up by the AP head.

Balance of the image size within print or slide format becomes more than just an aesthetic consideration with medical subjects. Distortions, or apparent distortions, may occur if the edge of the image coincides with, or lies near to, the edge of the format.

Presentation of medical photographs, whether in the case notes or in medical exhibits, should be a clean, well executed operation and not 'fussy', out of alignment or poorly stuck. Due consideration must be given to the colour of the mount, especially when presenting colour prints, (grey or pale green being the colour choice), and where a number of photographs with lettering are to be shown, a balance between the print size and the mount size must be struck. Mounts for case notes should contain the patient's full details, preferably typed, and in designing a mount for this purpose the method of retaining the photographs in the notes must be considered as well as the position of the prints on the mount in relation to the 'tethered' side, e.g. it may be desirable to design the mount so that prints are mounted at one side of the mount for easier access.

### 1.4.9 Management of the patient

(See also Section 2 Care of the patient)

#### (a) *Attitude*

A clinical photographer is not only concerned with obtaining a technically good picture, but must be able to do so without causing distress to the patient. Furthermore, if the patient feels relaxed and co-operative the photographer's task is much eased. One should always remember that not only may a patient be feeling ill, but that for many people a hospital is an unfamiliar place, full of strange equipment, much of which seems to be designed to produce discomfort or pain. The medical photographer must, therefore, have a sympathetic attitude and put the patient at ease from the moment he enters the department.

### (b) *Prepare the equipment*

When he comes to enter the studio, ensure that trailing wires and equipment are not left cluttering the floor to trip up the patient. Think through the complete photo session and have all the equipment that you need in a state of complete readiness so that you do not have to leave the patient in order to load a camera back or find some retractors.

### (c) *Prepare the patient*

Smile at the patient, welcome him by name and explain clearly what you are going to do and what you require of him. Assess what clothing and jewellery, etc. needs to be removed and tell the patient clearly what you would like him to remove. Unless there are strong reasons to the contrary, clothes, make-up, watches and other jewellery should never appear in a clinical photograph. Such exceptions would be where distress would be caused to the patient or where the clothes etc. were relevant to the purpose of the picture. If necessary, modesty can usually be preserved by the use of plain towels. Where all the clothing is to be removed, provide a dressing gown, and ask the patient to change into it prior to the actual photography.

### (d) *Good techniques:*

When a bright light has to be used, particularly on a patient's face, don't position the light first and then switch it on. It is less disturbing to switch on while the lamp is pointing away from the patient and then to turn it gradually towards the patient's face. Do not leave a hot lamp, such as a spotlight, pointing at a patient for an unnecessary length of time. You are not in the axis of the beam and may fail to appreciate its intensity. When using a flash source close to a patient's face, don't overtax the patient's tolerance. A view of both eyes followed by a close-up of each eye are three pictures. If these were colour transparencies required in quadruplet, you would be submitting the patient to twelve flashes close to his face. In such circumstances, it *may* be preferable to take a single shot of each view and then make duplicates from the transparencies.

When positioning patients, be quite clear in your own mind as to what you are trying to achieve, the exact angle and the extent of the view. If you are uncertain, the patient will find it difficult to follow your directions. It may be helpful to point to a spot on a wall for the patient to look at or to demonstrate the action you require in, for example, filming a patient's gait. Decisions concerning the choice of viewpoint and positioning of the patient are affected by two criteria. Firstly, the need to standardize so that comparable records can be made over a period of time, both in relation to one patient, and also to enable comparable pictures to be achieved in a series of patients. Secondly, the need to show the condition to its best advantage in a single view, so as to make a good 'teaching' picture. It may well be that the two criteria of a standardized record and the best possible single picture are not compatible, so that if both objectives are to be met, separate pictures must be taken. Work out a routine that you can follow so as to avoid unnecessary movements from camera to patient. For example, have both camera and lights ready aligned before starting – position the patient – adjust the lighting – then return to the camera for final adjustments and take the picture. Such routine is particularly important if the position required of the patient is uncomfortable for him to maintain for more than a short period. Remember that you are not dealing with a paid professional model.

Some positions, such as the extreme range of joint movement, may be impossible to maintain for more than a few seconds. In such cases, first ask the patient to demonstrate and form an estimate of the area to be covered by the camera and the exact viewing angle needed. Set up the camera, test again on the focussing screen, make any final adjustments required while the patient relaxes. The photograph can then be taken with confidence when the patient repeats the movement.

During the photography talk gently to the patient in a reassuring manner. If the session is to be long, explain each step as you go and check that your patient is not overtired.

If you need to touch the patient, e.g. to insert retractors or speculum, wash your hands and make certain you are using sterile equipment – it is important psychologically for the patient to know that you are scrupulously meticulous in this respect. (*See Section 5.6 for a detailed description*).

If you need to process the negative before the patient leaves the department, e.g. when doing a specialized technique such as infrared photography, make sure that the studio lights are turned off and that the patient is comfortable and not left where he may cause injury to himself. If in any doubt, an assistant should remain with the patient.

### 1.4.10 Requirements for standardization

Before deciding on a system of standardization a decision must be taken on the degree of accuracy which is to be achieved. At one end of the scale are routine pictures which need merely to look comparable when seen as a series. At the other end of the scale are pictures to be used for taking accurate measurements in, for example, pre-operative osteotomy planning or in somatotyping.

In the first case a routine procedure using a hand-held camera and capable of being followed by all members of a department would be adequate, whereas the latter would involve the meticulous use of measuring instruments, mechanical frames for positioning and the use of a large format camera.

A balance must be struck between the effort involved and the purpose of the pictures. However, a routine procedure itself saves time since decisions are largely pre-determined by a set of existing rules which can be followed by any member of the department. The clinical condition requires a certain view which in turn dictates a set scale of reproduction which then dictates a set exposure under known conditions. Every patient who attends for photography must be regarded as a potential candidate for serial recording, so it is imperative that the photographer not only uses a standardized technique but also keeps meticulous records of all the data necessary to repeat the result.

In any scheme of standardization, the following factors must be considered:

(1) Film emulsion, processing, printing and presentation
(2) Lighting and backgrounds
(3) Viewpoint
(4) Scale and perspective

(*1 and 2 have already been discussed*)

#### *(3) Viewpoint*

Antero-posterior (AP) and postero-anterior (PA) views are symmetrical viewpoints if both left and right sides of the body are to be included. Great care must be taken to position the camera centrally

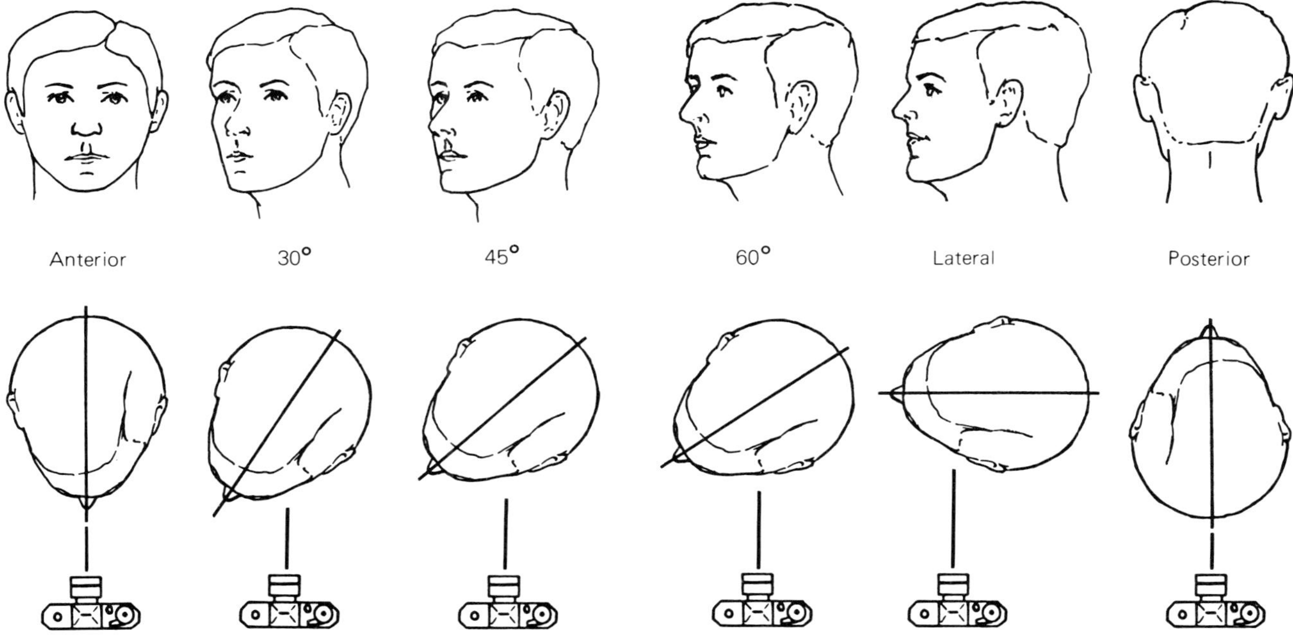


***Figure 1.6*** *A standardized series of views for photography of the head*

with its film plane parallel to the patient. Small variations in contour can sometimes only be detected by a comparison with the normal side so that if the camera is not positioned symmetrically error may easily be introduced. With lateral views an anatomical feature should be chosen to position centrally on the lens axis. For instance with a full head the external auditory meatus provides such a point while for a closer view of the face, the outer canthus of the eye is frequently used. Angled views are more difficult to standardize without going to the lengths of using a protractor but can sometimes be achieved by using the coincidence of two anatomical figures, such as the tip of the nose and the edge of the cheek.

A frequent error is to select too close a viewpoint. Many diseases are only revealed in relation to a surrounding area of normality. For example, an oil folliculitis of the forearms should be seen in relation to its absence on the upper arm. Too close a viewpoint may also give rise to difficulties in interpretation of a picture in which there are only slight and diffuse alterations in contour outline. The closer the picture 'frame' is to the contour of the subject, the more likely is any slight inaccuracy in camera symmetry to affect the observer's interpretation. A slightly more distant viewpoint will produce a good area of plain background against which subject asymmetry is readily seen. In general, it should be emphasized that the slighter the change, the larger the area of normal body contour which is needed to reveal it.

Comments on particular standardized viewpoints and their use are given throughout the sections on specialized clinical photography, but it is highly desirable to have a standard set of views for each particular area of the body you regularly photograph. It is recommended that you either have a standardization chart or you have example photographs of all the standard positions displayed on the studio wall (out of sight of the patient), or in a 'techniques' album, which you can compile for yourself. Whilst it is possible for you to devise all your own views it is desirable to consult the medical staff you serve to ascertain what standard views would be of most use to them.

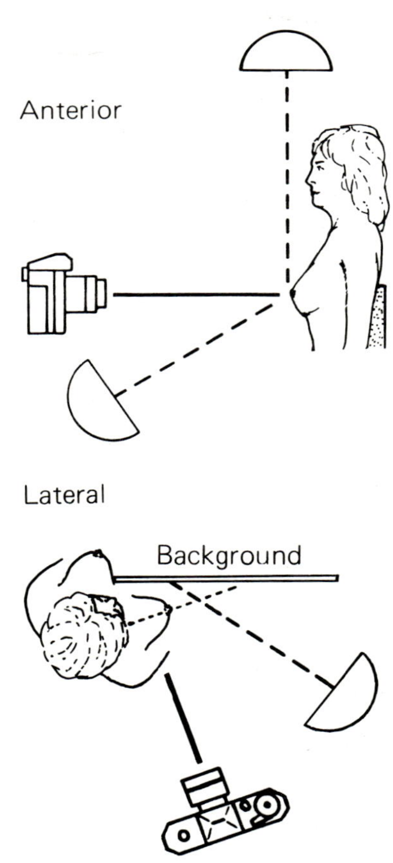


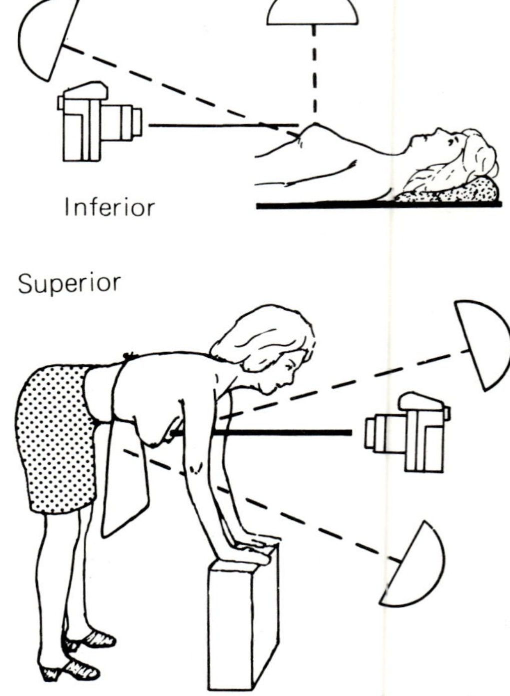


***Figure 1.7*** *A standardized series of views for the female breast would include anterior, lateral, superior and inferior views. Note the technique used in each case and that a lateral view of the breast is not necessarily a lateral to the body as a whole*

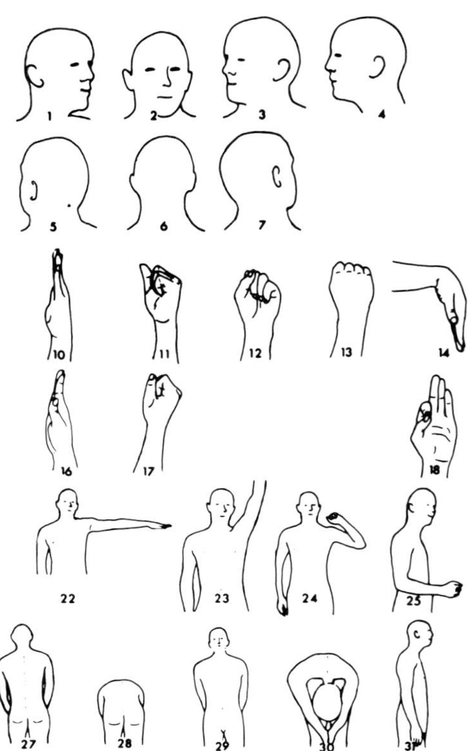


***Figure 1.8*** *An example of part of a chart showing standardized viewpoints; in this case from the Institute of Orthopaedics*

### (4) *Scale and Perspective*

Most clinical pictures can be taken to one of a range of fixed magnifications (these are in practice all fractions and therefore some prefer to use the term 'reduction scales'). One suggested set is the **'Westminster reproduction ratios'** given in the following table, but you could easily design your own system.

WESTMINSTER REPRODUCTION RATIOS FOR STANDARD ANATOMICAL REGIONS:

| | 35 mm slide | 13 × 18 cm print |
|---|---|---|
| Full length figure | 1:50 | 1:10 |
| Upper half-length | | |
| Lower half-length | 1:25 | 1:5 |
| Torso | | |
| Chest | | |
| Abdomen | | |
| Head and shoulders | | |
| Upper arm and shoulder | 1:15 | 1:3 |
| Forearms and hands | | |
| Thighs and knees | | |
| Knees and feet | | |
| Inguinal region | | |
| Face | | |
| Hands | 1:10 | 1:2 |
| Feet | | |
| Joints and neck | | |
| Any close-up | | |
| Fingers | | |
| Two eyes | 1:4 | 1:1 |
| Genitalia | | |
| Intra-oral | | |
| Ear | 1:2 | 2:1 |
| Tongue | | |
| Fingernails | | |
| Single eye | 3:4 | 3:1 |
| Big close-ups of lesions | | |

**Notes:**

(1) These recommendations refer to FINAL IMAGE SIZE, however derived.

(2) The scales are based on the largest convenient image size consistent with patient's records and the ability to mount more than one view on an A4 (297 × 210 mm) mount. Scales for 35 mm transparencies refer to the standard 24 × 36 mm format.

(3) Most of the areas will be contained in a 18 × 13 cm print. Exceptions are the upper height ranges of full and half-length figures.

(4) In the case of children up to the age of 2 years, divide the right hand figure by 2 when necessary, e.g. on full and half-lengths. Apply adult scales over the age of 2.

(5) Both lens-to-subject (principal plane) and lens-to-film distances must be checked in relation to these calculations.

(6) It is recommended that a centimetre scale (in the principal plane of focus) and an identity number be recorded on all negatives. This may even be desirable on some transparencies.

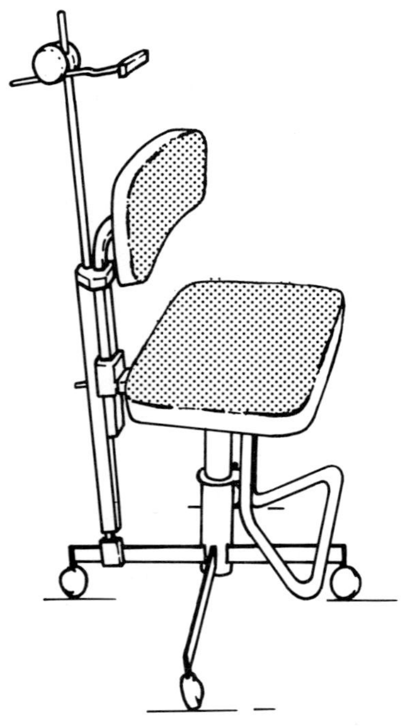

***Figure 1.9*** *A special studio chair with facilities for rotation and accurate location of anterior and lateral positions as well as a headrest*

Calculations needed to obtain a magnification factor involve both subject–camera distance and the focal length of the lens. Perspective is governed solely by the camera–subject distance (*see Section 22.1*), so that photographs taken at a specific magnification ratio are only strictly comparable if both these factors are identical. However, in practice, a slightly different combination of focal length and subject distance can be tolerated for the more distant views. At closer distances, such as when photographing a head, when m = 1/10 with a 35 mm camera, a focal length of at least double the diagonal of the picture should be used so that a more distant perspective can be maintained. This is particularly important with regard to the head, as the picture will include a considerable depth (i.e. from the tip of the nose to the back of the ear). Under these conditions small inaccuracies of camera – subject distance will result in obvious changes in perspective which would go unnoticed in a subject with less depth.

The conventional method of 'working to scale' is to present the camera distance according to the chart and then move the camera until the image is sharp. Most modern macro lenses are calibrated in reproduction ratios such as 1:10, 1:8, 1:4, etc. for working in this manner. Having pre-determined the scale of reproduction, and therefore the camera-distance, it is possible to fix the lights relative to the camera position. This can be achieved by using special brackets, or by the expedient use of a length of string attached to the light. For any one choice of emulsion therefore, each magnification will have a set *f*-number e.g. 1:15 = *f*/8, 1:10 = *f*/11 or 1:4 = *f*/22–32. This system is easy and convenient to use even by the most inexperienced staff; but does give a highly standardized end product.

### 1.4.11 The teaching transparency

Whereas standardization requires working to pre-determined rules, the teaching picture requires an understanding of the relevant visual pathology and the use of imagination to show as many facets as possible in a single picture. It can be very difficult for the clinical photographer (trained to produce highly standardized results) to forget the rules and tell a story with pictures. In some conditions such as contact dermatitis, the aetiology may need to be emphasized and an unusual positioning of the patient may be essential. An example would be a rubber dermatitis in an office worker with one lesion on the wrist over which he often slipped a rubber band and another on his calf caused by the rubber threads woven into the top of the socks. The story cannot be told by using standard views – it is necessary to show the rubber band *in situ* and to show the legs with one sock up and one down – perhaps a single picture showing the patient pulling up the socks. The same is true of any occupational disease. Pre-patella bursitis could be recorded by standardized AP and Lat views of the knees but an interesting addition would be a transparency showing the patient kneeling at his work of carpet laying. In orthopaedic conditions the limitation of movement can be revealed by showing the patient attempting to carry out a familiar action such as holding a cup. In diseases with a psychiatric element, the patient's facial appearance, demeanour and clothes may all contribute to the story that the picture has to present. In dermatitis artefacta for example, it is important to show that the lesions are all in areas accessible to the patient's own hands and that the middle of the back is free of disease.

If in doubt it is always better to take **both** the standard representational view and the imaginative teaching view. The latter does, however, require considerable knowledge of pathology.

## 1.5 CLINICAL PHOTOGRAPHY ON LOCATION

The general principles of clinical photography still apply when working on location in the ward or operating room, although it will be much more difficult to control the conditions of photography; the patient will be much less mobile and the equipment must all be portable. Trips away from the department can be very time consuming, so try to group together your visits to the wards, for example, so as to avoid unnecessary travel.

### 1.5.1 The ward

With this type of photography the patient is much more likely to be 'ill' and thus less able to co-operate, while the inadequate space available and obtrusive background objects will all cause difficulties. The photographer must time his visits to fit in with ward routine and an appointment should always be made by telephone before visiting the ward. The bed should be screened so that the patient has privacy. If possible, these screens should be neutral to avoid colour casts if they have to be close to the area being photographed. If you have to ask patients' relatives to leave the bedside do so politely and give them some indication of the time you will

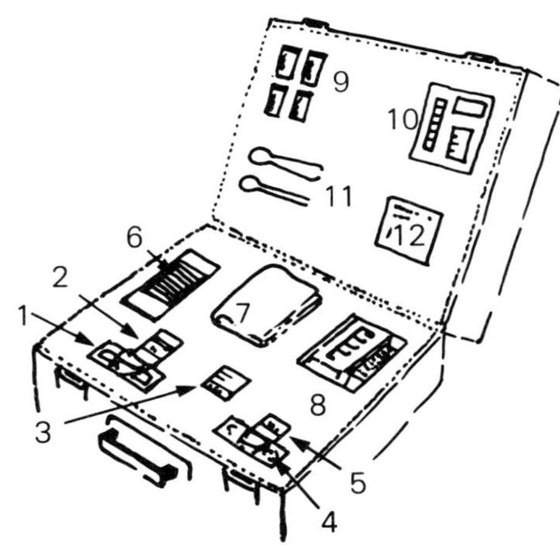


1 S.L.R. camera for colour work
2 105 mm macro lens
3 30 mm wide angle lens
4 S.L.R. camera for black & white work
5 55 mm macro lens
6 Bellows or extension rings
7 Green surgical towels
8 Portable electronic flash
9 Spare film
10 Standard grey card & colour wedges
11 Tongue depressors, retractors etc
12 Photographic record cards

***Figure 1.10*** *A portable suitcase loaded with all the equipment needed for clinical photography on location*

require. On arrival it is imperative to tell the nurse in charge that you are about to see the patient. Ask if there are any special features about the patient you are to photograph.

Before setting out for the ward, make sure you have all the equipment you will require. Most departments have a case with a portable camera and lenses (preferably 35 mm SLR) especially reserved for ward work. For dealing with small areas such as a forearm, a portable background such as a surgical towel can be taken. Otherwise considerable ingenuity will be required to keep backgrounds uncluttered. Because of the limited space available, full-length pictures will require the use of wide angle lenses. Illumination will generally be by portable flash-unit; since these do not have built-in modelling lamps be very careful to consider the nature of the background and possible reflections from gloss painted wall causing obtrusive highlights.

If necessary, ask a nurse to help you to turn a patient or hold a background. Wherever possible try to work with the patient on his bed – it is far more convenient for both of you. If you have to stand over the patient, on a bedside chair for example, make sure that you are firmly supported and that all equipment is secure. Before you leave the ward replace any furniture or equipment that you have had to move and inform the ward sister that you have finished. Complete any necessary documentation, e.g. patient record card before you leave the ward and forget the details.

### 1.5.2 The operating room

Surgical operations are carried out in a room (operating theatre) or suite of rooms especially designed for this purpose, and under sterile conditions. That is to say conditions which prevent or strongly inhibit the growth of germs. It is, of course, impossible to achieve totally sterile conditions in a general operating theatre but everything that can be made sterile is rendered so by various methods. In modern operating suites filtered positive pressure air conditioning is installed, thereby preventing, as far as possible, airborne infections from coming into the theatre. Each hospital has its own rules and regulations for theatre procedure. This section can only give general guidelines but the student is advised to contact the theatre administrator in his own hospital to discuss what particular regulations he should observe.

Two different categories of people work in operating rooms. There is the surgical team, all of whom are 'scrubbed' and therefore sterile, along with their instruments and apparatus. Working with them are non-sterile personnel, such as anaesthetists, some of the nursing staff and also theatre technicians. The medical photographer forms part of the latter group.

All drapes, gowns, trolleys, instruments and so forth are strictly sterile and must never be touched by anyone who is not themselves 'scrubbed-up' and dressed in sterile clothing. The photographer must understand that the 'non-touch' attitude is a vital part of theatre behaviour. If, by accident, a sterile trolley or gown is inadvertently touched by anything unsterile, this must be reported at once, so that sterile conditions can be re-established immediately. Before entering the operating theatre the photographer must change completely into special clothing and footwear, also a cap and mask. Hair, face and hands should be clean. It is usually sufficient if photographic apparatus taken to the theatre is wiped over with a damp cloth which has previously been soaked in disinfectant. This does not, of course, sterilize the apparatus but ensures that any dust adhering is removed. (Never take apparatus which has been used either in the post-mortem room or to photograph highly infectious materials directly to the theatre.)

It is generally preferable to photograph from the surgeon's viewpoint. This can sometimes be done over the surgeon's shoulder but on occasions it may be necessary for the surgeon to move so that the photographer can get close enough to take the photograph. (It is on both these occasions that great care must be taken not to brush against the drapes covering the patient, the instrument trolley or the surgeon.)

If serial still photographs (or cine film) are to be taken throughout the operation, the same viewpoint should be maintained wherever possible. Photographs taken from different angles can be extremely difficult to orientate, particularly if removal of part or all of an organ has taken place. Unless close-up views of a particularly small area are required, the scale of the photographs should remain the same throughout the series.

Care should be taken to see that there are no loose leads on any electrical apparatus, as sparks from faulty connections could cause an explosion. Always check with the anaesthetist that no explosive anaesthetic is being used, before photography commences. In the past, when ether and its derivatives were used extensively, the risks of explosions in operating rooms were considerable. Today the main anaesthetics in use are ethrane, fluothane, nitrous oxide and cyclopropane, all of which are administered in conjunction with oxygen. Of these only cyclopropane (which is used mainly in paediatric surgery) is explosive. If trolleys with rubber wheels are used they must be anti-static to prevent charges building up and causing sparks.

By experience, you will discover whether or not you need to alter your exposure to take account of any operating spotlight the surgeon may be using, whilst you are taking photographs. It is not generally necessary to do so, but you should be aware of the possibility of green casts appearing at wider operating apertures from the green line in the mercury vapour discharge tubes.

A 35 mm single-lens-reflex camera with flash attached as close to the lens axis as possible and hand held is the easiest system to use. Because the average size of the field to be covered is approximately 35 × 25 cm or under, the most suitable lens is a 100 mm (or 135 mm) with appropriate extension rings or bellows. Either of these lenses give comfortable working distance. Sometimes it will be impossible to approach the subject closely enough to obtain a satisfactory result, as for example, in open-heart surgery. On these occasions one can use a mirror mounted in the middle of the operating lamp and take the photograph from the side with a long telephoto lens. Ideally the mirror should be surface silvered and one must remember that the image will be laterally reversed.

It is very important to make certain that all attachments such as lens-hood, ring-flash and so forth are firmly attached and cannot fall off into the operating field. The photographer should adopt a routine of inspecting his apparatus for loose connections before he approaches the patient. It is particularly necessary in operating theatre photography to take with you all that you are likely to need for the job. Once you are in the theatre you cannot leave to go and collect say another lens without having to change your clothes on going, and on re-entering the theatre. Do not forget to take a photographic request form with you, so that you can fill in details of the patient's name, age, diagnosis, film used and so forth.

One problem which can occur in the operating theatre is condensation on spectacles and on camera lenses and viewfinders. This is due to the high humidity and warm atmosphere interacting with cold glass. The problem of spectacles can be overcome by wiping them with an anti-condensation fluid and by the use of face masks with a thin metal strip which folds round the nose and under the spectacle frame. Condensation will only take place on cameras and lenses if they are cold, so make sure that these are at room temperature before use.

Speed and accuracy in this work are essential. Whilst waiting to take photographs look at the operating field and try to orientate the anatomy and to decide what you are likely to be asked to photograph. Pre-set your apparatus and be ready to take your pictures as quickly as possible.

Any stool or steps that the photographer requires to use in order to obtain the right viewpoint should be absolutely rigid. Never attempt to stand on any 'made-up' piece of equipment, for the consequences of over-balancing are too serious to be contemplated. Grey or green drapes round the operating field are better than white. The latter when clean can cause flare and when they become blood stained can make the picture look more 'bloody' than is necessary. In orthopaedic surgery operations are carried out in a 'blood free field' i.e. a tourniquet is applied. This causes the tissues to appear white and lacking in contrast. It may be necessary to underexpose in the region of half to one stop in order to produce a more acceptably exposed transparency. Conversely in deep abdominal or chest incisions it may be necessary to open up half a stop, particularly if the field is especially dark in colour. In very 'bloody' fields, such as for example, an operation for pinning the femur, try to persuade the surgeon to cleanse the area so that bone and muscle may be easily differentiated.

The completed picture should contain only what was requested to be demonstrated and should not be cluttered with any unnecessary swabs, instruments, hands and so forth. The surgeon must be persuaded to remove these before photography – he will appreciate your advice when he sees the results.

### 1.5.3 The clinic

On occasions it may be necessary to go to the out-patient clinic to photograph a patient; as for example in documenting minor operative procedures, such as releasing fluid from a chalazion or setting a broken limb. Photography in the clinic is, however, generally unsatisfactory and wherever possible the doctor should be encouraged to send patients to the studio. The same problems that are found on the ward are found in the clinic – restricted space, poor background control and difficulty in lighting the patient adequately; the solutions are also the same. Clinics do rely on an efficient turnover of patients so one should not monopolize a consulting room for too long. Be quick but thorough - this is not like the ward where your visit may well provide a welcome diversion for the patient.

### 1.5.4 The post-mortem (or autopsy) room *(See also Section 15.1)*

To the new medical photographer this can be one of the most distressing kinds of photography – particularly if one has previously photographed the patient on the ward, or in the case of forensic pathology. Detachment comes with experience and the cadaver is no longer a person. Medicine would have progressed little if it were not for the efforts of pathologists investigating the disease process. The medical photographer should not touch the cadaver or fresh specimen – ask the pathologist or technician to move and orientate as necessary. The same rules apply as in operative photography: it is imperative that sufficient anatomy is shown to enable the viewer to orientate himself. Unlike the operating room the PM table rarely moves up or down so a sturdy pair of steps are an invaluable aid.

The principal difficulty is lighting. It is usually only possible to use a single hand-held flashgun, which is unsatisfactory in many respects. Specular reflections from the shiny/wet surfaces mask a good deal of important detail. Deep cavities, such as when working in the thorax or abdomen, are even worse – often requiring a ring-flash which then gives circular specular reflections all over the tissues. It is possible to overcome the problem by using 'crossed' polarizing filters: one over the camera lens, and one polarized at 90° to the first over the flash-head, but there is a serious loss of light and the result looks very 'flat' and lifeless. The best advice is to aim the flash such that the specular reflections do not overlie the important pathology. (A penlight torch taped to the flash-head can be a most useful aid in this task).

Backgrounds are also a problem in that the wet specimen 'leaks' fluid onto the background giving an unsightly appearance. One way of overcoming this problem is to use a 'wet' background e.g. a green surgical towel soaked in saline then stretched out on the floor or table. Although this reproduces rather dark it has the merit of not showing blood or other fluid leaks. After working in the PM room it is a wise precaution to clean your equipment with surgical spirit and change your white coat for a clean one. The risks of cross-infection are too serious to ignore this simple precaution.

## References

Antoniades, S. and Hochheimer, B. (1980). Developing films for high speed, high resolution and high gamma. *J. Biol. Photogr.*, **48**, 167-173

Berry, E.C. and Kohn, M. (1972). *Introduction to Operating Room Technology.* 4th edn. (New York: McGraw Hill)

Bowens, B.A. (1978). A simple method of including a one-millimetre grid in a photograph. *J. Biol. Photogr. Assoc.*, **46**, 13-14

Duguid, K.P. (1971). Remote photography of cardiac surgery via a membrane mirror. *Med. Biol. Illustr.*, **21**, 73-74

Ellison-Nash, D. (1973). *The Principles and Practice of Surgery for Nurses and Allied Proffessions.* (London: Edward Arnold)

Ericksson, S. *et al.* (1971). Photgraphic trauma. *Med. Biol. Illustr., **21**, 211–214*

Fletcher, R. (1969). Automatic theatre cameras. a review. *Med. Biol. Illustr.* **19** (Suppl.) 36-43

Gilson, C. and Parbhoo, S. (1981). Standardized serial photography in the assessment of treatment of advanced breast cancer. *J. Audiovis. Media Med.*, **4**, 5-10

Hansell, P. (ed.). (1979). *A Guide to Medical Photography.* (Lancaster: MTP Press)

Hansell, P. and Duguid, K. (1970). The use of membrane mirrors in surgical photography. *J. Biol. Photogr. Assoc.*, **38**, 176-178

Hansell, P. and Ollerenshaw, R. (1969). *Longmore's Medical Photography.* (London: Focal Press)

Kent, P. *et al.* (1978). Intra-operative photography – a sterile system. *Obst. Gynaecol.*, **52**, 365-368

Kodak. (1972). *Clinical Photography.* (Publication N. 3.) (Rochester, NY: Eastman Kodak)

Kodak. (1981). *Filters for Scientific and Technical Uses.* (Publication B.3.) (Rochester, NY: Eastman Kodak)

Maehr, C. (1975). Surgical photography through sterile bags. *J. Biol. Photogr. Assoc.*, **43**, 23

Marshall, R. (1957). Photographic background control. *Med. Biol. Illustr.*, **7**, 13–21

Marshall, R. and Marshall, B. (1975). Routine medical photography with 35 mm black and white film. *Med. Biol. Illustr.*, **25**, 115-119

McCausland, T. (1980). A method of standardization of photographic viewpoints for clinical photography. *J. Audiovis. Media Med.*, **3**, 109-111

Morris, M., Giannavola, S. and Williams, G. (1980). Techniques for photography of cardiovascular surgery. *J. Biol. Photogr.*, **48**, 159-162

Pearce, E. (1967). *Instruments, Appliances and Theatre Technique.* (London: Faber and Faber)

Ray, R. (1979). Surgical photography through a periscope. *J. Biol. Photogr.*, **47**, 133-135

Turner, B. (1977). Theatre photography – routine not ritual. *Med. Biol. Illustr.*, **27**, 159-162

Vetter, J. (1979). Standardization for the biomedical photographic department. *J. Biol. Photogr.*, **47**, 3-18

Vetter, J. (1980). Standardization for the biomedical photographic department. *J. Audiovis. Media Med.*, **3**, 44-53

Williams, A.R. (1979). Conversion of panchromatic to orthochromatic sensitivity by selective filtration. *Med Biol. Illustr.*, **27**, 185-186

## Practical projects

(1) Photograph the head and shoulders of a colleague in anterior and both lateral aspects, in colour and black-and-white. Then repeat the same photographs a few weeks later. Make a note of any difficulties you encounter and of all the factors you consider important in achieving a standardized result.

(2) Photograph a large subject, such as a full length human, against a black-and-white background in both colour and black-and-white. Take special note of the different lighting techniques needed to give a good result in each case.

(3) Photograph a human head in anterior aspect with 35, 50 and 135 mm lenses on 35 mm film. Produce a set of matching black-and-white prints with the inter-pupillary distance set the same. Make notes on your observations on the results.

(4) Photograph a reddish skin lesion (a) on panchromatic film, (b) on panchromatic film with a cyan filter over the lens. Produce a matching pair of black-and-white prints. Write notes on the results.

## Examination questions

Q.1 Describe fully the ways in which photography supports the medical profession, giving examples of techniques where appropriate.

Q.2 In a large teaching hospital, in what circumstances might it be advisable for non-photographic personnel to do their own photography instead of using central services.

Q.3 Provide lecture notes for a descriptive talk you might give to school leavers on medical photography as a career.

Q.4 'Photography may be used as a medical research tool': justify this statement.

Q.5 An outlying hospital wishes to do its own colour photography of surgical operations. The camera is to be operated by non-photographic staff. Discuss the desirable characteristics of the equipment that you would purchase for this purpose.

Q.6 Discuss the feasibility and merits of an appointment system for clinical photography.

Q.7 Discuss the factors which need to be considered when choosing backgrounds for clinical photography and describe how the choice of background will affect the choice of lighting technique.

Q.8 Discuss draping, surgical dressings, clothing and jewellery with respect to clinical photography.

Q.9 What parts do viewpoint and focal length play in the perspective rendering of the finished photograph? Describe ways of controlling perspective in standardized clinical photography.

Q.10 The production of serial records of a patient over a number of years is fundamental to medical photography. Discuss the general problems involved, illustrating your answer by reference to a particular disease with which you are familiar.

Q.11 Suggest working systems for achieving standardized results in black-and-white photography under the following headings:
(*a*) Reproduction ratios on negatives
(*b*) Intra- and inter-patient comparison
(*c*) Negative processing
(*d*) Printing and finishing.

Q.12 You are requested to make regular visits to wards in your hospital to take photographs of patients. State what equipment you would select for this purpose and give reasons for your choice. What additional problems would you expect to encounter with a patient who is barrier nursed.

Q.13 Discuss the problems involved in photography in the operating theatre. What risks exist and what action would you take to minimize these? What points would you discuss with the surgeon and his team to ensure maximum co-operation?

Q.14 The pathology department requires you to photograph extensive malignancies of the abdominal organs during a post-mortem. Describe fully your technique and any problems you may expect to encounter.

*Multiple choice (any of the statements may be true or false)*

Q.15 You are called to the operating theatre to take 35 mm colour transparencies during the course of a thoracotomy with mitral valve replacement:
(*a*) Once you have changed it is safe for you to come into contact with the surgeon and sterile trolleys.
(*b*) You can safely use an electronic flash as opposed to expendable flash bulbs in the presence of an explosive anaesthetic.
(*c*) If using a camera stand on rubber insulated wheels it should be earthed.
(*d*) A 5 cm wide-focussing range lens would be unsuitable for close-up pictures of suturing the valve.

Q.16 You have been taking serial colour transparencies with a 100 mm lens set at *f* 8 and the camera at 4 feet from the subject. This lens has been damaged and you must now use a 50 mm lens. However, you have available a 5 cm extension ring and a 2× converter. You can now achieve the same scale with the 50 mm lens and the 2× converter:
(*a*) But the extension ring must be used,
(*b*) With the camera at 4 feet from the subject,
(*c*) But double the camera exposure is required,
(*d*) But with the aperture set at *f*/8 the depth of field will be greater,
(*e*) But the perspective will be different.

Q.17 Whilst photographing a patient on the ward your usual flashgun which has a guide number of 40 with 25 ASA film (in feet) breaks down. You have to use a replacement gun with a guide number of 55.
(*a*) At 5 feet the exposure with the original flashgun was *f*/8 using 25 ASA film.
(*b*) At the same distance, and with the same film, the new flashgun requires an aperture of *f*/16
(*c*) Double the guide number means double the light output.
(*d*) Using a 0.3 neutral density filter over the head of the replacement flashgun will give it the same light output as the original.
(*e*) When using the new flashgun with film of 100 ASA it would have a guide number of 110.

Q.18 Perspective is an essential consideration in clinical photography:
a) Changing the focal length of the lens without altering the viewpoint changes both the image size and the perspective.
(*b*) Changing the object distance always changes the perspective.
(*c*) Altering the object distance without changing the focal length alters both the perspective and the image size.
(*d*) Two photographs of a patient at 1:10 magnification will have identical perspective whatever lenses they were taken on.
(*e*) The correct viewing distance for a 10″ × 8″ print from the whole of a 5″ × 4″ negative taken with a 6″ lens is 9″.

Q.19 Clothing in clinical photographs is generally unacceptable:

(*a*) To photograph a case of hypogonadism correctly the patient must remove all his clothes

(*b*) All the clothing may be left on for post-operative rhinoplasty photographs.

(*c*) In some cases of dermatitis it may be advantageous to have a photograph which includes some of the clothing.

(*d*) To record keratoconus correctly the patient must strip to the waist.

(*e*) The cine recording of a characteristic gait may be done fully clothed.

# Section 2
# Care of the patient and ethical considerations

**R.J. Lunnon** MPhil, FBIPP, FRPS, AIMBI, SBStJ
Director of Medical Illustration
Institute of Child Health and Hospitals for Sick Children

## 2.1 INTRODUCTION

It should never be forgotten that the main purpose of any hospital is the care and treatment of the sick. It should then follow that the most important consideration in patient photography is the patient himself. In subsequent sections, methods of photographing various conditions and diseases will be discussed and specialized techniques of photography explained. However, before these are tackled, the student must first try to gain an understanding of his patients and learn to assume a responsible attitude towards them.

You should understand that illness, combined with hospital surroundings and feelings of uncertainty as to what photography entails will make the patient need your care and reassurance to a much greater extent than he would if he were well. It is always wise to realize that your patient may sometimes be much more ill than he looks. Also that what you have been asked to photograph may not be the main cause of the patient's disease (e.g. the photography request form may ask for a lesion on the patient's ear to be recorded but he may be in hospital primarily for treatment of a heart condition). Try to cultivate an awareness of and concern for the patient that will become second nature to you, so that you may, for example anticipate the unexpected actions of children or very elderly people, in sufficient time to prevent an accident.

## 2.2 PATIENT MANAGEMENT

Every patient is an individual personality and may require a different approach in order to obtain his full co-operation. One may need firm authoritative handling while another responds better to the kindly reassuring manner.

You will learn, as you become more experienced, that patients with different diseases will require different handling. Take, for example, the advanced hypothyroid patient who may feel cold in a heatwave and slow in his movements while the hyperthyroid patient may be jumpy, talkative, and complain of the heat. These patients are not just being awkward and difficult, it is their diseases which produce these symptoms.

The patient's first impression of you is important. A smile is always welcoming as is a courteous greeting. Make the patient feel that you have plenty of time for him. It is very easy sometimes, in a busy clinic or if you are rushing to complete a task, to forget that you are photographing a person, not just a disease but a human being who is very probably apprehensive of you and of what he thinks you are going to do to him.

During a photographic session you are the one who knows what is going to happen, so it is up to you to give the patient sufficient information to reassure him that he will come to no harm in your care. Tell him what you want him to do, in simple terms. It is important that you speak clearly and explain precisely what you mean to the patient – this may mean speaking slightly louder than normal if your patient is old or hard of hearing. Never use medical 'jargon' to a patient. If you want him to do something complicated (e.g. eye movements to demonstrate strabismus) rehearse the movements with him before photography. Warn the patient if you are going to switch on bright lights or discharge an electronic flash. If you need to insert cheek retractors in order, for example, to demonstrate teeth more clearly, show these to the patient first and tell him why you are using them. This kind of approach to the patient, besides being the only reasonable way to behave towards other people, will pay enormous dividends in that you will have a relaxed and co-operative patient instead of one who is frightened, tense, and as a result, difficult to photograph.

Make a point of not having 'onlookers' while you are photographing a patient – his illness is to him a very personal thing and being photographed even more so.

Therefore, as much privacy as possible should be maintained. The only exception should be in the case of a chaperone (*see Section 2.9*). This intense personal concern with their illness will cause patients to ask your opinion of their condition. Never venture to do so; only the patient's own doctor is competent to do this. You can, however, be reassuring in a general way.

Medical photography is still a relatively 'new' profession and there is understandable ignorance about it with patients; confusion with radiography being particularly common. The patient may well ask 'why am I being photographed'. There are three possible answers you can give:

(1) 'The doctor wants a picture as part of your confidential medical records' or 'to help the doctor assess your treatment properly'.
(2) You can explain the value of the photographs for later comparison purposes.
(3) When the picture is obviously not for either of these, and the patient is intelligent, he will generally be satisfied if he realises the value to the hospital for treating similar cases, and its uses for the teaching of young doctors.

Always allow the patient privacy in which to undress and dress, and never hurry an ill patient. Help with dressing when necessary. During a photographic session, never leave the patient uncovered longer than is absolutely necessary, or ask them to remove more clothing than is required.

Never hurt the patient, no photography is worth causing such discomfort and distress to a patient that his progress may be affected in any way. If possible get the patient to take the required position himself, but if you have to position him yourself do so with tact and consideration. Some patients may be too ill to co-operate fully, in which case do the best you can while causing the least discomfort.

Never talk about the patient or his diagnosis in his hearing. When genitalia are to be photographed the least distress is caused if the work is undertaken by a photographer of the same sex as the patient. Allow the patient to wear a 'bikini' type garment (plain white material) in a full length picture if it is not necessary to record genitalia.

If patients' case notes are sent to you it is your responsibility to see that they are returned. Do not leave them where the patient can read them and do not give them to the patient personally to take with him. They should be given to the patient's escort, in a sealed envelope if necessary.

## 2.3 PATIENT CONSENT AND COPYRIGHT

Opinions vary widely on this subject but it is generally agreed that a clinical photograph is part of the patient's confidential medical records and its use for teaching or publication without the patient's consent would be a breach of medical etiquette. Many areas of the patient's treatment (e.g. giving a blood sample, having an X-ray or receiving prescribed medicines) are not subject to written permission, but some are (e.g. all surgical procedures involving general anaesthesia). Since it is usually difficult to maintain that photography is an essential part of the patient's treatment it is usual to obtain his written consent to photography (especially if the photograph is to be used for publication or teaching and the identity of the patient cannot be masked).

The back of the photography request form is a suitable place to include such words as 'I.........consent to being photographed, and I agree that the photographs taken may be used for the purpose explained to me by Dr.........'. This should be signed by the patient and requesting physician and dated. In the case of a child the parent or guardian should sign (the only exception to this might be the case of child abuse, or non-accidental injury, where a doctor's signature countersigned by the police or medical examiner may be sufficient).

The patient has a right to refuse to be photographed. If this happens you should always inform the requesting physician of the circumstances. If for any other reason you are unable to obtain the requested photograph you should also inform the doctor concerned.

Photography of the genitalia of young children is a problem legally. In England and Wales such photographs may be construed as pornographic and the qualified medical photographer could face prosecution even if he were in possession of a signed consent form. It is, however, unlikely that this will ever happen as this was not within the spirit of the Act when it was passed by Parliament.

Even where patients have signed a consent form the publication of medical photographs needs careful consideration – but, like all aspects of copyright, the situation is extremely complex. The laws of copyright, though similar in principle, may differ in detail in various parts of the world, so it is *imperative* that the student acquaint himself with the law locally.

In the United Kingdom the copyright is vested in the 'author' of the work concerned for a period of 50 years from the date of its first publication. The photographer is, however, not the 'author' of the work if he is using film and equipment owned by a medical institution. The copyright therefore belongs to the employing authority, e.g. the NHS or Medical School. In practice, though, the authority over the copyright of medical photographs is usually vested in the Head of the Medical Illustration Department. In theory, it would be possible to sell the reproduction rights to medical photographs on behalf of the employing authority; but there is another complication – that of medical etiquette. Because the photographs are part of the patient's confidential records they should not be published except with the permission of both the patient and his consultant, especially if the patient is recognizable in the photographs. If the picture just shows a close-up of a lesion then this formal procedure may be unnecessary, but care should be taken to ensure that the picture is really anonymous, for example, does it have a name or hospital number printed on the mount? Although doctors may appear to be 'commissioning' medical photographs when they sign a request form, in law they do not have either ownership or copyright of the resulting photographs.

## 2.4 ORGANIZATION OF WORKLOAD

It is most important to plan an appointment system which will avoid patients being kept waiting. Try to book in-patients at sensible regular intervals (e.g. 15–30 minutes) avoiding the times when you know you have busy out-patient clinics (e.g. dermatology, plastic surgery).

If sometimes a delay is unavoidable, then explain to the patient why he is being kept waiting, for example 'the photographer is with another patient at the moment'. If the delay is to be a long one ask the patient if he has to visit any other department, e.g. the pharmacy, or if he would like to go and have some refreshments.

Pre-arrange all the photographic equipment that you will require, before the patient enters the studio, then take your photographs as quickly as possible. People who are ill tire much sooner than healthy ones and you should never keep a patient standing or in a fixed position for any length of time.

Never turn a patient away if sent at a wrong or inconvenient time, and never allow the patient to become the butt of your annoyance over someone else's mistake. The department or its staff should never give the impression of inefficiency or indifference. Remember that if it were not for the patients you would not have a job.

## 2.5 CLEANLINESS

The care of the patient includes seeing that the photographic department is clean and tidy and that no unpleasant sights such as pathological specimens are visible. The staff should all wear clean white coats, hands should be washed before and after attending to any patient and long hair should be restrained from coming into contact with the patient. Sterile procedures, such as would involve the staff in 'scrubbing-up' and wearing a mask, gown and gloves, are not normally undertaken in the department but cleanliness is essential against infection.

Check the changing cubicle after each patient. The skin fragments from a patient with psoriasis or exfoliative dermatitis may not be infectious but they are a distressing site to any subsequent patient using the cubicle.

Equipment which has been used in the post-mortem or autopsy room, or animal house, must always be disinfected before being returned for use in the studio or taken to the bedside or operating room. It is an unwarranted risk to take a camera straight from an autopsy into a surgical operation.

If you are uncertain about the cleanliness of your department, or require advice on risks of infection, etc. consult the member of the pathology staff in your hospital who is responsible for the control of cross infection.

## 2.6 INFECTIOUS DISEASES

As a general rule patients suffering from infectious diseases should not be photographed in the department. Diseases such as varicella and typhus are usually isolated and 'barrier nursed', that is, they are surrounded with a 'barrier' of special precautions against the spread of infection.

Some contagious conditions such as impetigo, fungal infections and secondary syphilis will be seen in the department and precautions should be taken as follows:

(1) Arrange separate appointments at less busy times.
(2) Avoid unnecessary contact with the patient – use gloves.
(3) Use disposable material on seating and for backgrounds in contact with the patient.

Patients in hospital will often have a reduced resistance to infection and the effect on them may be greater than on a healthy person. Some patients so lack resistance that they are 'reverse barrier nursed' to prevent them being infected, e.g. patients with autoimmune deficiency diseases. As a general rule staff with colds and influenza should not be in close contact with patients but if this cannot be avoided a mask should be worn.

## 2.7 SURGICAL DRESSINGS

Dressings are often difficult and painful to remove and this is best done by a nurse in the ward or clinic before the patient comes to the department. A temporary dry dressing can be left in place to protect the lesion, which the photographer can remove simply and quickly, but carefully. The lesion should be re-covered with a clean dressing for the return journey.

## 2.8 ACCIDENTS

If anything untoward happens to a patient in your department, e.g. if he faints or is sick, always inform the patient's doctor or nurse. If he is an out-patient, do not allow him to go home until he has been examined by the medical officer on duty. Never presume that someone will look after the patient when he leaves your department; make sure yourself that he is all right. Find out from your administration whether there is an accident report form which has to be completed or any other additional action your hospital requires you to take. Make personal notes of the incident immediately after the patient has been placed under medical care. Such notes, which should be signed and dated, should be kept to serve as an 'aide memoire' should further investigation prove to be necessary.

Make sure you know the procedure that your hospital adopts in case of cardiac arrest and study closely the section on first aid and resuscitation. Your prompt action may save a life.

## 2.9 CHAPERONES AND ESCORTS

Widely differing views are held on this question and the best course of action is to avoid the problem altogether by using photographers of the same sex as the patient. It is always advisable for the medical photographer to have a chaperone present when photographing patients of the opposite sex, particularly when the patient has to remove clothing. The reasons for this are (1) supposedly, protection of the patient – but really to prevent any hysterical accusation of assault against the photographer; (2) it helps to lessen embarrassment to the patient (the chaperone can help the patient to undress and give assistance to stand and so on). Except in the case of very young children patient's relatives do not make suitable chaperones. If, as is common, the departmental secretary is used as the chaperone make sure she wears a white coat.

Each hospital has its own individual arrangements for escorting patients to and from departments. Your responsibility is to arrange for the safe return of the patient from your department, so find out from your administration how you should do this. The usual procedure is for hospital porters to escort patients except where the patient's condition is sufficiently unstable to warrant a qualified nurse to accompany him.

## 2.10 PHOTOGRAPHY AT THE BEDSIDE

Generally the main reason for deciding to photograph a patient in bed is because he is too ill to be moved to the photographic department. Those patients requiring complicated surgical dressings or having continuous uninterrupted treatment such as an intravenous drip, or the highly infectious case (consult with whoever is in charge of the patient as to what precautions you should take) may also be reasons for bedside photography. Often the photography of genitalia can be less distressing to the patient in the more familiar surroundings of the ward and with the nursing staff assisting where necessary.

When a decision has been taken to go to the patient's bedside always telephone the ward first to arrange a convenient time for photography. When you are with the patient, go about your business in a quiet and methodical manner. If the patient is very ill do not move him without first ascertaining that it is safe to do so and get a nurse to help you, or to do it for you. If the patient is in a ward or in a room with other people always screen him; he will not want his neighbours to see what you are doing. Do not uncover more of him than you need to do in order to get a satisfactory photograph. See that he is kept warm and when you have finished, see that he is comfortably settled again. Replace any furniture that you have had to move, such as the bedside locker and see that the patient can reach this should he need to. Again do all this quietly, loud noises when you are ill can be very disturbing. Finally when you are leaving the ward tell the sister in charge that you have finished with the patient.

## References

Cavallo, R. (1977). Copyright: what's the law? *J. Biol. Photogr. Assoc.*, **45**, 89-91

De Freitas, D. (1982). *A Brief Guide to Copyright in the United Kingdom.* (London: British Copyright Council)

Dornette, W. (1975). Biological photography and the law. *J. Biol. Photogr. Assoc,*. **43**, 78-82

Duncan, A. *et al.* (1977). *A Dictionary of Medical Ethics.* (London: Darton, Longman and Todd)

Gibbs-Smith, C. (1978). *Copyright Law Concerning Works of Art, Photography and the Written and Spoken Word.* (London: Museums Association)

Gillis, L. (1972). *Human Behaviour in Illness.* (London: Faber and Faber)

Gilson, C. and Green, P. (1984). Confidentiality of illustrative clinical records. *J. Audiovis. Media Med.*, **7**, 4–9

Hymers, R. (1972). *The Professional Photographer in Practice.* (Watford:Fountain Press)

Mathey, R. *et al.* (1972). *Fundamentals of Patient Centred Nursing.* (St. Louis, USA: C.V. Mosby)

Parry, W. (1972). *Communicable Disease* (London: English Universities Press)

Peters, M. (1978). The copyright act of 1976. Part 1. *J. Biol. Photogr. Assoc.*, **46**, 31-43

Peters, M. (1978). The copyright act 1976. Part 2. *J. Biol. Photogr. Assoc.*, **46**, 46-54

Roper, N. (1973). *The Principles of Nursing.* (Edinburgh and London: Churchill Livingstone)

Stevens, G. (1978). Medical photography, the right to privacy and privilege. *Med. Trial Tech. Q.*, **24**, 456-464

Tarcindale, M. (1980). Medical photographer's role in protecting a patient's right to privacy. *J. Biol. Photogr.*, **48**, 183-185

Weed, L. (1969). *Medical Records, Medical Education and Patient Care.* (Cleveland, USA: Case University Press)

Williams, B. (1979). Home Office report of the committee on obscenity and film censorship. (London: HMSO)

## *Practical projects*

(1) Make sure you understand the difference between 'infection' and 'contagion'. In a good medical dictionary look up the following communicable diseases and make notes on them:– Actinomycosis, Brucellosis, Diphtheria, Epidemic parotitis, Encephalitis lethargica, Erysipelas, Gonorrhea, Hepatitis, Herpes simplex, Herpes zoster, Impetigo contagiosa, Infectious mononucleosis, Meningitis, Ophthalmia neonatorum, Pediculosis, Pertussis, Poliomyelitis, Psittacosis, Rubella, Rubeola, Scabies, Scarlet fever, Syphilis, Tinea, Tuberculosis, Typhus, Variola.

(1) Students in tropical and sub-tropical countries should also look up the following:– Amoebiasis, Bilharzia, Cholera, Filariasis, Lassa fever, Leishmaniasis, Leprosy, Malaria, Rabies, Trachoma, Trypanosomiasis, Typhoid fever, Yellow fever, Yaws.

(2) Study carefully the medical photography request/consent form used in your department – could it be improved upon? If so design an improved form.

(3) Request your microbiology department to culture some dust samples taken from the studio floor – photograph the results according to the principles outlined in Section 15.

(4) Ask a ward sister (when she is not too busy) to explain the complete daily routine of a ward – you might even persuade her, and your head of department, to allow you to spend a day on the ward. Take special note of the timetable of events and of 'who does what'.

## *Examination Questions*

Q.1 What is barrier nursing? Describe the circumstances in which it would be employed and how it would affect your photographic technique.

Q.2 Explain the difference between contagion and infection, illustrating your answer with descriptions of at least two examples of each.

Q.3 Write brief notes on the care of the following patients in your department:
(*a*) A patient with language difficulties
(*b*) An elderly, partially sighted lady
(*c*) A teenage girl with vulval warts
(*d*) A patient who declines to be photographed.

Q.4 Describe the circumstances where it would be appropriate to use a chaperone. Explain fully all the factors to be considered in selecting a chaperone.

Q.5 What steps do you think should be taken to secure a patient's permission to be photographed and what approach would you take in the event of a refusal? Discuss the question of copyright in relation to the publication of such photographs.

*Multiple choice (any of the statements may be true or false)*

Q.6 A patient with an immuno deficiency disease is being reverse barrier nursed and you are asked to produce colour photographs of a skin rash:
(*a*) Sterile green surgical towels would make a suitable background.
(*b*) You may enter the patient's room with you photographic equipment but must clean it afterwards with neat alcohol.
(*c*) You must scrub and wear protective clothing before entering the room.
(*d*) All propective clothing used in the patient's room must be sent for safe disposal after photography.
(*e*) It is not safe for a female photographer to photograph this type of patient in case she is in the first three months of a pregnancy.

Q.7 You have been requested to take photographs of lesions on the genitalia of a member of the opposite sex and you are the only photographer available. You would:
(*a*) Tell the patient of your anxiety and apologize for the situation.
(*b*) Ensure that the patient's consent form is properly signed.
(*c*) Ask a colleague of the same sex as the patient to act as a chaperone.
(*d*) Ask the patient to wear rubber gloves when they are retracting the labia or prepuce.
(*e*) Line up your camera and lights on the clothed patient then ask them to quickly slip off their underclothes for photography.

# Section 3
# Organization of the photographic department

**A.R. Williams**, MPhil, FBIPP, FRPS, FBPA, AIMBI.
Head of Medical Illustration and Teaching Services
Charing Cross Hospital and Medical School, London

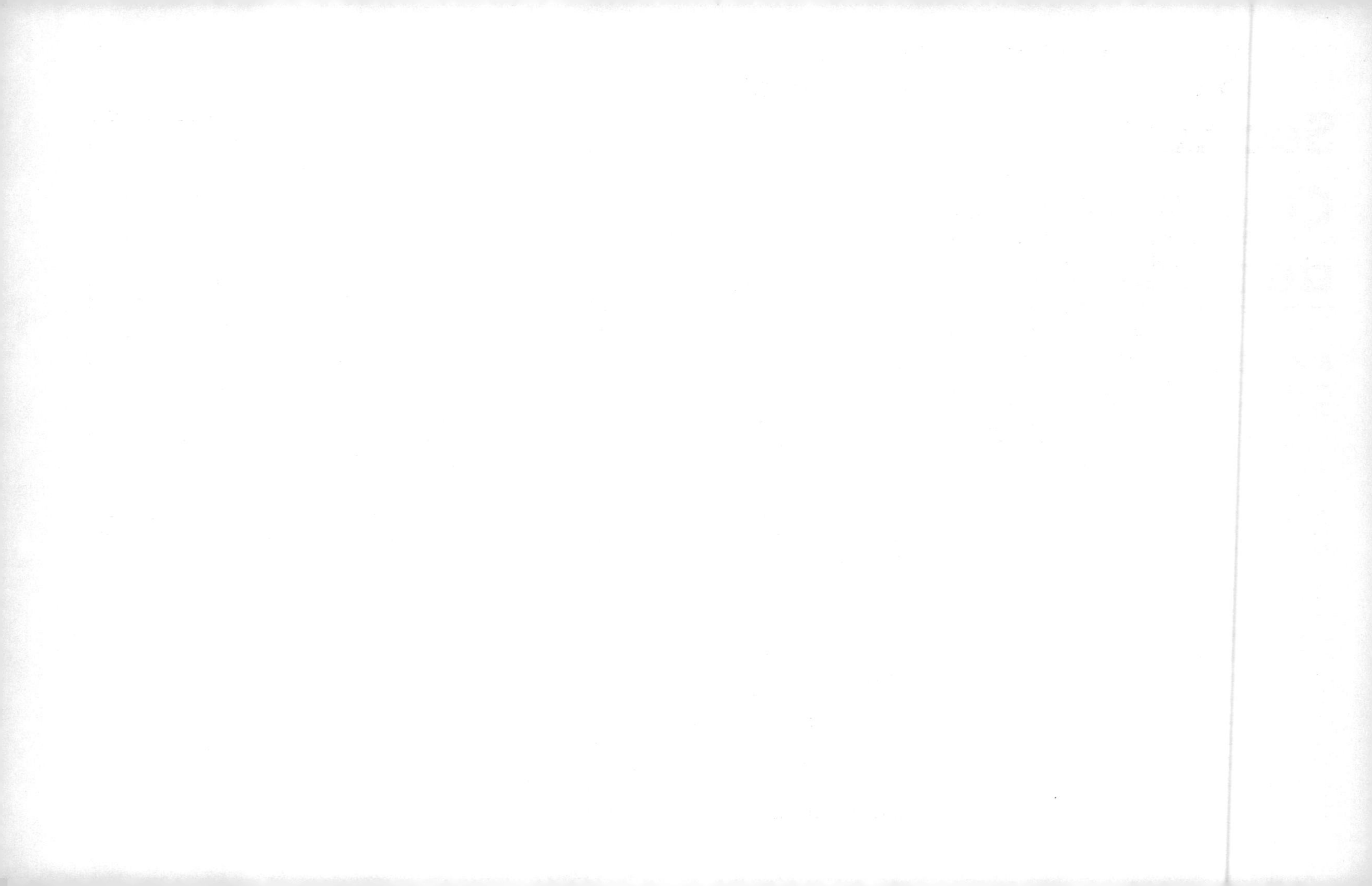

## 3.1 INTRODUCTION

Organization of a photographic unit within a hospital is undertaken with a number of points in mind. Apart from the basic function, which is to produce medical photographs expediently, the department has to have an efficient and comprehensive filing system so that photographs can be easily located; the administration of the unit should be organized so that stocktaking, ordering and costing are built into the routine; the department must establish good working relationships with other departments and their staff; a chain of responsibility must be clearly known. The relationship of the department to the general hospital administrative structure is also a most important feature of the organization but one which will vary considerably between hospitals.

## 3.2 ACCOMMODATION

Departments of medical photography vary considerably in physical size, number and variety of staff, types of work undertaken and the quantity of work. All these factors affect the size and extent of the accommodation which may be new, newly designed conversion of an old building, or a longstanding department. There are certain basic requirements for a small department which are necessary even though the staff comprises only one photographer. To this basic accommodation may be added further rooms for additional techniques and members of staff. Basic accommodation should comprise at least a studio, negative and print darkrooms, dressing cubicle, WC (including washing facilities) and office space which should include finishing and transparency mounting facilities. Larger units need a special technique studio for setting up apparatus for non-clinical photography, or for jobs requiring a special set-up which cannot be left in the clinical studio, or indeed may be unsuitable for that room. The clinical studio may need extending to incorporate individual fixed set-ups for dental, ophthalmic photography, cinematography, etc. Further techniques and reprography will require accommodation of considerably

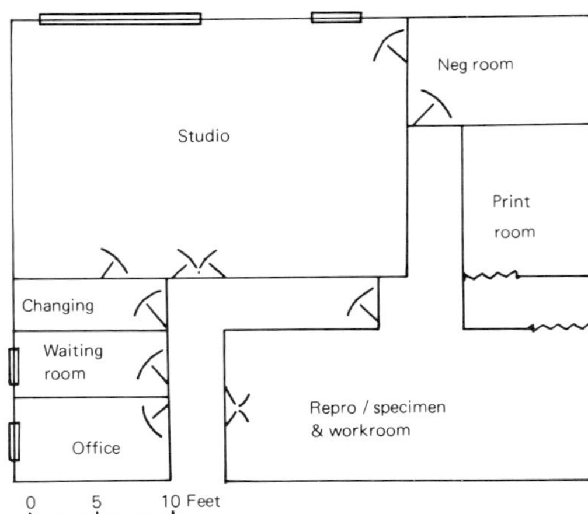


***Figure 3.1*** *A typical layout for a small medical photography department with perhaps two photographers*

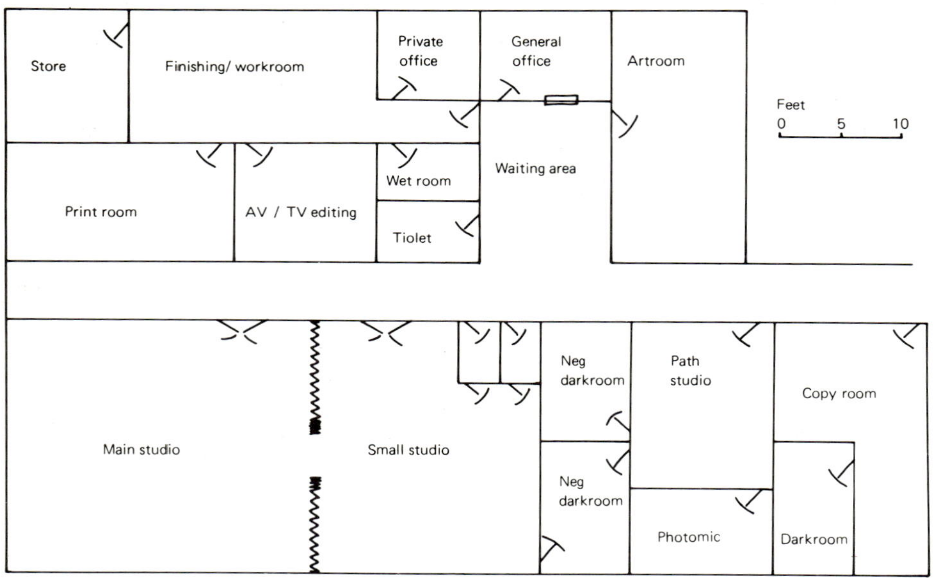


***Figure 3.2*** *A medium-sized department suited to a busy district general hospital with perhaps six photographic staff*

greater variety. Specific examples include rooms for photomacrography and photomicrography, copying techniques, reproduction of radiographs, colour processing, sound recording, film editing, offset litho services, graphic services, exhibition space and a preview room, workshop and storeroom. Such an extensive layout must include proper office space for the secretary to operate effectively and will also include space for a pictorial library, a film library, negative storage and indexing systems. A private office is necessary for the head of department. In most cases separate rooms or cubicles are necessary for each of the above processes. Self contained areas are also necessary for fixed set-ups where apparatus is reserved for one specific task, but in some instances open-plan working space with movable partitions is more adaptable to changing requirements of a department.

### 3.2.1 Arrangement of space and traffic flow

Provision of sufficient space for a variety of techniques demands the arrangement of rooms into a layout providing easy access, good traffic flow and a straightforward sequence of operations. The main entrance, reception area, waiting room, studio and changing cubicles should be close together so that patients are moved as little as possible as mobility may be difficult for them. Access to patient areas should be wide enough to accommodate wheelchairs, beds and stretcher trolleys. Stairs or curbs of any kind must not impair access to the department from other areas of the hospital or within the department itself. It is important that toilet facilities exist for patients (a WC, wash-hand basin and disposable towels) and this should be designed for use of disabled persons in wheelchairs. Separate toilet facilities should exist for the departmental staff preferably as part of the staff rest

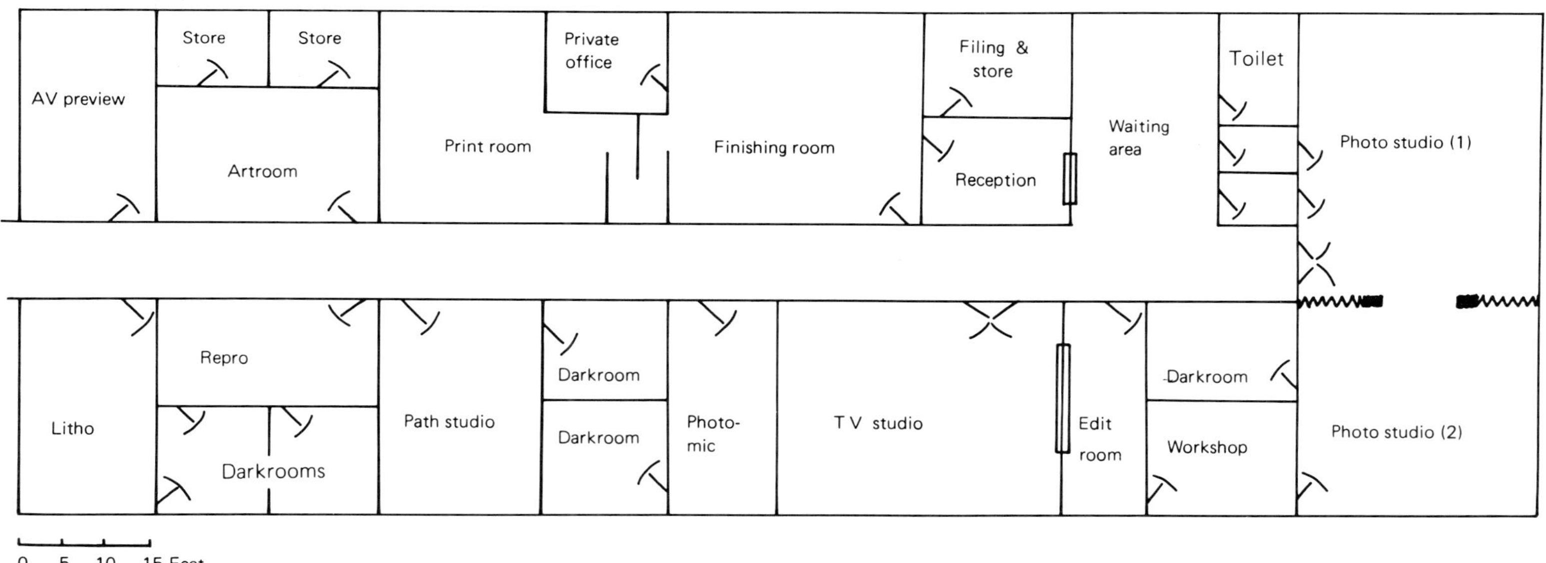


***Figure 3.3*** *A large university department suitable for up to twenty staff*

room facilities. A variety of chairs should be provided in the waiting room as children, elderly people and the disabled may require special seating.

Organization of traffic flow of staff, patients and various types of work as it proceeds through a number of processes is important. A logical progression of work from room to room is essential, for example, exposed films having been processed in the negative room should be collated with the patient identifying strip or negative bag and together with instructions for printing be passed through into the adjacent print room. A communicating hatch or door from the print room to the finishing and mounting room means that these processes can be continuous. Studio space should also be near to the processing rooms. Due to the nature of the work it is important that 'patient areas' and the space in which the photographic production and filing takes place are strictly separated. Patients cannot then be disturbed by morbid specimens or other unpleasant sights which are often part of the medical photographer's work. Also confidentiality of the patient's records is preserved in that they are unable to see other patients' photographs. Much of the design of a medical photographic department follows standard practice for the planning of photographic facilities in general. Mention will be made here of facilities which are peculiar to the *medical* department. The relevant Health and Safety legislation, e.g. the Health and Safety at Work Act (1974) in the UK, must be borne in mind when designing or modifying departments as this affects virtually every aspect of the unit.

### 3.2.2 The studio

Safety of the patient while being photographed requires a number of design features which are specifically necessary. The studio floor needs to be of a non-slip material, but allowing easy manoevrability, of apparatus and cleansing. Electrical sockets and controls both of the mains and electronic flash units should be inaccessible to children. Lighting cables, boom stands and hot lamps are all potentially dangerous. Sufficient room height should be provided (e.g. 11 feet or over) as overhead suspension of lighting leaves the floor free of encumbrances.

The Department of Health (UK) has issued *Building Note No. 19* which relates to Departments of Medical Illustration and a minimum specification is given for technical apparatus, furnishings and fittings. Floors, chairs, patients' couches and tables should be suitable for regular cleaning with antiseptic. Special containers should exist for clean and soiled linen, rubber gloves, retractors, mirrors and other items in regular use in the studio. According to the individual hospital requirements, facilities may be necessary for the management of patients with dressings. A sink with hot and cold water, soap and scrubbing brush is essential. A small autoclave for the sterilization of instruments, or facilities for soaking in a germicidal solution should be provided. Coloured backgrounds for still photography and sufficient background for filming gait must be available.

### 3.2.3 Darkrooms

Floors should be washable and a floor drain is necessary in each room. Benches may be topped with laminated plastic or polyvinyl which are suitable for regular wiping down with a damp cloth. Darkroom layout differs little from designs used in general practice and such plans may be seen in the relevant Kodak publications.

### 3.2.4 Finishing and other rooms

Floors of these rooms must be suited to wheeled equipment but could be cork, polyvinyl or thermoplastic tiles. Maximum bench, drawer and cupboard space is essential and benches should be topped in laminated plastic or polyvinyl or wood finished in polyurethane. Adequate cupboard and shelf space is essential.

### 3.2.5 Specimen room

Space for camera and lighting set-up must be supplemented by facilities necessary to prevent infection such as impervious bench tops which can be swabbed down with antiseptic. Dissecting boards and a large sink are necessary for handling specimens. Also a separate wash basin and towel must be provided with elbow operated taps. If this room is used for photomacrography and photomicrography this apparatus may need to be mounted on an anti-vibration bench. Facilities for sterilizing instruments used in handling specimens must be provided and these instruments kept strictly for use in this room only.

### 3.2.6 Office space

Adequate space for day books, office equipment and all the necessary items for library activities of a department, should be ensured, i.e. a slide viewer, index textbooks, etc. Telephones should be within easy reach of the secretary who should also be in close contact with the reception and waiting area; with an intercommunicating window or hatch.

### 3.2.7 Reception and waiting area

This space should be large enough to accommodate wheelchairs or even a stretcher and be made to look as attractive and welcoming as possible. Carpet or carpet tiles add to this appearance as will a non-institutional form of decoration.

### 3.2.8 Storeroom

A cool, lockable storeroom is necessary for all departments, however small, and should house a refrigerator to store colour film. Adequate shelving of wall or stand variety is essential.

## 3.3 SUPPLY AND SERVICES

### 3.3.1 Electrical

All photographic rooms and offices will require an adequate number of power points. A guideline would be to provide twice as many points as necessary to connect all intended apparatus. Distribution of power points is equally important, e.g. background areas must be avoided and points grouped for easy access. It is important that isolating switches, centrally located, be incorporated so that all apparatus can be doubly isolated when the staff go home. This system is a useful safeguard against fire which can be caused by several items in the department e.g. mounting irons, lamps, driers. The only exception to this isolation switching will be for the refrigerator and possibly for charging points used for flash accumulators. Do not underestimate total power requirements for your department – sufficient ring mains must be provided. As a rough guide you will need four amps of electrical current for every kilowatt of power needed (on a 240 volt mains supply). Switched power points for all apparatus should be positioned at bench level or higher. Sockets mounted near floor level are undesirable but ceiling mounted sockets with remote switching may avoid trailing cables. Darkrooms must have suitable cord operated switches for all lighting. Voltage control units are essential for colour printing darkrooms and desirable for the whole department. Local safety regulations will always apply and must be adhered to.

### 3.3.2 Water

Hot and cold water supplies should follow normal design patterns. It is essential that processing rooms have thermostatically controlled water as well as the hot and cold supplies. Filters are usually required on supplies to automatic processors – it is quite surprising to see how much 'debris' is present in a hospital water supply.

### 3.3.3 Gases

Nitrogen burst agitation for black-and-white-and colour processing is commonplace and provision for this supply from a central source may be possible. Compressed air is useful in medical art studios, finishing rooms and print rooms, for driving air brushes and cleaning guns.

### 3.3.4 Ventilation

Adequate air changes throughout the department are necessary. The consulting architect or hospital engineer will be able to give advice. The studio should be kept at a higher temperature (about 23 – 25 °C) because of the need for patients to undress. Again filters may be necessary to prevent excessive dust formation.

## 3.4 COMMUNICATION WITHIN THE DEPARTMENT AND HOSPITAL

The department must be connected to the internal and external hospital telephone systems. Ideally, calls should be intercepted by the secretary and provision of distribution points to other rooms is essential. Take care that telephones with 'cue lights' are not fitted in darkrooms.

An intercom system is also essential for the large department and in some cases beneficial to small departments where the rooms are physically spread out. The master control should be situated at the secretary's desk and ideally photographers should be able to respond to calls without having to push buttons with wet hands.

In a large department it is also desirable to have 'key' staff, such as the duty clinical photographer, on the hospital radiopaging or bleep system, so that they can be reached when out on location around the hospital. A great deal of time and effort can be saved in this way.

## 3.5 SECURITY

Photographic apparatus is popular, usable and saleable. A hospital is a public building accessible to all. It is necessary to take steps to ensure that the equipment is safe both during and out of working hours. Consult the hospital security officer – burglar alarms, security gates and other devices may be necessary. A carefully kept inventory of all equipment should be maintained and in particular the serial number, model number and peculiarities (special appearance) noted. It is worthwhile having all valuable items such as cameras and lenses marked with their ownership; either by engraving, or by indelible UV fluorescent dye. Check what insurance cover exists in the institution for your equipment – there may be none!

## 3.6 STAFF

It is the responsibility of the Head of Department to interview and engage staff in consultation with the hospital administration. All matters regarding conditions of employment, health, safety and welfare of staff are chanelled through the Head of Department. The student must familiarize himself with local or national conditions of employment and the relevant industrial and trade-union law.

Types of staff may include medical photographers, medical and graphic artists, copy photographers, photographic and off-set printers, photofinishers, projectionists, secretary/receptionists, photomicrographers and other specialists. If a film or television unit is included, camera and studio staff, electronic engineers and producers may be required. Most categories of staff may be graded as trainee, non-supervisory and supervisory personnel.

### 3.6.1 Personnel selection

Good selection means finding the right person for the job. Errors can be very costly – perhaps even impossible to rectify. There are several important stages:

(1) Analysing the job –. a critical analysis should be undertaken to establish if the job still exists, and what is involves or should involve, i.e. the job content.

(2) Listing personal requirements/qualities – what qualities and skills are necessary to perform the job? What personality, attitudes and interests will fit the candidate for the organization? It will then be possible to draw up a job description from (1) and (2).

(3) Publication of the vacancy – choose the media carefully. Advertisements should be designed to ensure that only suitable applicants apply. They should explain what is involved and who should apply; they should be based on the job description.

(4) Assessment of applicants – from the application form make a careful selection of the best candidates (do not shortlist too many), then call for interview. During the interview always ask open-ended questions, probe deeper to establish the background in more detail and also future aims. Avoid multiple questions, reproof, mannerisms and assumptions. Establish interests, attitudes and leisure activities. Establish skills and personality by asking, for example, what aspect of their present job they enjoy/find difficult. Clarify any details necessary by further questions about the organization/job. Conclude the interview by thanking the candidate and let him know how long he will have to wait for a result. After the formal interview it is highly desirable for the candidate to meet his immediate superior and to see the department – one can sometimes learn a great deal about a candidate in this informal setting.

(5) Decide on the best candidate, take up references and offer the post subject to a satisfactory health check and references.

### 3.6.2 Chain of command

Staff generally appreciate being left to get on with their work and enjoy a measure of responsibility and freedom so it makes good sense to delegate some managerial tasks down a chain of command. Figures 3.4 and 3.5 shows how a large, and a small, department might be organized into a tree of responsibility. Each higher level of the pyramid brings with it an increasing level of responsibility, greater technical skill, but less involvement in day-to-day photography. The Head of a large department will, for example, spend most of his time on administrative work, the chief will be largely responsible for day-to-day organisation of the unit, the senior photographer will spend 50% of his time supervising and checking photography and 50% undertaking it, the basic grade medical photographer will spend all his time doing photography but may help by monitoring say film stock, whereas the trainee will only perform photography in a largely supervized capacity. It is important for every member of staff to understand what his responsibilities are and it is usually best to have a detailed job description available to help in defining the duties. Examples of job descriptions for chief, senior and basic photographers in a large university department are given for reference in Appendix 3.1.

### 3.6.3 Training and instruction

The introduction of either new staff or new procedures and techniques will involve senior photographers in training and instruction. Do not attempt to teach too much at once – break large jobs into several small tasks. *Tell* the trainee what to do, then *show* him, then get him to *attempt* the task, then *review* what he has learnt. Encourage new or junior staff to keep a comprehensive notebook on the various techniques and procedures used in the department. Encourage the trainee to ask questions and get him to explain what he is doing as he attempts the task. Try to make all your instructions clear, indicate a source of help in case of problems, and tell him where to find all the necessary equipment and materials.

In a large department undertaking a wide variety of techniques it is useful to have a departmental 'procedure manual' or 'techniques book' with full details of all the approved procedures, such as lighting arrangement, film choice, typical exposures, processing conditions, and a sample finished product.

'Algorithms' or 'Logical trees' can be

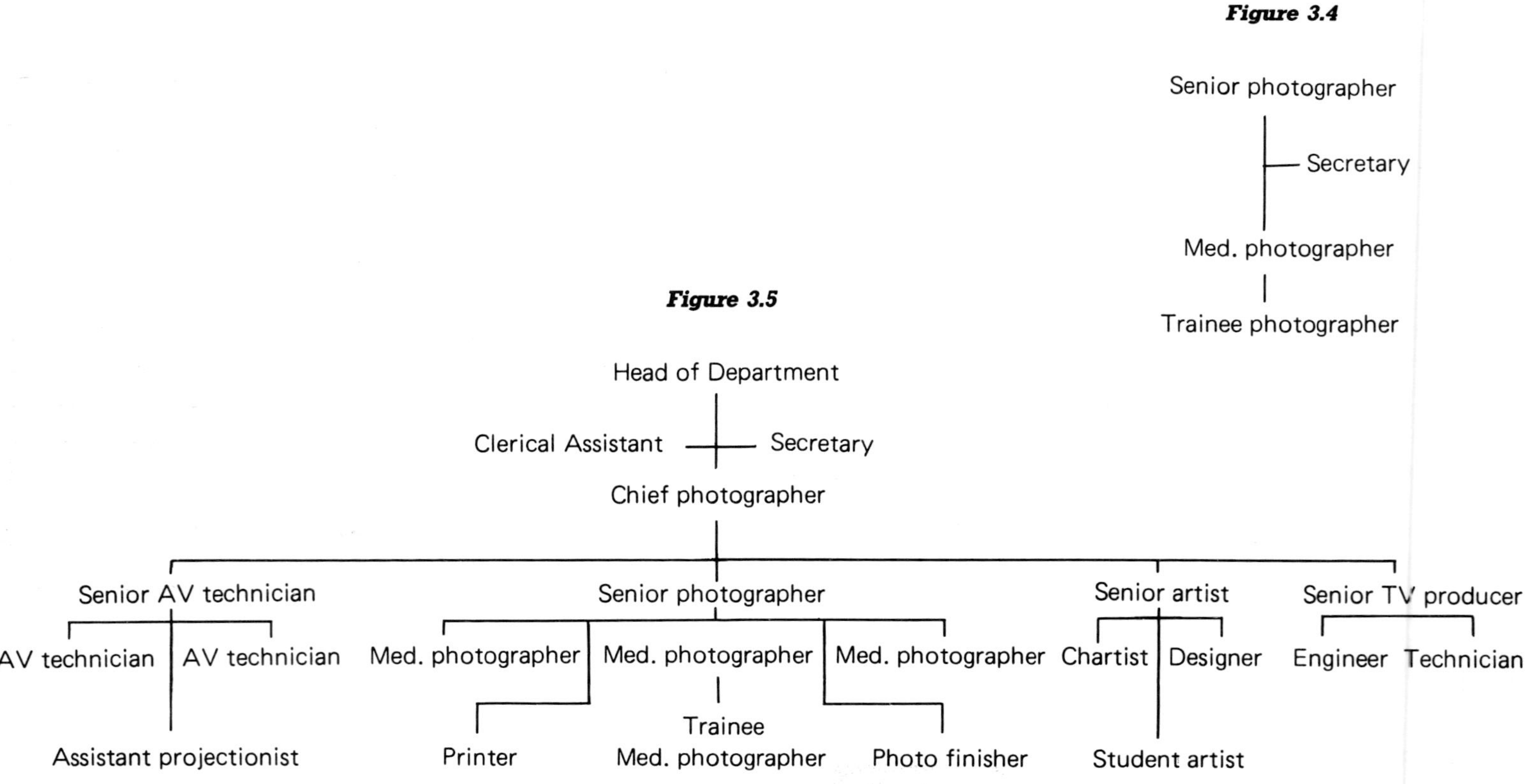


***Figure 3.4*** *Organizational structure for a small department*
***Figure 3.5*** *Organizational structure for a large university department*

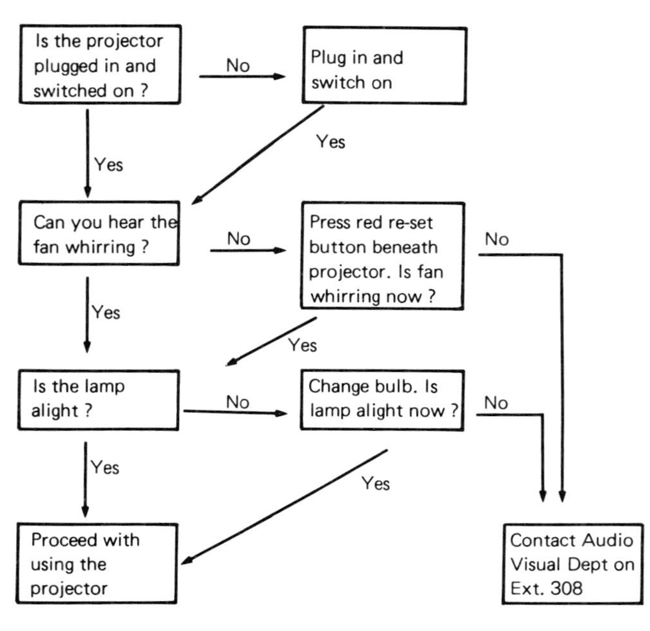


***Figure 3.6*** *An example of an algorithm or logical tree*



| | U V direct | U V fluorescence | I R clinical | Bone fluorescence | Scoliosis-Moire | Dr Jones plates | Schlieren | Photo-optical gaits | Phase contrast | X polarisation | Interference | |
|---|---|---|---|---|---|---|---|---|---|---|---|---|
| Mark | ▲ | ▲ | | ▲ | | ▲ | | | ■ | ■ | ■ | |
| Charles | | | ■ | | ■ | ■ | | | | | | |
| Mandy | | | | | | | | | | | | |
| Tony | | | ▲ | | ▲ | | ▲ | ▲ | | | | |
| Hazel | ■ | ■ | ▲ | ■ | ■ | ▲ | | ▲ | ▲ | ▲ | ▲ | |
| Andy | ▲ | ■ | ■ | ▲ | | | ▲ | ■ | ■ | ■ | ■ | |
| Liz | | | | | ■ | ■ | | ■ | | | | |
| Paddy | ■ | ■ | ▲ | ■ | ▲ | ▲ | ▲ | ▲ | ■ | ■ | ■ | |

KEY
▲ Good
■ Some experience

***Figure 3.7*** *A sample training plan for special photographic techniques*

useful for jobs which are rarely undertaken or for particularly complex tasks which have to be performed by inexperienced photographers. They consist of a series of questions with yes/no answers which lead to a single action or result for each given set of conditions.

A training plan can also be very useful in a large department, to show the current 'status' of staff, and when used in conjunction with a holiday leave planner enable one to cover all types of photography throughout the year. Such a plan lists all the staff and all the specialist tasks performed in the department with some provision for indicating which staff can perform what jobs.

### 3.6.4 Sickness and annual leave

The law and rules and regulations for these two types of absence from work vary considerably so the medical photographer should acquaint himself fully with the system as it applies locally. From an administrative point of view it is essential to have some kind of leave chart or year planner with all the staff leave marked on it (peak periods of work may also be recorded here). An accurate and confidential record of the annual leave and sick leave taken by each individual should also be kept by the Head of Department.

## 3.7 ADMINISTRATION

### 3.7.1 Organizational structure

It is important for the medical photographer to appreciate where his profession fits in relation to health care in general. In the UK the National Health Service (NHS) was established in 1948 to offer a high standard of medical care to all, irrespective of means. The service is broadly classifed into three areas:

(1) Community care – involving caring for the patient in his own environment, e.g. at work or home. Public health inspectors, health visitors and general practitioners (family doctors) all work in this area.

(2) Primary health care – based on an extensive network of general medical practitioners (GPs), each of whom is assigned a number of patients on a geographical basis. Many diseases are treated entirely by the GP.

(3) Secondary or specialist health care – provided by district general hospitals and specialist clinics staffed by doctors who have specialized in one or another branch of medicine. It is almost exclusively within this area that the medical photographer is employed. Many of these hospitals will have been designated as 'special teaching hospitals' and will work closely with attached medical schools and schools of nursing. Patients may either be seen as 'out-patients' when they attend clinics, or as 'in-patients' when they are admitted to a ward.

Within the hospital itself there are various categories of staff:

(a) Specialist medical staff, such as surgeons, physicians, pathologists and radiologists. The most senior specialists are known as 'consultants' and below them are senior registrars who have usually obtained fellowships of the relevant colleges and are awaiting appointment to consultant status. Next down in line is the registrar who is gaining specialist knowledge and experience and studying for higher qualifications. Lowest in the team is the house officer who is a junior doctor gaining experience within a hospital before embarking on a career as a specialist. He is frequently resident in the 'house', i.e. the hospital.

(b) Nursing staff, such as nurse managers, ward and theatre sisters, state registered nurses, state enrolled nurses and nursing auxiliaries. Their role is to assist the medical staff in treating the patient and to provide a comfortable and caring environment for the patient.

(c) Paramedical staff, such as biochemists, chiropodists, dieticians, pharmacists, physicists, laboratory technicians, social workers, occupational therapists, orthoptists, physiotherapists, radiographers and speech therapists. It is to this group of workers that medical photographers belong.

(d) Administrative staff, such as planning, building, equipment and finance officers, medical secretaries and many other clerical staff associated with the proper management and co-ordination of services.

(e) Manual and auxiliary workers, such as engineers, laundry workers, caterers and cleaning staff who provide the services necessary for the smooth running of a hospital which is like a large hotel devoted to the sick.

It will be appreciated that the medical photographer is a very small 'cog' in a very large and complex piece of 'machinery' but nevertheless his work may extend into any of the areas outlined above and he will meet all those categories of staff mentioned. It should always be remembered that the whole system only exists to make the patient healthy again, and that the 'consultant' has absolute power over what may or may not be done to his patient.

The Head of Medical Illustration should be responsible to the management through one of the following channels:

(i) A divisional committee (e.g. In the UK – the NHS cogwheel structure)
(ii) A special photographic subcommittee
(iii) The Dean of the medical school
(iv) A hospital administrator or management team.

The correct and most efficient method is for the Head of Department to be a member of the appropriate committee so that he can directly represent the department. In a medical school it is important that the Head of Department should sit on the appropriate academic and organizational committees if he is to fulfil his function, i.e. Academic Board, Teaching Sub-Committee, etc. It is important also that the department should not be under the control of any specific discipline within the hospital as the service should be available to all medical and scientific staff on an equal basis.

### 3.7.2 Organization of work

How work is organized within the department is dependent upon the size. The smaller the department the easier the organization. Some departments organize the routine tasks so that a job is carried out from start to finish by one member of staff. While this may be advantageous in some respects, in larger departments a 'production line' can handle a larger quantity of work. Large departments, however, are not without their problems. As the unit becomes more complex and sophisticated, the department's objectives become obscured. Tasks are not automatically directed towards meeting today's needs. Complexity attracts sophisticated procedures and tight systems of control. As a result, staff do not develop as expected and their seniors see a need for even tighter control. This tight control is resented since employees expect more recognition as individuals. Resentment reduces the display of ability and more control is then seen to be necessary. This

'vicious circle' is easily established in a busy department where photographers are constantly working under the stress of multiple deadlines. Not only does the Head of Department find difficulties in planning and motivating, but he may be tempted, as as result of day-to-day pressures, to concentrate on today's targets and ignore the requirements of the clients. The effective manager must:
**Plan** – targets of work, resources available, ability of staff, need for training, new techniques and systems, etc.
**Organize** – work and people to give the most efficient service
**Direct** – staff and effort; this involves *delegation*
**Control** – workflow to even out seasonal peaks and troughs, etc.
**Check** – quality and quantity of output, etc.
**Maintain** – standards of work, etc.

### 3.8 INDEXING SYSTEMS

A comprehensive index system must always be devised so that negatives, prints, transparencies and films can be stored and retrieved quickly. Access to photographs taken in the department must be achieved from various points such as:

(1) Date photograph was taken
(2) Photographic index number
(3) Hospital registration number
(4) Patient's name
(5) Diagnosis
(6) Consultant's name

The minimum requirements of a suitable recording system are: A day book in which jobs of all types are entered in date order, giving the details mentioned above and also including production and costing details where necessary. This book is the key to the whole system. A record card which shows all the patient's details, itemized photographic instructions, and dates of follow-up photographs should be filed in alphabetical order of patient's surname.

It is essential that a filing system for prints and transparencies be established in any hospital but especially one with a teaching commitment. A disease index system, such as the International Classification of Diseases (WHO) will enable the photographic department to produce quickly all its photographs on a particular disease or topic. Each disease is allocated a numerical reference number which is unique and the slides and prints are all filed in numerical order according to the codebook. Retrieval of the available photographs on any one topic is, therefore, easily achieved. To be of real value though there must be a comprehensive system of cross-referencing between related diseases and symptoms. 'Finger clubbing' for example, must be cross-referenced with, say, carcinoma of the lung. Complex cross-referencing and retrieval can be aided by either a punch card or computer based system.

A file for negative storage in safe and dust-free conditions is a necessity and must be arranged in photographic number order. The photographic index number may be derived in several different ways:

(1) Each negative given a number (1, 2, 3, 4, etc),
(2) Each patient given a photographic index number which may be used:
(a) together with the date of each negative
(b) with a letter as a suffix or prefix to identify each negative or type of photograph (i.e. patient's number 3537, first black-and-white negative 3537A, second 3537B, etc.). Colour transparency given prefix C (fix transparency C3537A) and X-ray transparency given prefix X (X3537C).
(3) Each negative given a number

which indicates the year/month/day/negative number of that day (i.e. Year – 83, Month – 06, Day – 22, Negative that day – 15, would be negative number 83062215 immediately identifying it as the fifteenth negative taken on the 22nd June 1983).

It is always advantageous to have all the negatives taken of one patient in one place, i.e. under one number. Methods (1) and (3) above distribute negatives taken of one patient on different occasions throughout the negative file. Method (2) keeps them together which is time saving where follow-up photography over a period is the routine.

## 3.9 PRODUCTION CONTROL

Administrative processes in the department will require documentation, which although time consuming is necessary for steady progress of the work. The number of documents should be kept to the minimum, and the data should be arranged in a logical sequence so that a minimum of entering is necessary. Records may include:

(1) A request card for clinical photography bearing details of the patient, his diagnosis, views to be taken and the purpose for which they are required.
(2) A non-clinical request form bearing full details of the job requirements.
(3) A film control sheet with the frame by frame account of content.
(4) A patient record card with full details of each photographic session and the work undertaken.
(5) Production – itemised list showing number of negatives, prints, etc., produced.
Progress control – a quick means of identifying the stage that any particular job has reached Costing – a means of arriving at a cost for any job.
(6) Publication/copyright release – to document photographs released for publication – this may also involve patient consent.

Number (6) may be combined with (1) and (2) and with some thought (1) can be combined with (4).

There is a variety of ways of monitoring the point a job has reached in the system. One method is to use an envelope or folder, into which the various components are placed, e.g. negatives, prints, colour slides, etc. and onto the front of which is clipped the request form. These folders are then placed on special shelves in the work-room which might be designated 'awaiting negatives', 'awaiting printing', 'awaiting colour', or 'awaiting mounting', etc. The job folders themselves are then telling the observer where they have got to in the system. Also the quantity of folders on any one shelf identify backlogs in, say, printing, Another system of control utilizes small marker tags which have written on them details of the job and then get moved around a special display board as the job progresses. In a very small unit it might be sufficient to write a note of which jobs are in the darkroom on a white board in the finishing area.

## 3.10 FINANCIAL CONTROL – COSTS AND COSTING

Financial adminstration of a department is the duty of the departmental head. Methods differ, but in those departments which are not self-supporting there will usually be budgets for (1) staff salaries, (2) maintenance items (stock, repairs, postage) and (3) capital items (new equipment, furnishings, etc). Overheads such as heating, electricity, water and cleaning may be off-costed to the department but possibly will be carried on the hospital's budget for these items.

One specific problem of the photographic department in regard to expenditure is that the number of requests for work (and their complexity) is variable and needs careful supervision. For instance, a new member of the medical staff may request regular filming sessions for his patients. This would mean a considerable increase in the annual running cost. Therefore, special budgets may have to be sought when long running or particularly expensive projects are undertaken.

A costing system may need to be implemented in order to charge for work done in the department. This may be necessary for two reasons: (a) To apportion total departmental costs between two or more authorities, e.g. hospital, medical school, or research funds; (b) To charge individual jobs to other departments, grants or individuals.

In the UK, costing systems have been introduced comparatively recently mainly for the purpose of apportionment of costs between employing authorities. Most departments work on a fixed annual budget which is based on the previous year's figures and is designed to provide 'minimum level' service. In departments where charges are made the system may be one which includes profit, in which case the department would operate along commercial lines (this is not uncommon in the USA and can have positive benefits). In other establishments the charges recover the total or part of the costs. In each case calculation is based on labour, materials, and overheads. Whatever the system or purpose for which it is introduced there can be no doubt that to cost medical photographic work is an expensive and time-consuming activity and should be kept within a simple framework. Possibly the easiest system to administer is one based on 'unit costs'.

Each particular end-product, for example a duplicate colour transparency, is assigned a 'unit cost' based on the time taken to produce it and the relative cost of materials used. A duplicate colour transparency might be three units whilst a colour transparency of a microscopic histological section might be eight units. The price of a single unit is fixed annually based on the true cost of labour and the real costs of materials. The unit values for each product remain constant but the unit cost can be reviewed as often as necessary. To supply a client with an invoice, one only has to summate the number of units he has consumed, then multiply by the current unit value to obtain a monetary costing. If all the jobs in a large department are to be costed it will often require a clerical assistant or microcomputer to assist in the task.

## 3.11 SUPPLIES AND STOCK CONTROL

Methods of ordering stock differ considerably. Some departments write their own orders, others require orders to be countersigned by an administrator, but often the orders are handled by the hospital supplies department. Purchasing officers now exist in many hospitals and can obtain the best prices for ordered goods. Bulk purchasing by hospital or universities can also make considerable savings.

Careful control of stock using stock record cards or sheets will ensure that a minimum holding stock is kept of items in regular use. Monthly orders can then be placed to 'top up' the stock. Changes in usage of particular items should be anticipated so as to avoid waste. Delivery notes should be checked against stock delivered and invoices checked against delivery notes. Checks should also be made to see that photographic materials are not out of date especially when specific items are infrequently used. Over-ordering or inadequate rotation of stock on films and papers can cause serious loss of image quality.

## 3.12 PROVISION OF REFERENCE MATERIALS

The Head of Department should ensure that adequate reference books are available. These may be in two forms, (1) Published works, (2) Departmental data books.

Published books should include:

A dictionary of medical terminology and a standard dictionary.

Medical textbooks appropriate to the work of the department.

An atlas of anatomy, e.g. Gray's Anatomy, Ciba collection.

Textbooks on applied photography, scientific applications, photomicrography, etc.

Technical and scientific journals applicable to the subject, e.g.

*Journal of Audio-visual Media in Medicine,*

*British Journal of Photography,*

*Journal of Biological Photographic Association, etc.*

All the major manufacturers' technical data books.

Departmental handbooks should be made up to give:

(1) Examples of all standardized clinical photographs taken as routine for any particular diagnosis plus technical details.
(2) Full technical details of all standardized and special set-ups for non-clinical photography.
(3) Technical data on manufactured goods, i.e. equipment catalogues, price lists, technical information and so forth.

## 3.13 THE USE OF COMPUTERS

The introduction of inexpensive, compact, but powerful microcomputers is having a considerable impact on the way medical illustration units are administered. Applications are wide-ranging and varied; they include:

(1) Finance – producing invoices and statements and keeping financial records of all types.
(2) Photo library – indexing, allowing comprehensive cross referencing with very fast recall time.
(3) Process control and replenishment – of, say, colour transparency processing machinery.
(4) Monitoring work flow – with all jobs being documented solely on the computer as they progress through the department. At the end of the month the analysis of production figures is provided almost instantaneously.
(5) Patient records – details of patients and the photographs taken can all be stored on a computer database.
(6) Research calculations – e.g. in photogrammetry a computer can be used to calculate volumes and surface areas from photographs.
(7) Documentation – of all types, e.g. the production of slide labels or mailing labels for sending out work.
(8) Wordprocessing – for all departmental correspondence and mailings.

The equipment which is available to perform these tasks changes almost daily – in general getting smaller, cheaper and more powerful all the time. The student should familiarize himself with any particular system available within his own institution and be aware of the functions that such a microcomputer can perform.

## References


Armstrong, R. (1969). Managing your photographic department. *J. Biol. Photogr. Assoc.*, **37**, 81-87

Atkinson, J. (1983). Experience with a microcomputer in a medical illustration department. *J. Audiovis. Media Med.*, **6**, 15-16

Bernstein, L. and Rosalyn. S, (1980). Interviewing – a guide for health care professionals.

Breadmore, R.G. (1973). *Organisation and Methods* (McKay: Teach Yourself Series)

Caliendo, M. (1981). Aid to hiring non-technical photo-department staff. *J. Biol. Photogr.*, **49**, 27-30

Cockburn, N. (1982). Slide retrieval systems – a pharmaceutical industry approach. *J. Audiovis. Media Med.*, **5**, 27-29

Cooke, S. (1981). Microcomputer application for camera, lighting, and device control. *J. Biol. Photogr., **49**, 53-54*

Fulwiler, D. (1982). Charge-back audiovisual system for a small department. *J. Audiovis. Media Med.*, **5**, 135-136

Giannavola, S. (1983). Low cost microcomputers. *J. Biol. Photogr.*, **51**, 27-30

Gilson, C. (1976). Experiences in planning and commissioning a new department of medical illustration. *Br. J. Photogr.*, **123**, 802-804

Gilson, C. and Collins, J. (1982). Use of a microcomputer in a department of medical illustration for retrieval of clinical teaching slides. *J. Audiovis. Media Med.*, **5**, 130-134

Hawkins, C. and Dee, T. (1973). The department of medical illustration; use and abuse. *Med. Biol. Illustr.*, **23**, 74-77

Hedley, A. and Morton, R. (1976). The clinical slide library: a valuable learning resource in continuing medical education. *Med. Biol. Illustr.*, **26**, 203-207

Irvine, R. (1976). Court appearances and the biophotographer. *J. Biol. Photogr. Assoc.*, **44**, 21-23

Johnson, A. (1969). *Organisation and Management of the Hospital Laboratory.* (London: Butterworths)

Klosevych, S. (1981). Cost recovery for instructional resources – boon or bane? *J. Audiovis. Media Med.*, **4**, 49-51

Kodak. (1978) *Photolab Design.* (Publication K-13) (Rochester, NY: Eastman Kodak)

Kodak. (1980). *Ideas for the Applied Photography Studio.* (Publication K-1) (Rochester, NY: Eastman Kodak)

Loudon-Brown, R. (1976). *A Guide to the Whitley Councils.* (London: IMBI)

Lund, R. (1981). Total cost recovery in a University photographic department. *J. Audiovis. Media Med.*, **4**, 23-25

Lunnon, R. (1974). Costing medical illustration. *Med. Biol. Illustr.*, **24**, 10-13

Renner, W. (1979). Circumventing the law of diminishing returns. *J. Biol. Photogr.*, **47**, 123-126

Siertsema, J., *et al.* (1980). Storage and retrieval of slides and angiograms. *J. Audiovis. Media Med.*, **3**, 92-93

Stenstrom, W. (1976). Management involves everyone. *J. Biol. Photogr. Assoc.*, **44**, 47-49 *Chapter 4*

## Practical projects

(1) Obtain a copy of DHSS Building Note 19; then use it together with the Kodak publications on studio and darkroom design to plan an imaginary department for a 600 bed general hospital. Look up approximate prices for the photographic equipment you will require and make a note of the total cost.

(2) Using realistic values for time and materials, cost out two typical 'end-products' from your department, e.g. a diazo slide and a 'line' print of a graph.

(3) Familiarize yourself with any classification system for clinical transparencies, e.g. the International Classification of Diseases. See for yourself how the slides obtain a classification number from a primary diagnosis. Try classifying some slides and also retrieving some specific diagnoses.

(4) If your department does not have a microcomputer, find one that does and make certain that you appreciate the *types* of job it can perform. (There is no point in familiarizing yourself with any one particular system – unless of course you intend to use it).

## Examination questions

Q.1 Suggest a staffing structure for a medical illustration department serving a hospital group of 1000 beds with an associated medical school and a school of nursing. Indicate by *outline* job descriptions the role of each staff member and lay out a hierarchical array indicating lines of responsibility within the department.

Q.2 You are asked by your administration to cost out the various end-products of your comprehensive departmental service. How would you tackle this exercise?

Q.3 Discuss the cost factors involved in setting up and running a medical photographic department in a 400 bedded non-teaching hospital. Indicate the approximate costs under general headings.

Q.4 Describe fully the system of documentation and information retrieval you would recommend for a new illustration department serving a teaching hospital group.

Q.5 What qualifications and experience would you expect in:
(i) A trainee medical photographer
(ii) A supervised medical photographer
(iii) An unsupervised medical photographer?
Describe how you would like to see the training of medical photographers organized.

Q.6 Produce a sketch design for a medical photographic department to serve a general hospital (non-teaching) of 600 beds – the unit to be sited on the ground floor. Give reasons for the positioning of the necessary rooms.

Q.7 Discuss fully the place of computers in medical photography.

Q.8 Describe a filing system for negatives, prints and transparencies, suitable for a department employing three photographers and a secretary, and serving both a hospital and a medical school.

# APPENDIX 3.1

**Example job descriptions for photographic staff in a large university department.**

## Chief Medical Photographer (Deputy Head of Department)

*General*

The post is on the scale of Chief Medical Laboratory Scientific Officer of the Whitley Council and salary and terms of service are as laid down for that grade. Additionally the School makes a special payment for the added responsibility of being Deputy Head of Department.

The Chief Photographer works as a practising medical photographer within the department, but additionally is reponsible for the day-to-day running of the department as a whole. He is directly responsible to the Head of Medical Illustration and Teaching Services and supervises all the other technical staff within the department. Control of basic grade staff is achieved through the four senior technicians who act as 'section leaders' for the art, photography, audio-visual and television services.

Hours of work are 9.00 am. to 5.30 pm. Monday to Thursday, 9.00 am. to 5.00 pm. Friday, with one hour for lunch between 12.00 am. and 2.00 pm. Inevitably the senior nature of this post demands considerable flexibility over hours of work.

Annual leave is 20 working days plus statutory and customary holidays as defined by the medical school.

*Qualifications*

It is expected that the holder of this post will possess a qualification at graduate level in medical photography and must have had extensive experience in one or several of the specialities in medical illustration.

He must be recognized as having the highest level of ability in medical photography and is expected, therefore, to have achieved the standard of Fellowship of the relevant professional body.

He will have had considerable experience in a supervisory capacity and a record of continuing research and development in medical photography. He should be capable of the work outlined in the job descriptions of all the staff under him – and indeed will be required to do it to meet the deadlines of the department on occasions.

The Chief Medical Photographer must be of smart, professional appearance, able to communicate effectively orally and in writing with all the staff, have a mature outlook and the ability to inspire confidence and competence in the department's staff. He must be discreet, supportive and versatile and able to act reliably on his own initiative. He will at all times be a model example to the staff.

*Job Content*

Under the direction of the Head of Department the Chief Photographer is responsible for the day-to-day running of the department. Broadly speaking the work falls into the following categories:

1. *Management of the Department*

This involves, for example:

1.1 Stock control of all departmental consumables, ordering new stock and monitoring usage.

1.2 Selection, ordering, testing and maintenance of all equipment for departmental use.

1.3 Processing of all departmental orders and invoices, keeping internal financial records.

1.4 Maintenance and organization of all internal charging as directed by Head of Department.

1.5 Liaising with technical and clerical staff to ensure comprehensive departmental records are kept accurate and up-to-date, including a clinical slide and print library.

1.6 Quality control – ensuring that the standards of production of artwork, photography, audio-visual programmes, television and projection all meet those defined by the Head of Department.

1.7 Ensuring proper co-ordination of art, photography, audio-visual, television and teaching services provided by the department – keeping the Head of Department informed.

1.8 Monitoring, checking and organizing the work-flow in all the sections. Liaising with

section leaders to re-locate staff and work as necessary to maintain a high quality efficient service.
1.9 Assigning the priorities defined by the Head of Department to work on a daily basis.
1.10 Liaising with commercial organizations, e.g. processing laboratories to ensure adequate provision of necessary services.
1.11 Examination of work methods, developing and installing new techniques and procedures where necessary.
1.12 Implementation and maintenance of appropriate departmental policies written by the Head of Department.
1.13 Liaising with section leaders over the testing and selection of the best possible materials and processes for the department's use.
1.14 Ensuring ethical standards in the fields of clinical work and copyright, as defined by Head of Department, are maintained.

## 2. *Supervision of Staff*

This involves, for example:
2.1 Advice, encouragement and support of all staff in work activities, further education and research.
2.2 Training of all staff in every respect of the work, including technical and professional performance and medical knowledge.
2.3 Organization of staff within the department, via the section leaders, to meet the demands placed upon it, on a day-to-day basis.
2.4 Checking staff performance and behaviour; correcting where necessary by support, training and discipline (liaising with section leaders and Head of Department).
2.5 Ensuring health, safety and welfare of the department's staff at work by, for example, monitoring the handling of pathological material, and maintaining all codes of safety. Informing the Head of Department immediately of potential hazards.
2.6 Ensuring good staff relationships by fair treatment, positive encouragement and recognition of extra effort; and by listening to the ideas of section leaders.
2.7 Acting as an effective communications channel between section leaders and Head of Department.

## 3. *Specialist Advisory Work*

This involves, for example:
3.1 Advising all staff on the appropriate audio-visual media to be used for any given situation.
3.2 Advising all staff on the research applications of advanced photographic techniques.
3.3 Consultation and advice on the preparation of material for input into the department, e.g. art-roughs, television scripts, booklet texts, typed tables for slides, etc.
3.4 Advising all staff on the visual presentation of data, including preparing illustrations for publication, thesis or report.
3.5 Consultation and advice with all staff over the provision of DIY facilities, e.g. routine photomicrography, theatre cameras, endoscopes, psychiatric television recording, etc.
3.6 Advising all staff on the appropriate use of 'outside' illustration services, e.g. freelance artists, commercial laboratories and film companies, etc.

## 4. *Advanced Photographic Work*

This involves, for example:
4.1 Complete familiarity with all specialist still-photographic techniques – advising and training staff where necessary.
4.2 Complete familiarity with all specialist medical photographic techniques – advising and training staff where necessary.
4.3 Complete familiarity with all cinematographic techniques and the lighting/photographic aspects of television – advising and training staff where necessary.
4.4 Complete familiarity with all photomicrographic techniques – advising and training staff where necessary.
4.5 Practical work in the above four sections, being responsible for the whole process.

The Chief Photographer will also perform all aspects of the Head of Department's job description in his absence and undertake any relevant duties as may be specified by the Head of Department from time to time.

## Senior Photographer

*General*

The post is on the Senior Medical Laboratory Scientific Officer scale and equates to the grade of Senior II Medical Photographer on the Whitley Council scale (UK).

The Senior Photographer works as a qualified medical photographer within the department, but additionally is responsible for the day-to-day running of the photographic section, and supervises all photographic staff. He reports to the Chief Photographer and is responsible to the Head of Department. Liaison with other technical staff is via the senior technicians in each section of the department.

Hours of work are 9.00 am. to 5.30 pm. daily, Monday to Thursday, 9.00 am. to 5.00 pm. Friday, with one hour for lunch between 12.00 and 2.00 pm. but inevitably the nature of this post demands flexibility here.

Annual leave is 20 working days plus statutory and customary holidays as defined by the medical school.

*Qualifications*

It is expected that the post-holder will have 'City and Guilds 745 Advanced Photography' and 'IIP Basic Medical Photography' certificates, or their recognized equivalents, and a recognized higher qualification such as 'IIP Medical Finals' or 'Higher Certificate in Medical Photography'.

The Senior Photographer is expected and encouraged to work for the Fellowships of the relevant professional organizations – the Associateships are, therefore, prerequisites for the post.

At least three years experience on a qualified grade is required.

The Senior Photographer should have above average technical skill, mature outlook, good appearance and the ability to inspire confidence and competency in the photographic staff.

*Job Content*

*1. Management of Photographic Section*

This involves, for example:
1.1 Monitoring and checking work-flow within the section, allocating staff and resources as appropriate to meet the targets set by the Head of Department.
1.2 Checking all photographic work, at its various stages of production to ensure it meets the quality and quantity standards desired.
1.3 Consultation and advisory work in connection with the appropriate choice of communication medium, and all aspects of the photographic presentation of information to medical, scientific and nursing staff.
1.4 Design and preparation of photographic aspects of exhibitions, tape – slide programmes, booklets, television and cine films; including layouts, scripting story-boards and costing.
1.5 Planning, organizing and developing the work procedures of the section. Devising, wherever possible, standard techniques and keeping a comprehensive techniques book.
1.6 Research into, testing and selection of the best possible materials and processes for the section's use. Advising senior staff accordingly.
1.7 Research into, testing and selection of the most suitable equipment for section use.
1.8 Responsibility for ensuring maintenance and general up-keep of all photographic equipment and facilities within the department.
1.9 Stock control of all consumables within the photographic section, preparing orders for senior staff.

*2. Supervision of Photographic Staff*

This involves, for example:
2.1 Checking staff performance and behaviour; correcting where necessary by support, training and discipline.
2.2 Training of all photographic staff in every aspect of the section's work including technical and professional performance and medical knowledge.
2.3 Organization of staff within the section to meet the demands placed upon it, on a day-to-day basis.
2.4 Advice, encouragement and support of photographic staff in work activities, further education and research.
2.5 Ensuring health, safety and welfare of the section's staff by developing appropriate techniques for handling pathogenic material and arranging, via the Head of Department, for

appropriate prophylactic innoculations.
2.6 Ensuring good staff relationships by fair treatment, recognition of extra effort, and listening to the ideas or problems of basic grade staff.
2.7 Acting as a communication channel between junior staff and senior policy makers.

*3. Advanced Photographic Work*

This involves, for example:
3.1 Specialist still photography for medical and biological research including: Schlieren photography, high-speed photography, slow-motion and time-lapse photography, equidensitometry, photo-elastic stress analysis, autoradiography, photogrammetry, densitometry, holography, microphotography, chronocyclography, periphery, panoramic and orthographic cameras.
3.2 Specialist medical photographic procedures including photoendoscopy (fixed rod and fibre optic), fluorescein angiography, slit-lamp and photokeratography, infrared and ultraviolet – both reflected and fluorescence, somatotyping, transillumination techniques, etc.
3.3 Cinematography; surgical, medical and scientific, 16 mm and 8 mm, optical, magnetic or silent, including: scripting, lighting, photography, logging, animation, editing, special effects and titling, sound-track recording and transfer, and the use of laboratory facilities.
3.4 Photomicrography and photomacrography, in all forms and at all powers, including techniques such as dark-field, phase contrast, polarization, ultraviolet, interference, and epi-illumination. A knowledge of the photographic aspects of electron microscopy.
3.5 A working knowledge of the photographic aspects of related imaging processes, e.g. television, reprography including the process camera and autoscreening, thermography, nuclear track recording, radiography, etc.
3.6 Research into the application of advanced photographic techniques to solve problems in clinical diagnosis, research and publication.

The Senior Photographer will also undertake any relevant duties as may be specified by the Head of Department from time to time.

## Medical Photographer

*General*

The post is on the scale of Medical Laboratory Scientific Officer of the Whitley Council (UK) and the salary and terms of service are as laid down for that grade.

The Medical Photographer works as part of a team of photographic staff reporting to the Senior Photographer, and responsible ultimately to the Head of Department.

Hours of work are 9.00 am. to 5.30 pm. Monday to Thursday, 9.00 am. to 5.00 pm. Friday, with one hour for lunch between 12.00 and 2.00 pm. As with all jobs within the health care environment some flexibility is necessary here. Extra time worked is given back as time off in lieu.

Annual leave is 20 working days plus statutory and customary holidays as defined by the medical school.

*Qualifications*

It is expected that the post-holder will have 'City and Guild's 745' and IIP Basic Medical Photography' certificates (or recognized equivalents). Every encouragement is given to work towards higher qualifications.

*Job Content*

Essentially the work falls into the categories below. At all times the word 'photography' implies the complete process from taking the request and discussion with the client, through loading film and cameras, processing, printing, mounting, numbering, labelling and keeping records, to sending out the finished product. Each photographer is responsible for his own work from beginning to end.

*1. Clinical Photography*

This involves, for example:
1.1 Photography of patients of all types and ages, in the studio, in black-and-white or colour, still or cine, for record, teaching, research or publication. Being in sole charge of the patients in their care.
1.2 Photography of patients as above but on location, e.g. in the operating theatres, wards, delivery rooms, clinics or post-mortem rooms.
1.3 Photography of medical, nursing and surgical procedures.
1.4 Specialist diagnostic photography such as: fluorescein angiography, or ultra – violet fluorescence photography.

*2. Pathological Photography*

This involves, for example:
2.1 Photography of pathological, surgical, anatomical or forensic specimens, fixed or fresh, in the studio, or on location.
2.2 Photography of culture plates – bacteriological and mycological immunoelectrophoresis patterns, sedimentation and agglutination tests, agar diffusion plates, chromatograms, etc.

*3. Research Photography*

This involves, for example:
3.1 Photography of laboratory animals and experiments.
3.2 Specialist photography such as photomicrography, photogrammetry, ultraviolet or infrared photography, time-lapse or high-speed cinematography (this advanced work will often be undertaken under the supervision of the senior photographer).
3.3 Photography of CRT displays or experimental equipment.

*4. Reprographic Photography*

This involves, for example:
4.1 Production of teaching tansparencies from drawings, books, graphs, charts, tables radiographs, ECG and EEG traces, etc. in colour, line, tone, tinted or diazochrome forms.
4.2 Production of prints, in black-and-white or colour, for publication or display, of the material mentioned in 4.1.
4.3 Duplication of trannsparencies or prints for widespread distribution.
4.4 Production of overhead projection transparencies.

*5. General Photography*

This involves, for example:
5.1 Portraiture, passport and ID photography.
5.2 Public relations photography, including occasional press, sports and social photography.
5.3 Industrial and commercial photography, including, for example buildings, equipment and apparatus, food layouts and instruments.
5.4 Photography for exhibition and display,

booklets, tape–slide and television programmes.

*6. Other Activities*

These involve, for example:
6.1 Assisting the Senior Photographer in stock control, testing and selection of materials, and equipment, and provision of supplies.
6.2 Helping to keep proper departmental and patient records, and departmental slide and print libraries.
6.3 Helping to maintain all photographic equipment and facilities in clean and working order.
6.4 Organising and liaising with photographic laboratory services under the direction of the Chief Photographer.
6.5 Other relevant duties as may be specified by the Head of Department from time to time.

*Personal Qualities*

The Medical Photographer should have a sympathetic but firm attitude with patients, good appearance and the ability to communicate effectively with medical staff. The ability to work cheerfully and effectively as part of a team under pressure to meet constant deadlines is necessary.

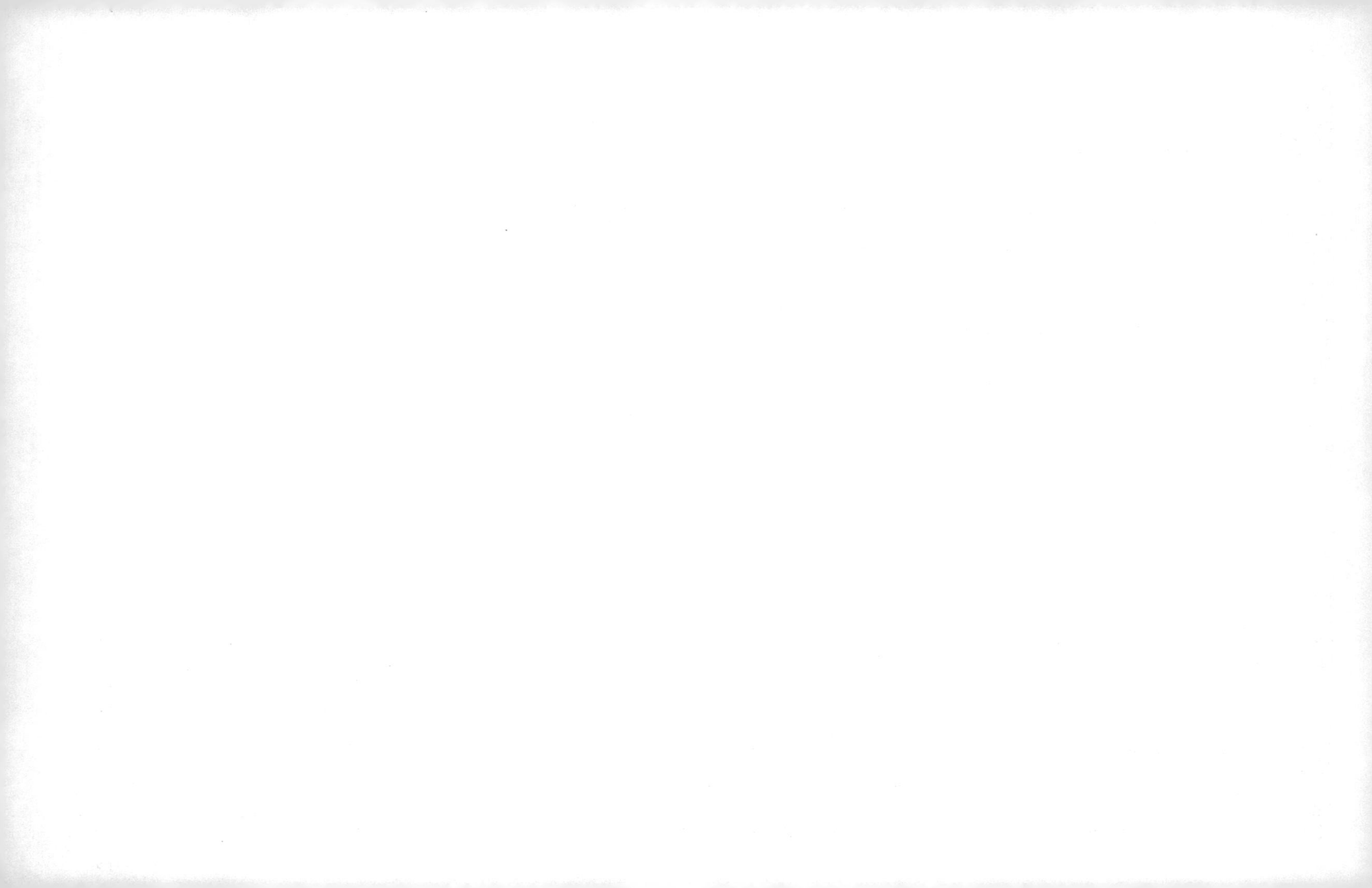

# Section 4
# First aid and resuscitation

**A.R. Williams**, MPhil, FBIPP, FRPS, FBPA, AIMBI
Head of Medical Illustration and Teaching Services
Charing Cross Hospital and Medical School, London

## 4.1 INTRODUCTION

Too often it is assumed that because one works in a hospital environment it is not necessary to learn first aid. In actuality the opposite applies – it is essential for all paramedical staff to be familiar with first aid procedures – your studio may be several minutes away from professional help. In any event you have a responsibility as a health care professional to the community at large to be able to help in an emergency situation.

The whole subject of first aid is too large to be adequately covered in this text, which inevitably is orientated towards the incidents most commonly met by the practising medical photographer. The student is strongly advised to undertake some form of formal training such as the short courses run by the St. John's Ambulance Association or the International Red Cross Society.

As a medical photographer, patients in your care will expect you to cope with an emergency situation – make sure you can justify their confidence.

## 4.2 THE PRINCIPLES OF FIRST AID

First aid is the skilled application of accepted principles of treatment on the occurrence of an accident or in the case of sudden illness, using facilities or materials available at the time. It is the approved method of treating a casualty until he is placed, if necessary, in the care of a doctor. Except in very minor cases, remedial treatment is the province of the Medical Practitioner. However, you may be the only person in a position to save life. If action is delayed until a doctor arrives, in some situations the patient may be dead.
The aims are:

(1) To sustain life
(2) To prevent the condition being aggravated
(3) To relieve pain and make the patient comfortable, and
(4) To obtain medical aid, or promote recovery.

## 4.3 AN APPROACH TO THE SUDDEN EMERGENCY

(1) Keep calm
(2) Assess the situation
(3) Send for help
(4) Establish a diagnosis
(5) Give immediate and adequate treatment
(6) Dispose of the casualty, e.g. to Ward, Accident and Emergency department etc., and
(7) Document the incident.

### 4.3.1 Keep calm

Try to act in a logical and systematic way despite the trauma and confusion of the incident. Take charge of the situation, give confidence to the conscious casualty – talk to him, listen to him and reassure him – decide on your priorities.

### 4.3.2 Assess the situation

First, check to see if there is any continuing danger to your patient, or yourself, e.g. from electricity, poisonous fumes etc. If so either remove the danger (e.g. put out the fire, switch off the electricity, etc.) or carefully remove the patient from the danger area.

Secondly, check if there is any immediate danger to life,

*Respiration* – is there any failure of respiratory function? Check the airway is clear and if necessary start artificial respiration.
*Cardiac activity* – is the heart beating? If not start external cardiac massage.
*Haemhorrage* – check for serious bleeding and control it – raise the part if possible or use pressure dressings.

Next, assess what other assistance is needed and how it might best be obtained. Will it be best to send for medical aid or to send the patient to it?

Lastly, assess what other less urgent problems there may be, e.g. fractures, minor cuts, etc.

### 4.3.3 Send for help

This may mean simply calling for assistance from a colleague in the department, but may also mean asking a bystander to telephone for an ambulance in the case of a roadside accident.

Work out what medical aid is required and how best it can be obtained. For example, once the patient is made safe from immediate danger, will it be best to send for medical aid or to send him to it? Remember, if you do have to telephone for assistance give the exact location, the number and approximate age of casualties, the nature of the accident and your assessment of the injuries/diagnoses.

All major hospitals have cardiac arrest teams accessible via special telephone numbers or 'bleep' numbers – make sure you learn your local one by heart. You may need it one day and there will not be the time for looking in telephone directories.

### 4.3.4 Establish a diagnosis

Use all your senses to obtain the maximum information about your patient – look, speak, listen, feel and smell.

(1) *If the casualty is conscious*
*Look* at the patient and the situation that surrounds him. Ask him if he has pain and where it is, examine that part first. Ask him what happened and if there is anything else wrong. Handle injured areas gently but firmly. Make sure there are no other injuries that the patient is unaware of. Examine the casualty carefully–starting with head and neck, then moving down over spine, trunk, upper limbs, lower limbs – comparing left to right sides as you go.
*Check* colour of skin, nail beds, eyes and inside eyelids, nature of breathing and its odour, if any, the pulse rate, noting strength and rhythm, the body temperature.
*Remove* only the minimum amount of clothing consistent with treating the injuries.

(2) *If the casualty is unconscious*:
The task will be more difficult and extra attention to detail will be necessary.
Establish that breathing and pulse are present (if not, immediately institute resuscitation procedures – see below), and note the rate and character of both and any changes with time. Examine over and under the casualty for bleeding – stop any serious bleeding before proceeding any further (bear in mind the possibility of internal bleeding). Try to establish the cause of unconsciousness by checking:
*breathing* – rate, depth, regularity, odour;
*pulse* – rate, character;
*skin* – colour, temperature and condition;
*eyes* – pupils, inside eyelids;
*head* – for injury, bleeding from nose or ear; and
*whole body* – for external signs of possible internal injury.

### 4.3.5 Give immediate and adequate treatment

Although it will have seemed a very long time to you the first four steps of the plan may only have taken seconds if you have been working efficiently. Now comes the time to start treatment – the details of which will be found in the rest of the section.

Remember, however, to give the appropriate treatment gently and quickly in a confident manner. Nothing inspires greater confidence in a casualty than calmness and efficiency coupled with words of reassurance and encouragement. Remember also that the casualty may overhear remarks not intended for him. Listen to the casualty's comments or requests. Many who are seriously injured will ask for water – it is not advisable to give it. Do not keep asking the patient how he is feeling. Once treatment has been given keep a careful watch on the casualty until assistance arrives. A good measure of common sense is necessary on every occasion.

### 4.3.6 Disposal of the casualty

After you have carried out treatment and depending on the seriousness of the injuries the casualty may be:

- Allowed to go home and seek medical advice if necessary.
- Taken to a nearby house or shelter to await the arrival of a doctor.
- Handed over to a doctor, nurse or other qualified person.
- Sent to hospital by ambulance.
- Transferred from your department to the accident and emergency unit, coronary care unit, or operating theatres as required.

Never send home, or leave unaccompanied, a casualty who has been unconscious for even a short period.

### 4.3.7 Document the incident

Your responsibilities do not end with sending the patient away. You must make full and accurate records of the event and your action.

If the incident happened in your department:

- Fill in the appropriate accident form/incident report for your institution.
- Inform the hospital administration, the ward or department where the patient came from and the patient's consultant.
- Write out a full record of the incident and the treatment/action you took. If necessary take statements from your staff who may have been involved.
- If the accident involved faulty equipmentservices inform the appropriate department immediately, and later in writing.

If the incident happens outside the hospital environment:

- Take the name and address of the casualty and of any witnesses or others involved in the incident. Give this information to the police (a) so that next of kin can be informed, (b) in case of any subsequent legal action.
- Write out a full record of the incident and the treatment/action you took, keep it safe in case you are ever called upon to explain the incident, e.g. if the casualty subsequently dies.

## 4.4 SUDDEN LOSS OF CONSCIOUSNESS

This is probably the most common situation that the medical photographer will have to deal with. It can be the most dangerous or the most innocuous of states, and your action must depend upon accurate assessment of the likely diagnosis.

### 4.4.1 Syncope (fainting) and shock

This is caused by a sudden fall of blood pressure due to nervous action caused by fright, mental shock, pain, standing for a long time, etc. This is the commonest

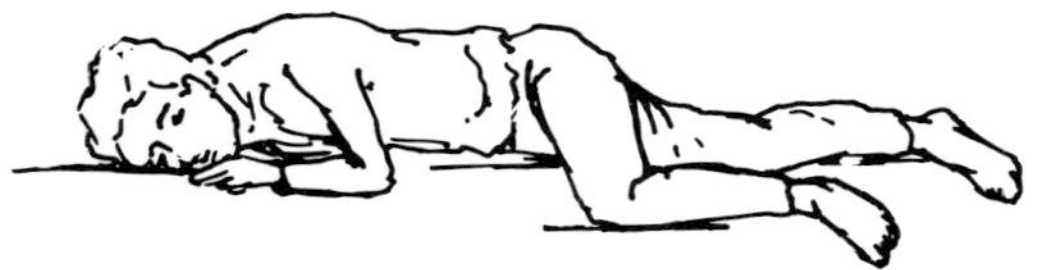

***Figure 4.1*** *The recovery position ensures that the casualty maintains an open airway. With the head and neck extended the tongue will not occlude the trachea and vomit or blood will drain safely away*

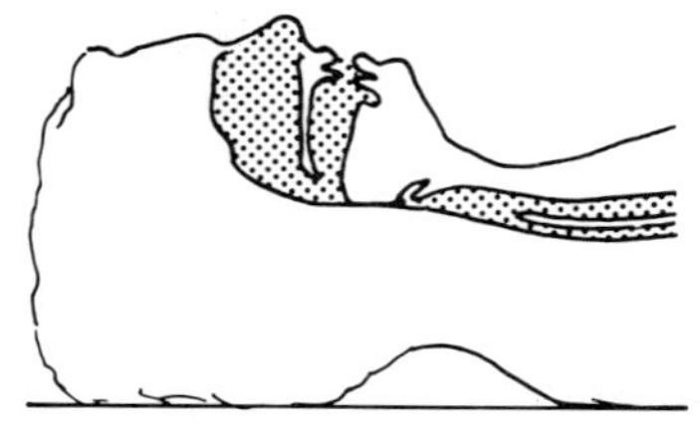

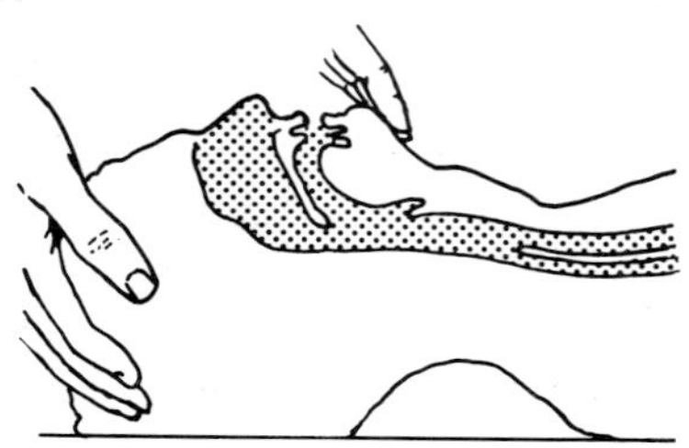

***Figure 4.2*** *When the chin is allowed to drop the tongue falls back to occlude the airway – this must be prevented*

form of loss of consciousness and can often be induced just by the sight and smell of hospital equipment.

The patient feels pale, clammy, dizzy then staggers and ultimately falls.

Recumbent patients do not faint. Lie the patient down on a couch to do your work whenever practicable, and you think there may be a risk of fainting.

*Treatments:*

Impending faint – sit the patient down with his head between his knees, tell him to take deep breaths.

Actual faint – put the patient on his side into the lateral 'coma' or 'recovery' position (Figure 4.1). Elevate the feet slightly, loosen clothing, sponge face with cold water.

Never support the unconscious patient in an upright position, either sitting or standing – his heart may cease to beat or he may choke to death.

Never force fluid (brandy, tea, etc.) into a patient's mouth while he is unconscious, you may choke him.

### 4.4.2 Coma – more serious loss of consciousness

This is caused by:

Physical agents – electrical, traumatic concussion;
Medical – diabetes, cerebral vascular accidents, epilepsy, etc.
Asphyxia – suffocation, coal gas, drowning;
Cardiac arrest; or
Drugs – overdose or allergies.

Whatever the cause the approach to the problem is the same:

#### *(1) Are the patient's air passages obstructed?*

If yes – clear out the mouth and extend the head to open the airway. Push the chin forward, (Figure 4.2); the most common form of airway obstruction is for the tongue to occlude the trachea. If a child has a foreign body (e.g. a coin) which is obstructing the airway, hold it up by the ankles and gently thump his back until the object drops out. If the foreign body is not obstructing the airway, do not attempt to remove it, particularly if it is irregular (e.g. a toy soldier) or you may do a great deal of harm. Lie the patient in the recovery position and obtain medical assistance.

***(2) Is he breathing?***

If yes – turn the patient on his side into the recovery position. Call for medical assistance. Keep the airway clear allowing saliva, blood etc., to drain out of the corner of the mouth.
If no – start expired air ventilation, preferably mouth-to-nose, mouth-to-mouth, or Holger–Nielson methods, or if available, use the AMBU respirator bag or a Brooke airway (see below). **Seconds count – Move quickly.**

***(3) Is his heart beating?***

Feel for the major pulses – the carotid (neck) or radial (wrist) are the most reliable (Figure 4.3).

Is he pale or cyanosed? (For coloured patients check nail beds or inside lower eyelids.)
Are his pupils dilated?
If the heart has stopped, elevate the legs and start external cardiac massage (see below).

If the heart has stopped beating the brain will be irretrievably damaged after about 4 minutes unless expired air ventilation and external cardiac massage are started and maintained. **seconds count – move fast**.

If you are alone, institute a cycle of one breath of expired air ventilation, ten strokes of external cardiac massage, and so on. If working with an assistant, one breath to every five strokes of external cardiac massage.

### 4.4.3 The recovery position

In order to prevent asphyxia it may be necessary to turn a casualty when lying on his back into the recovery position. This can be done as follows:

(1) Kneel beside him and place both arms close to his body.
(2) Turn the casualty gently onto his side (this is most easily achieved by grasping the clothing at the hip).
(3) Raise the upper arm until it makes a right angle with the body and flex the knee.
(4) Gently draw out the underneath arm to extend slightly behind his back.
(5) Flex the undermost knee slightly.

Placing the limbs in this configuration provides the necessary support to keep the casualty comfortable in a position where the airway will be kept free from vomit or other obstructions (see Figure 4.1)

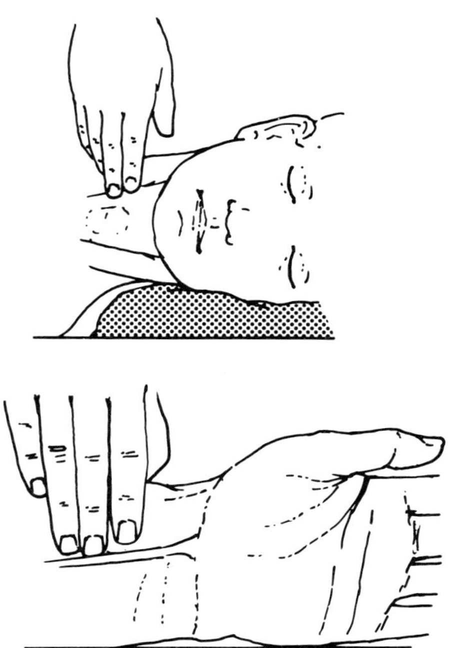

***Figure 4.3*** *The two most useful pulse detection points – the carotid and radial arteries*

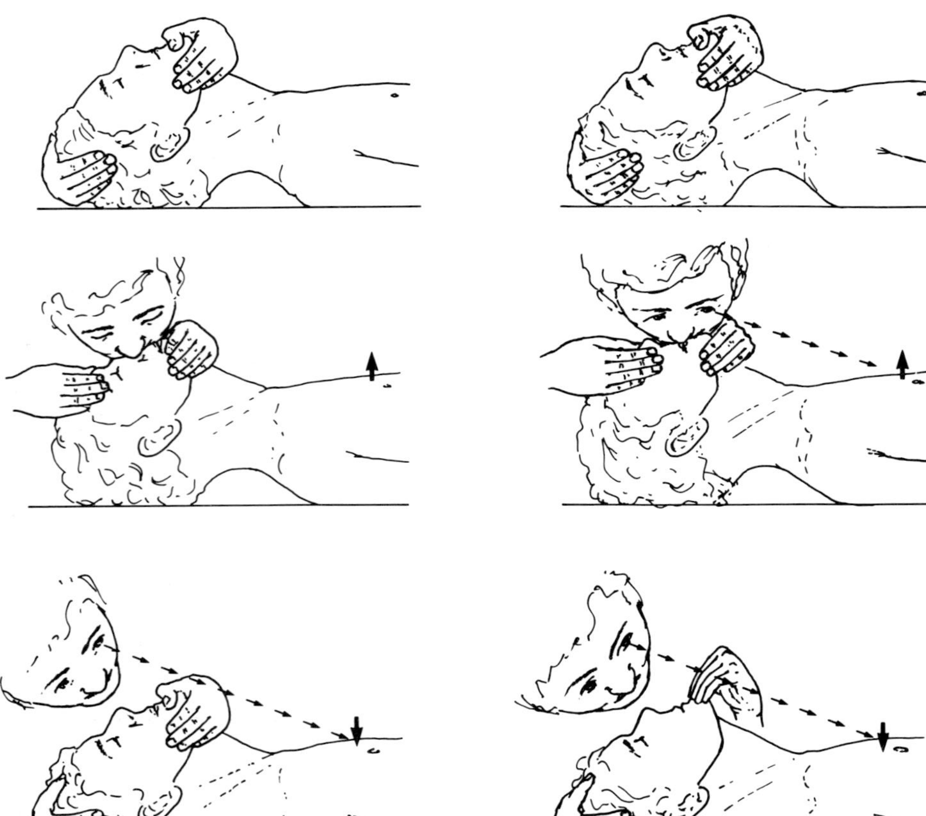

**Figure 4.4** *Mouth-to-nose respiratory resuscitation*

**Figure 4.5** *Mouth-to-mouth respiratory resuscitation*

## 4.5 RESPIRATORY RESUSCITATION

Expired air ventilation (mouth-to-nose, or mouth-to-mouth), sometimes called the 'kiss of life' is superior to and supersedes other first aid methods of respiration. It works because expired air contains sufficient oxygen to act as useful inspired air for the patient. It can be used by almost all age groups and in almost all circumstances except:

- when there is severe injury to the face and mouth,
- when the casualty is pinned face down,
- or when vomiting interferes with respiratory resuscitation (vomiting often occurs when breathing is re-established and consciousness is returning).

The patient's lungs are expanded by air blown into the patient's mouth or nose. The lungs deflate by elastic recoil of the lungs and chest wall.
The various methods of artificial respiration are:

### 4.5.1 Mouth-to-nose (preferable) – Figure 4.4

Clear nose, mouth and throat of debris,
Extend head and push jaw forward to open airway,
Take a deep breath,

Spread lips widely over nose – close patient's mouth,
Blow steadily,
Watch chest expand,
Stop blowing and remove lips from nose, and watch chest deflate.
If you follow these instructions, the rate will be 12–16 times a minute which is ideal.

### 4.5.2 Mouth-to-mouth (alternative) – Figure 4.5

As for mouth-to-nose except pinch the nose and blow through the mouth.
**N.B.** Do not blow too hard, or after the chest has fully expanded the oesophagus may be opened allowing the escape of stomach contents. With small infants, blow into mouth and nose at the same time.

### 4.5.3 The 'AMBU' respirator bag

Apply the mask to the patient's face – make sure there is no leak. Squeeze bag and watch chest expand.
Stop squeezing and allow bag to expand again while chest deflates – there is no need to lift the mask from the face.
Repeat the process.

### 4.5.4 The 'Brooke' airway

Insert the airway over the back of the tongue with notched air shield fitting round nose.
Press shield firmly over mouth, pinch nose and blow down airway to expand lungs.
Stop blowing to allow chest to deflate.
Repeat process.

### 4.5.5 The Holger–Nielson method, Figure 4.6

Useful where the face or mouth are particularly damaged or where ingestion of liquid poisons is suspected.
Place the casualty face down with arms overhead and elbows flexed so that one hand rests upon the other.
Turn casualty's head to one side, so that the cheek rests on his uppermost hand.
Clear nose, mouth and throat of any debris.
Kneel on one knee at casualty's head and put the foot of your opposite leg near his elbow.
Place your hands on his back just below the shoulder blades.
Rock forward with elbows straight until arms are approximately vertical, exerting steady pressure on casualty's chest.
Grasp his arms just above elbows and rock backwards raising his arms until resistance is felt at the casualty's shoulders.
Release casualty's arms.
Repeat 12 times a minute – each phase of compression and expansion to last 2.5 seconds.

## 4.6 EXTERNAL CARDIAC MASSAGE

External cardiac massage works on the principle of compressing the heart between the sternum and the vertebral column thus squeezing blood into the arterial circulation.
**N.B.** The pressure must be applied in the correct place (lower third of the sternum) otherwise serious damage may be done to the ribs, lungs, spleen, liver, etc.
The method is as follows: (See Figure 4.7)

- Institute artificial ventilation (external cardiac massage is useless without artificial respiration).
- See that the patient is supine on a firm surface.
- Identify the sternum between the sternal notch (between the medial ends of the clavicles) and xiphisternum.
- Place the palm of one hand on the lower third of sternum and the second hand on top of the first.
- With arms straight exert downwards

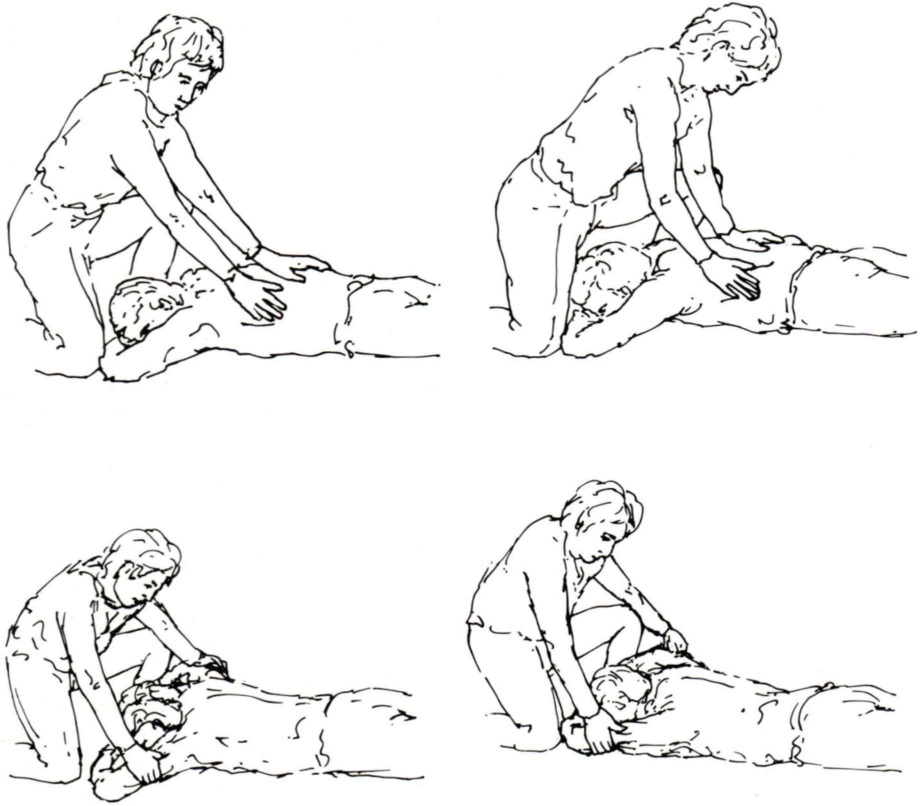

***Figure 4.6*** *The Holger-Nielson method of artificial respiration*

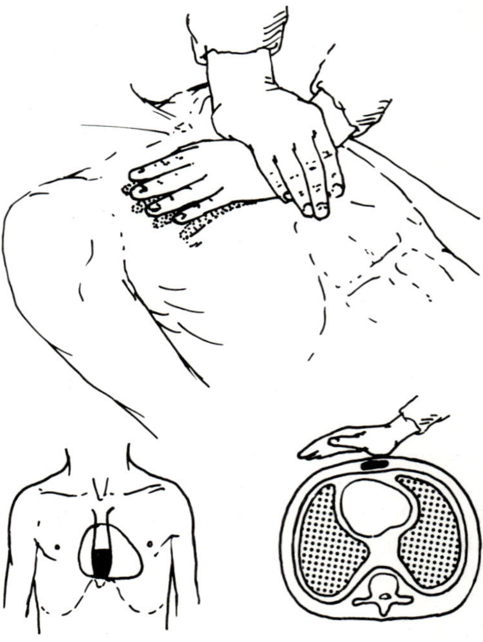

***Figure 4.7*** *External cardiac massage*

pressure with the palms being careful not to press on the ribs with the fingers.
- Press the sternum 2–4 cm towards the backbone (the pressure required is the equivalent of about 30 kg on your bathroom scales).
- Relieve pressure and allow sternum to return to the original position.
- Time your action to give approximately 50–60 beats per minute.
- Watch for returning colour and contraction of pupil and ask a colleague to monitor the carotid pulse by palpitation.

**N.B.** Children will require much lighter pressure – place one hand behind the back and the palm of the other over the lower third of the sternum. For infants use two fingers in the same position. The rate should be increased correspondingly to 80 or even 100 times per minute.

Watch for returning spontaneous respiration or pulse beat, but do not stop artificial ventilation or external cardiac massage until both are of satisfactory volume. In the absence of medical aid, continue resuscitation for at least 1 hour, and then stop only if artificial ventilation and cardiac massage make no difference to the colour of the patient.

*Remember.* In respiratory arrest it is safe and wise to commence artificial respiration while breathing appears to be failing. In cardiac arrest external heart compression should not be started unless you are satisfied that the heart has stopped beating. If in doubt as to whether the casualty is clinically dead give treatment until qualified medical staff arrive.

## 4.7 HAEMORRHAGE

The results of severe blood loss are similar to those of shock, i.e. pallor, cold clammy skin, fainting, weak rapid pulse, restlessness and thirst, shallow breathing accompanied by yawning.

Almost all external bleeding can be stopped by firm pressure on the wound with a clean pad, elevation of the affected part and subsequent firm bandaging.

Do not attempt to remove dirt or debris from a wound – this is best done under anaesthesia.

Tourniquets are rarely necessary and may be dangerous if applied incorrectly, they can cause congestion and increase bleeding.

Lie the patient down with the trunk horizontal and elevate the legs to increase the blood supply to head and trunk.

Internal bleeding is evidenced by the general symptoms described above, possibly accompanied by coughing or vomiting of blood, blood exuding from the ear canal, or nose, or blood appearing in the urine. Lie the patient down, keep him calm and warm, obtain medical assistance immediately. Frequently monitor pulse and breathing rate.

Bleeding from the nose occurs spontaneously in some patients (epistaxis). Support the patient in a sitting position with head slightly forward, pinch the soft part of the nose closed. Apply a cold pad to the bridge of the nose. Tell the patient to breathe through the mouth.

Varicose veins burst easily when knocked and bleeding may be sudden and severe. Apply immediate pressure to the bleeding point, lie the patient down and raise the leg. Apply a firm dressing.

## 4.8 HEART ATTACKS

In general a severe reduction in the blood supply to the muscular wall of the heart.

*Angina pectoris* – over-exertion brings on an acute attack of pain in the chest which often spreads to the left shoulder and arm. Attacks are relieved by rest and usually last only a few minutes.

(**N.B.** Patients who are prone to angina often carry glyceryl trinitrate tablets which are useful in preventing attacks but not treating them.)

*Coronary obstruction* – a blood clot suddenly occludes a coronary artery and

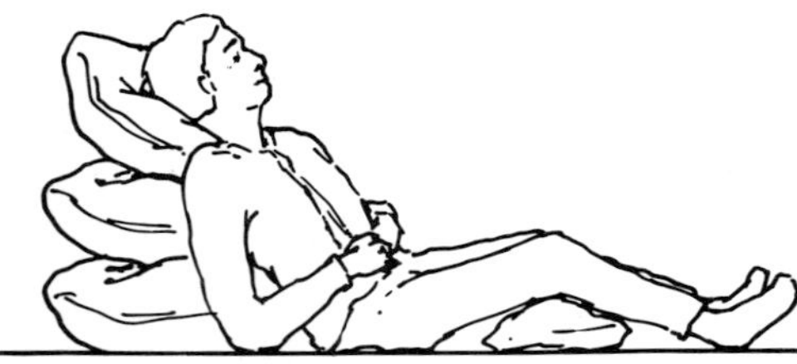

***Figure 4.8*** *The semi-recumbent position*

the patient is gripped by excruciating pain behind the sternum and upper ribs. Rest is essential but may not ease the pain. Cardiac activity may stop altogether. Treatment – do not move the patient unnecessarily.
Place into the semi-recumbent position (Figure 4.8); laying the casualty flat may prevent respiratory activity.
Loosen clothing.
Monitor cardiac and respiratory function until medical help arrives.

## 4.9 BURNS AND SCALDS

It is necessary to treat the local injury and also generally for shock. The seriousness depends upon many factors – most important being area and depth. An extensive superficial burn will be more painful than a small deep one. The area of most burns including clothing, is usually sterile and every effort should be made to keep it that way.

*Burns caused by heat (wet or dry)*

- If clothing is alight extinguish by rolling patient in fire blanket, white coat, etc.
- If minor burn – cool with cold water, the reduction of heat is most important.
- Apply light clean dressing.
- Make the patient comfortable.
- Give cold fluids by mouth if conscious.
- Obtain medical aid.

**DO NOT**

- touch the burn,
- remove charred clothing or debris, or
- apply any kind of grease, jelly, etc.

*Acid or alkali burns*

- Flood with water immediately, dilute the chemical as much as possible (specific antidotes may be provided for this).
- Apply a dry dressing.
- Make the patient comfortable.
- Obtain medical aid and try to establish the nature of the corrosive chemical involved.

## 4.10 FRACTURES

Although patients with fractures need less urgent attention than say asphyxia or cardiac arrest they will all need professional medical attention, and the fracture can be potentially very serious. The aim is to support the injured limb to prevent further damage (complex bandaging and splinting are beyond the scope of the present text).

Broadly, fractures are classified as:

### (1) *Closed and not distorted.*

Handle with great care, always support the limb with one hand on each side of the fracture.
*Legs* – bandage together and/or support with improvised splints, well padded. Also put padding to separate knees and ankles.
*Arms* – support in a sling, use improvised splints.

### (2) *Open or compound and/or distorted.*

Do not attempt to 'set' the fracture or reduce the deformity.
Great damage, especially to arteries and nerves, can be caused by allowing movement.
Support in the deformed position with suitably padded splints or with cushions/pillow.
Lie the patient down, head lower than the feet.
The pain of the broken ends of the fracture rubbing together can cause shock.

## 4.11 DIABETES MELLITUS

### (1) *Insulin coma*

Diabetic patients may collapse from hypoglycaemia caused by excessive exercise, insufficient food, or accidental overdose of insulin. Symptoms are pallor, profuse sweating, rapid pulse, shallow breathing, confusion and faintness. (The longer a patient has been on insulin the less evident are warning symptoms for hypoglycaemia).

### (2) *Diabetic coma*

Hyperglycaemia caused by insufficient insulin or excessive food intake can also cause coma. Here the symptoms are dry skin, flushed face, deep breathing – with the breath smelling strongly of ketones.

*Treatment* – If it can be established that the patient is suffering from hypoglycaemia, do not hesitate to give sweetened drinks or sugar lumps.

## 4.12 EPILEPSY

Epileptic patients may experience fits at any time, which may be of two types – 'petit mal' or 'grand mal'. The aim of first aid is to prevent the patient, who has no control of himself, from receiving any injury and to keep his airway clear.

*Petit mal* – patient becomes pale with fixed, staring gaze, not conscious of surroundings. Attack is brief and should be treated as syncope.

*Grand mal* – The true epileptic fit, with sudden loss of consciousness, followed by rigidity and cyanosis then muscular convulsions possibly accompanied by incontinence, lastly followed by a quiet relaxed phase. On regaining consciousness the patient is confused, distressed and exhausted – he may fall into a deep sleep. Protect the patient from injury – do not attempt to restrain him. If the opportunity arises place something soft between the teeth – to prevent damage to the tongue. In the coma phase place into the recovery position to prevent choking.

## 4.13 INFANTILE CONVULSIONS

These sometimes occur in infants and babies as a result of raised temperature from any cause. There may be twitching of muscles, rigidity and congestion of the face and neck.
*Treatment* – loosen all clothing, ensure adequate supply of air, place child in recovery position, start tepid sponging, reassure the parents.

## 4.14 APOPLEXY (CEREBRAL VASCULAR ACCIDENT – STROKE)

There is a sudden loss of use of a limb, sometimes with slurred speech and other signs of severe brain damage, due to a ruptured cerebral vessel. Usually occurs in middle-aged or elderly patients suffering from high blood pressure. Treat generally as for coma.

### References

Anonymous (1982). *First Aid – the Authorised Manual.* (London: St. John's Ambulance Association)

Procter, N. and London, P. (1977). *Principles of First Aid for the Injured.* (London: Butterworths)

### *Practical projects*

(1) With a colleague practise the movements required for placing a casualty in the recovery position.

(2) Practise taking carotid and radial pulses on colleagues.

(3) Try to obtain a model torso for practising mouth-to-mouth respiration and external cardiac massage (e.g. 'Resusi Anne') – a school of nursing may be able to help. Practise until you have perfected both techniques.

(4) Find out your Departmental policies on first aid and cardiac arrest. Check the location of the first aid box and its contents, and commit to memory your cardiac arrest team 'call out' number.

(5) Ask your Head of Department or Administrator for a sample accident form – make yourself aware of the information which will be required after any incident.

(6) Enrol for any short course on first aid which may be run locally by, for example, St. John's Ambulance to obtain your first aid certificate.

### *Examination Questions*

Q.1 A patient collapses whilst you are photographing him in your studio. Describe how you would assess the situation, treat the patient and document the event.

Q.2 A 59 year old female patient with severe varicose veins knocks her leg on your studio camera stand and starts to bleed profusely. Describe *fully* the actions which you would take in this situation.

Q.3 You enter your studio to find a colleague slumped over the studio 'strobe' (high power electronic flash). Describe fully the actions which you would take.

Q.4 Discuss the potential health hazards in a department of medical photography and the steps you would take to reduce them.

*Multiple choice (any of the statements may be true or false)*

Q.5 A patient collapses whilst being photographed in your studio:

(*a*) You would immediately start cardiac massage.
(*b*) Sit the patient comfortably and call for help.
(*c*) Start mouth to-mouth respiration immediately.
(*d*) Check the patient's pupils first.
(*e*) Place the patient supine with a pillow under his head.

# Section 5
# Photography in dentistry, orthodontics and oral surgery

**M.K. Johns**, FIMBI, ARPS
Deputy Director of Medical Illustration
Institute of Child Health and Hospitals for Sick Children, London

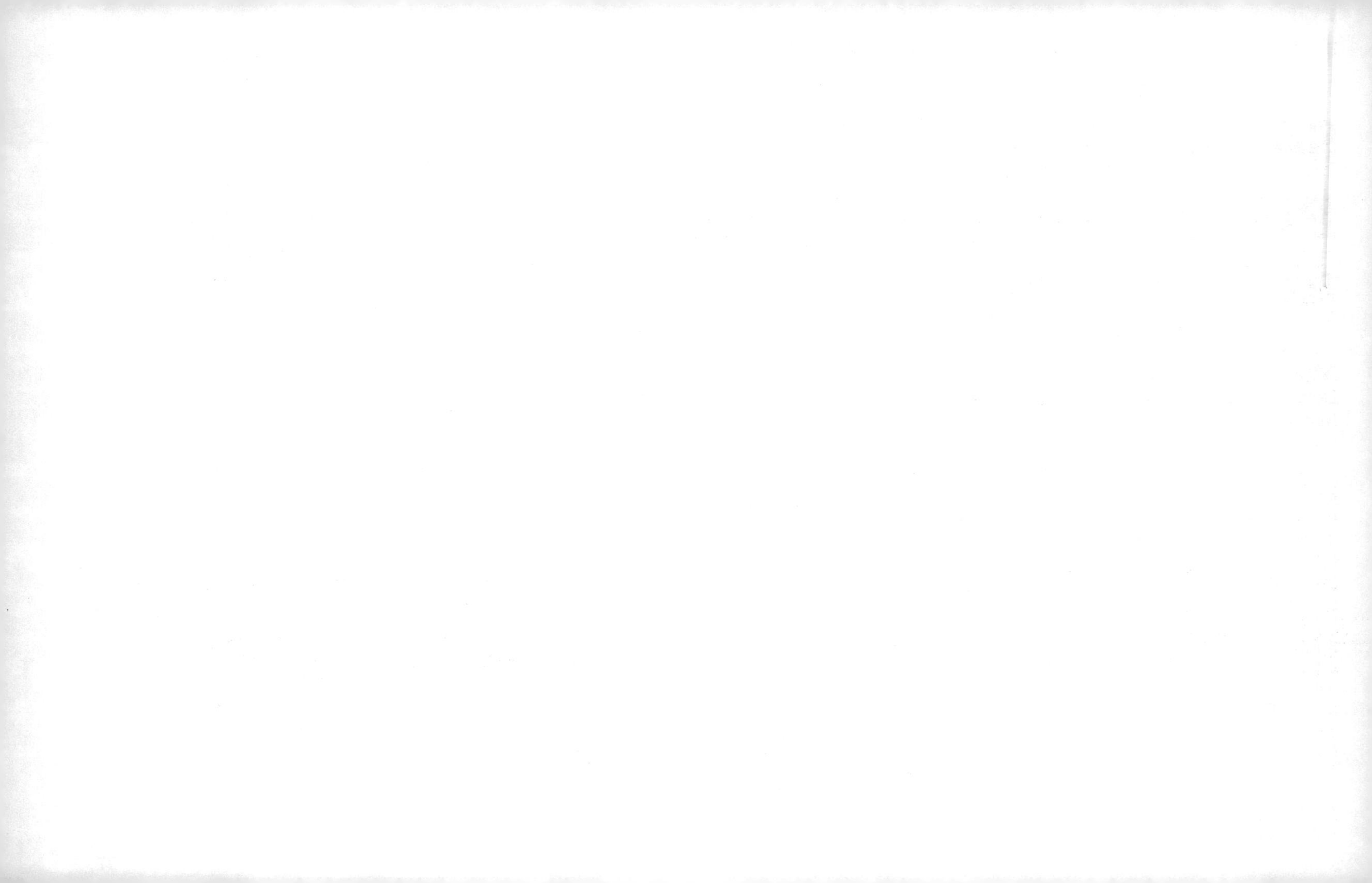

## 5.1 INTRODUCTION

The work of the dental surgeon is, like, medicine, divided into general practice and specialist surgery. The general dental practitioner is concerned mainly with 'conservative' dentistry (preserving and repairing teeth); whereas the specialist dental surgeon undertakes orthodontic treatment, maxillo–facial and related plastic surgery, in addition to general dental work. Conservative dentistry is all performed 'in the chair'.

The photographer working in these fields will be concerned primarily with the teeth, the oral cavity and the face. As well as working in the studio, he may be called on to work at the chairside during routine dental procedures (e.g. fillings, minor oral surgery, inlays, orthodontics, crown and bridge work, etc.) or in the operating theatre to record more major oral surgery (e.g. extraction of impacted wisdom teeth, maxillary or mandibular osteotomies, etc). All the general guidelines for clinical photography apply in this area.

## 5.2 ANATOMY

The structure of the teeth should be understood, as should their development in the child and adult through deciduous (primary) to permanent teeth. In addition the photographer should understand the anatomy and physiology of the face with particular reference to the bony structure and the musculature.

### 5.2.1 Specialist terminology

In common with all branches of medicine there is a range of specialized terms, some anatomical, some pathological, used in dentistry and oral surgery. In a good medical dictionary *look up* the following terms, and *make notes* on their relevance and meaning. Accretion, Alveolar abscess, Alveolus, Anodontia, Antrum, Apical, Aphthous ulcer, Buccoversion, Candida, Caries, Cementum, Cingulum, Concrescence, Dentine, Enamel, Enameloma, Epulis, Exostosis, Fauces, Frenum, Gingivitis, Glossitis, Gnathion, Hutchinson's teeth, Impaction, Leucoplakia, Ludwig's angina, Malocclusion, Mesiodens, Mesognathic, Micrognathia, Microdontia, Moulage, Odontocele, Odontolysis, Periodontitis, Prognathism, Ranula, Resorption, Sialadentitis, Stomatitis.

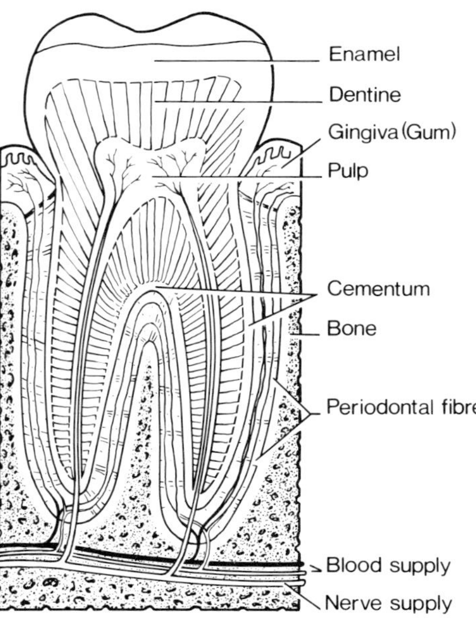


***Figure 5.1*** *Longitudinal section through a generalized tooth*

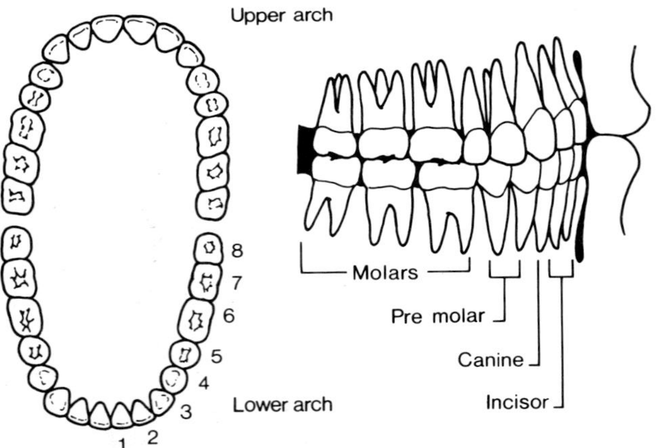


***Figure 5.2*** *Primary or deciduous teeth*

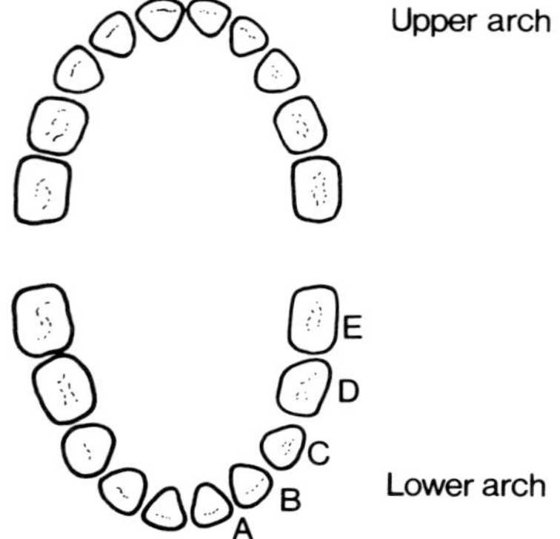


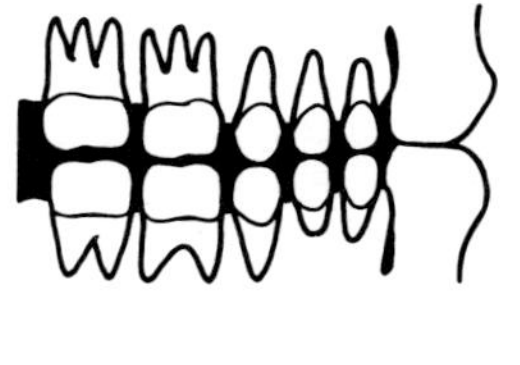

***Figure 5.3*** *Adult or permanent dentition*

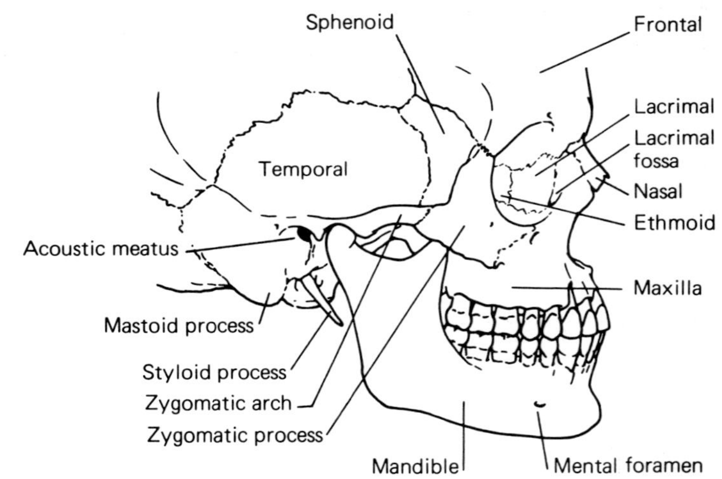


***Figure 5.4*** *The bony structure of the face and jaw*

### 5.2.2 Annotation of teeth

The international reference chart for primary or deciduous teeth is:

| *R* | E D C B A | A B C D E | *L* |
|---|---|---|---|
| | E D C B A | A B C D E | |

and for permanent teeth:

| *R* | 8 7 6 5 4 3 2 1 | 1 2 3 4 5 6 7 8 | *L* |
|---|---|---|---|
| | 8 7 6 5 4 3 2 1 | 1 2 3 4 5 6 7 8 | |

example: the upper right premolar would be symbolized as 4|
Each tooth has five 'aspects' or 'surfaces': mesial, distal, buccal, lingual, and occlusal.

## 5.3 STANDARDIZED PHOTOGRAPHY

With the possible exception of certain aspects of operative dentistry and oral surgery, photographs should be carefully standardized in terms of both *scale* and *lighting* in order that serial records can be satisfactorily obtained. Many dental patients will become regular visitors to a photographic department over the course of their treatment, which in the case of orthodontics may last several years. Subject areas may be grouped as follows:

(1) *Head and neck.* Various AP lateral and ¾ views may be required, and can be accommodated comfortably at a scale of 1:8 on 35 mm film.

(2) *Intra-oral views*

(a) anterior teeth:

| 4 3 2 1 | 1 2 3 4 | (1.2) |
|---|---|---|
| 4 3 2 1 | 1 2 3 4 | |

(b) ¾ teeth:

| (8 7) 6 5 4 3 2 1 | 1 2 | or left (1.2) |
|---|---|---|
| (8 7) 6 5 4 3 2 1 | 1 2 | |

(c) upper incisors: 2 1|1 2 (1:1)

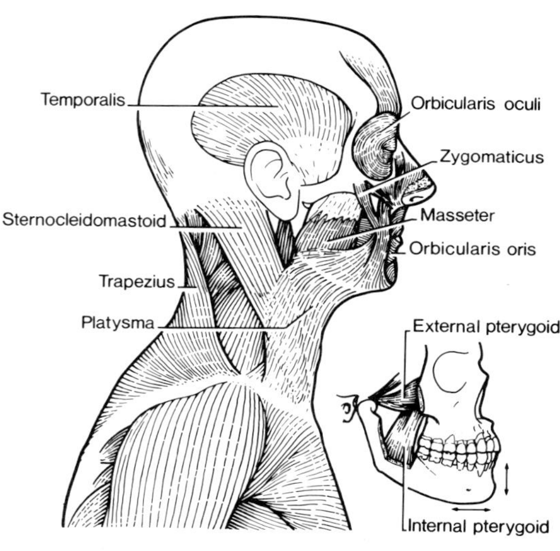


**Figure 5.5** *The muscles of the head and neck*

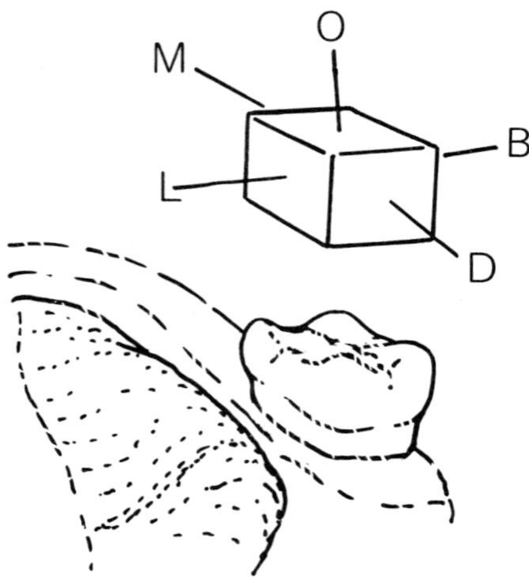


***Figure 5.6*** *The five 'aspects' or surfaces of a tooth. The lingual surface is adjacent to the tongue whereas the buccal surface is adjacent to the cheek. The occlusal surface is that which contacts the other set of teeth for chewing*

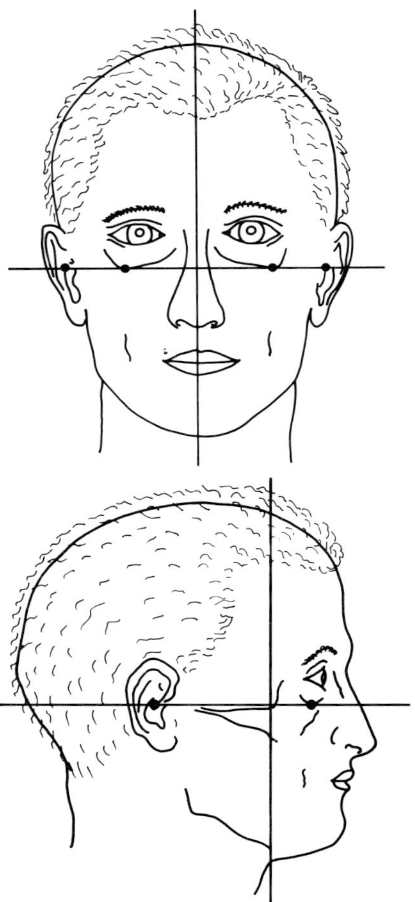

***Figure 5.7*** *The Frankfurt horizontal*

(d) single tooth or equivalent area (2:1)
(e) mirror views of palate and/or upper arch, lower arch, or any other directly inaccessible area to scales as above.

Various authors have proposed standard sets of views for dentistry and indeed orthodontists themselves have been the keenest. Perhaps the most common set of views for comparative photography are the so-called BEGG views, named after an orthodontist. These are:

(i) AP, face,
(ii) Left and right laterals of face,
(iii) Left and right ¾ views of face,
(iv) Anterior teeth in occlusion (4+4)
(v) ¾ teeth in occlusion (6+2) (2+6) and
(vi) Lateral teeth in occlusion (8 + 1) (1 + 8).

It is most important to standardize viewpoint in comparative dental photography, particularly in photography of the face to show jaw deformity. The patient should always be orientated so that a line drawn from the lower orbital margin through the external auditory meatus is horizontal – the so-called Frankfurt horizontal. The film plane should be at right angles to this line, and the principal ray of the lens at the same level.

Many dentists and surgeons will want to differentiate between views taken with the mouth at rest and in occlusion. Correctly, 'occlusion' means biting together with the back teeth (molars) even if this means a malocclusion of the incisors – the 'open anterior bite' often photographed for orthodontists. The patients will usually adopt a compromise 'compensatory' bite if asked to bite the teeth together naturally. Removable appliances in the mouth should normally be removed before photography, unless there is a specific request for the photographs to be taken with appliances in position to demonstrate their effectiveness.

## 5.4 EQUIPMENT

### 5.4.1 Cameras

For all routine work, conventional camera systems will suffice, although the portability and ease of use at close-range of the 35 mm SLR will make it the camera of choice. A lens of long focal length (100–135 mm for a 35 mm camera) should be selected to minimize perspective distortion. The lens of choice will be a macrolens which because of its extended focussing mechanism can produce magnifications of up to 1:1 without the use of bellows or extension rings and has its aberrations corrected for close-range work. Small working apertures (*f*/22–*f*/32) are required in order to obtain sufficient depth of field.

### 5.4.2 Lighting

Electronic flash is the lighting of choice, using a studio flash set-up for head and neck views. There are two schools of thought about the most suitable light source for intra-oral photography. Some workers use a ringflash for all this work, but this gives a very flat result with minimal shadows (which may be misleading when photographing the front teeth to demonstrate protrusion, for example), while other workers favour a single small portable flash unit mounted on a bracket on the lens. Various suitable brackets which allow the flash source to be rotated around the lens are commercially available, and have been described in the literature. An alternative espoused by some is to combine a single flash-head for directionality with a ringflash for softening the shadows and lighting cavities. An 'Anglepoise' type lamp to provide illumination for focussing intra-oral views is a valuable addition to the lighting equipment.

### 5.4.3 Retractors and mirrors

Lip retractors to hold the lips clear of the gingival margins are commercially available from most dental equipment suppliers. These should be used in all intra-oral photography – in general good intra-oral photography needs good retraction. There are various types of retractor available including:

(1) Self retaining full mouth retractor, which is constructed from a shaped section of thin walled large tube. Usually metal, they can be steam sterilized, but cannot be tolerated by many patients.

(2) Moulded acrylic or plastic side retractors, which can be moulded into any size or shape, are more popular with patients but cannot be autoclaved. Because they are in two parts there is also the temptation to ease off the tension on retraction during photography causing 'lip-sag' in the middle.

(3) Steel-rod retractors, marketed in the UK as the 'Martin lip retractor'. They consist of a high tensile stainless steel thin rod, available in four sizes from child to large adult mouth, which springs open to hold the lips well clear of the gingiva. They are well tolerated

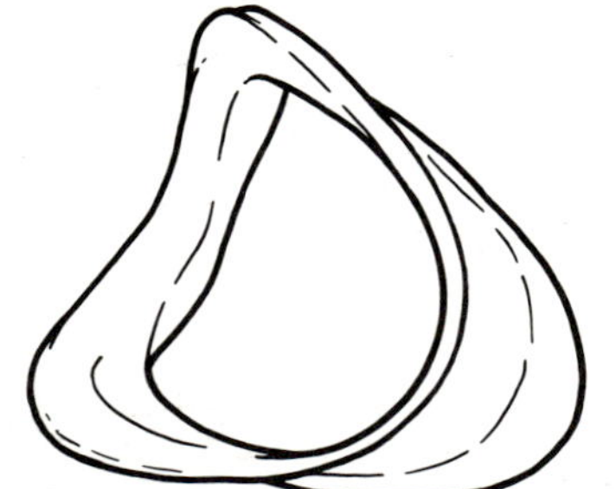
***Figure 5.8*** *Full mouth retractor*

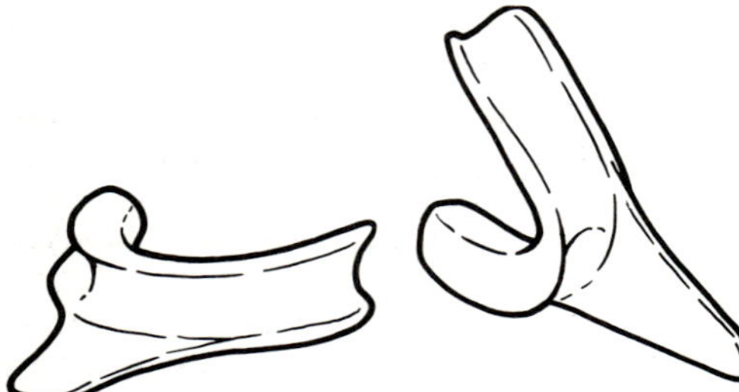
***Figure 5.9*** *Acrylic side retractors*

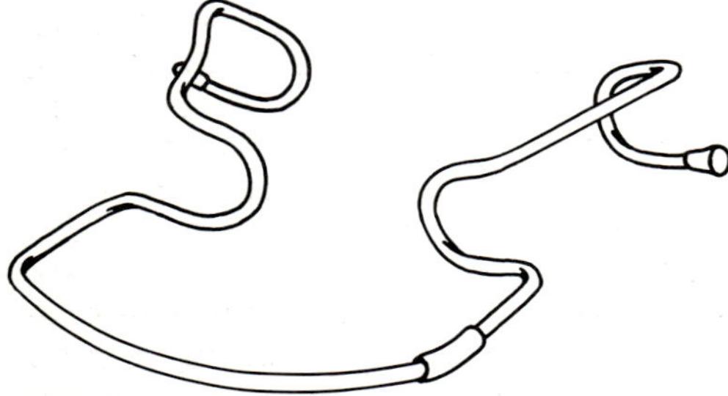
***Figure 5.10*** *Steel-rod retractors*

by the patient and have the advantages of being self-retaining and suitable for autoclaving.

Mirrors of various sizes and shapes, made of either surface-silvered glass or polished stainless steel, will be required to visualize the palate or tongue and upper or lower arch form, as well as for buccal views of the molar teeth. Optical glass mirrors are superior, but they cannot be autoclaved and chemical sterilization soon ruins the surface. Polished steel are more robust and can be steam sterilized, and if kept in good condition can be very good optically. A recent introduction favoured by some is the vacuum coated plastic mirror.

### 5.4.4 Other equipment

Wooden spatulas will be required to control or depress the tongue – these should be discarded immediately after use.

If a great deal of intra-oral work is to be undertaken then a proper dental chair which reclines and has a good headrest will be an asset – as will a spray/suction unit for cleaning the area to be photographed in close-ups.

A piece of glass plate larger than an adult tongue (with ground edges) will be found invaluable for recording distribution of lesions on the tongue, e.g. geographical tongue. The glass is pressed flat onto the extended tongue – making photography and lighting easy.

## 5.5 THE PATIENT

Patients in this category of work will vary in age from the young child to the old age pensioner, but they will all share a fear of the dental chair – reassurance is the key word. In all dental photography it is imperative to 'secure' the patient's head properly – at the very least a headrest is required. Retractors can be frightening for a child and difficult to insert in an adult – if necessary use a spare set to demonstrate on yourself. It is good practice to warm dental mirrors under the hot tap prior to use to prevent the patient's breath condensing on them during photography. For *dental* photography it is not necessary to remove any clothing (but have tissues available for the patient to mop up saliva); for *maxillo–facial* surgery you must remove clothing down to shoulder level (shoulder flaps may be used later on the jaw). Do remember that many dental conditions are painful and that extra effort will be required from the patient to obtain a good photograph.

## 5.6 INFECTION CONTROL

The oral cavity is always heavily contaminated with potentially pathogenic organisms, and there is a real danger of infecting either yourself or other patients unless special precautions are taken. Unfortunately it is not always easy to see which conditions are hazardous. An acute ulcerative gingivitis may be relatively harmless, whereas an innocuous red spot on the lip may be herpes simplex and easily transmitted to another patient. There are three principal ways of spreading infection:

(1) Patient's mouth to photographer's fingers, when inserting retractors etc.
(2) Patient's mouth to patient's mouth by poor sterilization of retractors.
(3) Airborne infection from patient to photographer.

Always use rubber gloves if the patient is suspected of having any oral infection, and always wear a mask if there is a risk of airborne infection, e.g. a TB ulcer.

All instruments, mirrors, retractors, etc. used in a patient's mouth must be properly sterilized. Ideally steam sterilization is the method of choice, and this may either be done by the Central Sterile Supply Department of the hospital or locally in the department using a small autoclave such as 'The Little Sister'. Unfortunately, plastic retractors and glass mirrors cannot be steam sterilized, so the use of a cold disinfectant solution, such as chlorhexidine with a 0.1% solution of sodium nitrate as a corrosion inhibitor, is recommended. (These disinfectants are not effective against spores and viruses.)

## 5.7 SPECIALIZED TECHNIQUES

There are a number of specialized photographic techniques used in dental recording and the student is advised to be familiar with these, in outline if not in detail.

### 5.7.1 Osteotomy planning

There is often a requirement prior to major oral surgery (e.g. osteotomies) for life-size photographs of the face to be prepared for planning purposes. The surgeons will cut these photographs to mimic various surgical procedures in an attempt to forecast their effect on the soft tissues of the face. These photographs are usually required to be matched to lateral radiographs taken of the patient in a cephalostat and are most conveniently printed onto large film so that the combination of photograph and radiograph can be cut and assessed on a light-box. Perspective distortion must be reduced to a minimum and many photographers prefer to use a large format camera for these applications to obtain sufficient quality. Accurate positioning of the patient and absolute standardization of technique are imperative.

### 5.7.2 Macrophotography of gingivae

The condition of the gingivae, including blood supply, is of great interest to the dental research worker and there will be a requirement to photograph at high magnifications. The principles and practice of macrophotography are dealt with in Section 16 and more detail on dental applications can be found in the references. The principal difficulties are positioning the patient so that he does not move (depth of field being almost non-existent) and lighting the subject. A special 'bite block' moulded especially for each patient may be used for positioning and electronic flash directed by fibre-optics will usually solve lighting problems. With an accurate bite-block it is even possible to undertake time lapse studies of the gingivae over periods of days or even weeks, to monitor and measure tooth eruption for example. Others have reported using photogrammetric techniques (*see Section 22*) at high magnifications to assess gingival swelling.

### 5.7.3 Ultraviolet photography

Normal dental enamel fluoresces strongly under ultraviolet rays, whereas plaque or prosthetic materials do not. Ultraviolet fluorescence techniques can therefore be very useful for differentiation of what to the eye are identical white substances. Some compounds that are taken up by developing teeth, e.g. tetracycline antibiotic, fluoresce strongly under UV. Reflected ultraviolet photography can also be useful for detailed examination of the surface of the enamel for such effects as mottling. The techniques of ultraviolet photography are dealt with in Section 19. and the specialist applications to dentistry are covered in depth by the references.

### 5.7.4 Measurement of dental models

The storage of plaster impressions of patients' dentition is very wasteful of space and methods of accurately photographing them, so that they might be destroyed, have been described in the literature. The techniques for photographing these white models are covered in Section 24.

## References

Adams, C. (1968). *Dental Photography* (Bristol: John Wright)

Callender, R. (1972). Observation of the capillary structure of the human gingiva. *Med. Biol. Illustr.*, **22**, 238-244

Callender, R. (1975). A photographic survey of the human mouth. *Br. J. Photogr.*, **122**, 24-26

Callender, R. (1977). An ultraviolet camera system for intra-oral photography. *Med. Biol. Illustr.*, **27**, 113-115

Callender, R. (1983). Photography and the study of the mottling of tooth enamel. *J. Audiovis. Media Med.*, **6**, 57-59

Clark, M. *et al.* (1977). Photocephalography for evaluation of tissue relations in mandibular surgery. *J. Oral Surg.*, **35**, 319-320

Dervin, E., Gore, R. and Kilshaw, J. (1976). The photographic measurement of dental models. *Med. Biol. Illustr.*, **26**, 219-222

Dodge, C.A. (1969). Clinical dental photography. *J. Maxillofac. Orthoped.*, **26**, 22-26

Fanibunda, K. and Hill, B. (1981). Facial photoradiography: practical considerations. *J. Audiovis. Media Med.*, **4**, 95-98

Freehe, C. (1965). Dental photography. *J. Biol. Photogr. Assoc.*, **33**, 160-164

Gibson, H.L. (1968). Depth of field in oral photography. *Dent. Radiogr. Photogr.*, **41**, 42-44

Hill, B. and Geddes, D. (1975). A photographic approach to recording pre-carious changes on teeth *in situ*. *Med. Biol. Illustr.*, **25**, 79-88

Johanson, G. and Lindenstam, B. (1961). Dental evidence in identification: photographic registration of the dentition and a method of rapid identification. *Acta Odonto. Scand.*, **19**, 101-119

Kaiser, D. *et al.* (1978). Intra-oral photographic survey. *J. Prosthet. Dent.*, **40**, 457-460

McCarty, G. (1976). Intra-oral infrared colour photography of radiotherapy patients. *J. Prosthet. Dent.*, **35**, 327-331

Morgan, W.J. (1979). Hazards in intra-oral photography. *Br. J. Photogr.*, **126**, 891-892

Morgan, W.J. (1980). Retraction for intra-oral photography. *Br. J. Photogr.*, **127**, 867-869

Phillips, J. (1978). Photo-cephalometric analysis in treatment planning for surgical correction of facial disharmonies. *J. Maxillofac. Surg.*, **6**, 174-179

Rogers, G. (1971). Standard views in oral photographic practice. *Med. Biol Illustr.* **21**, 134-141

Thomas, P. (1975). The photography of irregularly shaped objects. *Br. J. Photogr.*, **122**, 1059

Tyldesley, W. (1978). *A Colour Atlas of Oral Medicine.* (London: Wolfe Medical Publications)

## ***Practical projects***

(1) Photograph the complete set of BEGG views using a colleague as a model. Ensure the correct use of retractors to prevent lip sag or bulge.

(2) Photograph both ¾ views of the anterior teeth in occlusion,
(*a*) With a single light source, and
(*b*) With a ringflash.
Note the effects on modelling produced by the two light sources.

(3) Use a ringflash, retractors and tongue spatula to photograph the uvula and pillars of fauces.

(4) Photograph the anterior part of the hard palate, along with the lingual surface of the upper incisors, using a suitable mirror.

(5) Photograph the interstitial area of 76 from the buccal aspect at a magnification of ×2. Make notes on any special problems encountered.

(6) Practise putting retractors in and out of your own mouth – note the effects of different types and sizes of retractor on degree of retraction and on comfort.

(7) Photograph several colleagues' faces anteriorly in monochrome. Then print the negatives (*a*) correctly, (*b*) 'flipped over', and cut the prints down the midline of the faces. Then mount each set of photographs as (i) normal, (ii) two left sides butt-mounted, (iii) two right sides butt-mounted. Take note of the degree of facial asymmetry present in normal subjects and the usefulness of this simple technique.

(8) Produce four full head views of a traumatic repair, dental osteotomy or orthodontic patient in a medium of your choice:
- front and left lateral views before surgery,
- front and left lateral views after surgery.

## Examination questions

Q.1 Describe fully the equipment and techniques you would use to photograph the teeth of teenage children routinely.

Q.2 Give a brief description of the retractors, mirrors and spatulae required for comprehensive dental photography and outline two common methods of sterilization for such instruments with their advantages and disadvantages.

Q.3 Write concise notes on four of the following:

(*a*) Photoradiography for osteotomy planning,
(*b*) Infection control in intra-oral photography,
(*c*) Lighting the oral cavity,
(*d*) Photographic measurement of dental models,
(*e*) Ultraviolet photography of teeth, or
(*f*) hotomacrography of the gingiva.

Q.4 Outline the relative merits of the ring-flash and the single flash-head for dental and intra-oral photography. Illustrate your answer with examples of medical conditions suitable for each lighting technique.

Q.5 Describe fully three diseases which give rise to mucosal lesions in the oral cavity under the following headings:

(*a*) The visible signs of disease,
(*b*) The cause,
(*c*) Special handling the patient may need, and
(*d*) Other views you may need to take to record the condition fully (apart from the intraoral views).

*Multiple choice questions (any of the statements may be true or false)*

Q.6 The orthodontist requires a set of 35 mm colour transparencies of a patient with malocclusion:

(*a*) Some form of lip retraction will be necessary.
(*b*) A palatal mirror will be required.
(*c*) A ring-flash would be the lighting of choice.
(*d*) You would ask the patient to bite together with his front teeth.
(*e*) A long focal length lens would be ideal.

Q.7 You are taking intra-oral colour photographs on 35 mm film with a 10 cm lens and a small light source mounted alongside the lens. If instead you use a 5 cm lens but keep the scale the same then:

(*a*) It will give a greater depth of field when used at the same *f* number.
(*b*) It will allow a greater working distance.
(*c*) More of the inside of the mouth will be seen in a single picture.
(*d*) One must stop down more.
(*e*) The field of view will be more easily illuminated.

Q.8 A 1:1 magnification 35 mm colour slide is required of a lesion on the lip:

(*a*) Using a 50 mm lens, extension tubes of 50 mm are required.
(*b*) The extension required can be calculated by multiplying the focal length by the magnification.
(*c*) A supplementary lens could be used with advantage.
(*d*) An increase in exposure by a factor of ×2 is required.
(*e*) Reversing the 50 mm lens on the extension tubes will give the same magnification but with better aberration correction.

# Section 6
# Photography in dermatology

**S.J. Robertson**, BA, ABIPP, ARPS, AIMBI
Director of Medical Illustration
Institute of Dermatology and St John's Hospital
for Diseases of the Skin, London

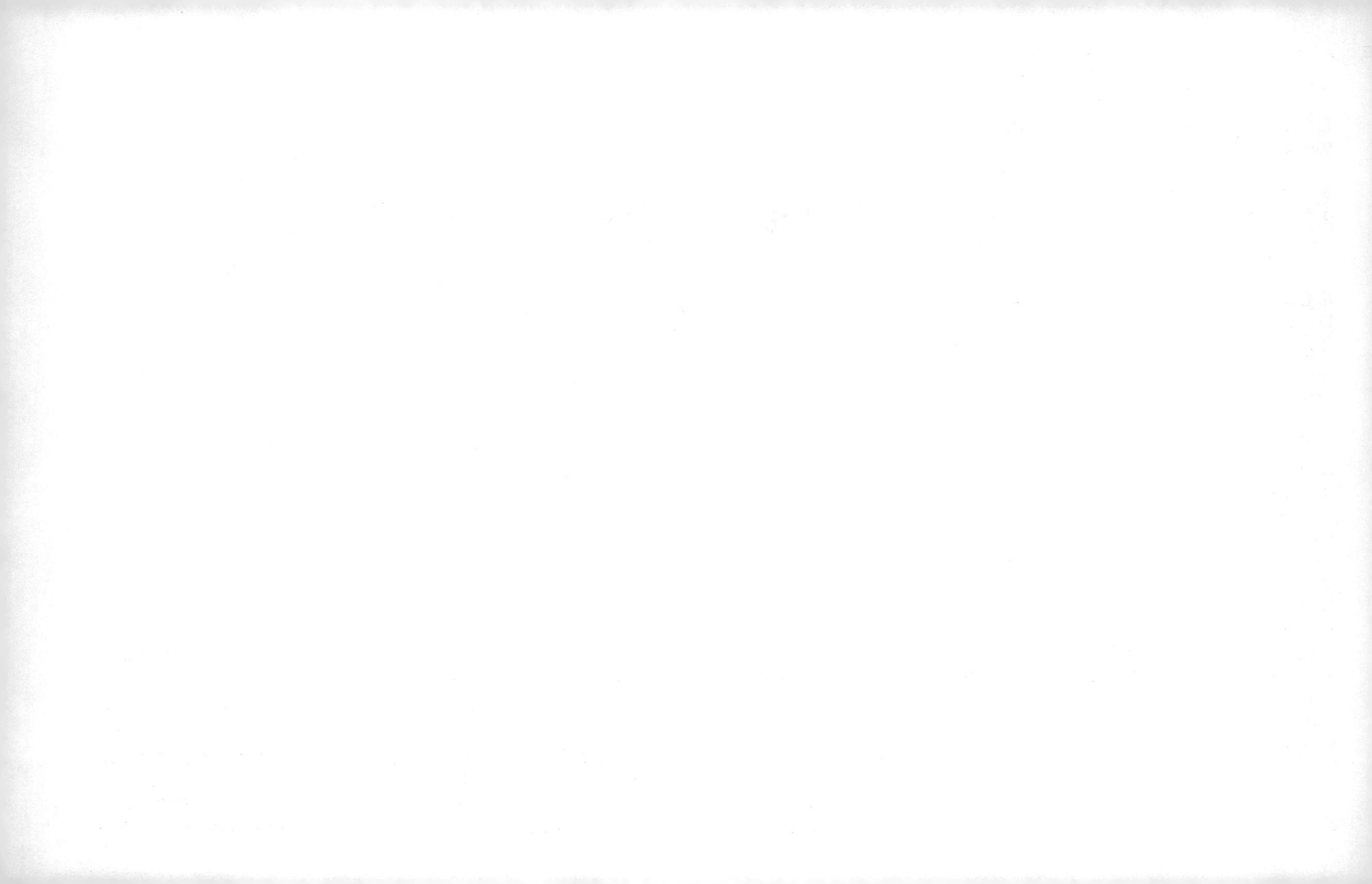

## 6.1 INTRODUCTION

Dermatology is the study of diseases of the skin, but also includes those diseases affecting the appendages (hair and nails) and the mucous membranes of the mouth, anus and vulva. As diagnosis in dermatology is largely dependent upon visible signs, the photograph is a very valuable recording medium for any or all of the following: teaching, patient records, publication and clinical research. In fact, photographs are probably of greater value to the dermatologist than to any other medical specialist. It is immensely useful in the monitoring of chronic conditions to include photographs in the patient's notes; before a lesion is excised its appearance should always be recorded; for the teaching of post- and under-graduate medical students, GPs and nurses, clinical transparencies are essential. For these reasons, it is usually the dermatologists who send the most patients to be photographed and are the most exacting in their demands. As dermatologists, they have a keen visual sense and are often quite capable photographers. Hence, working with them can be both demanding and rewarding.

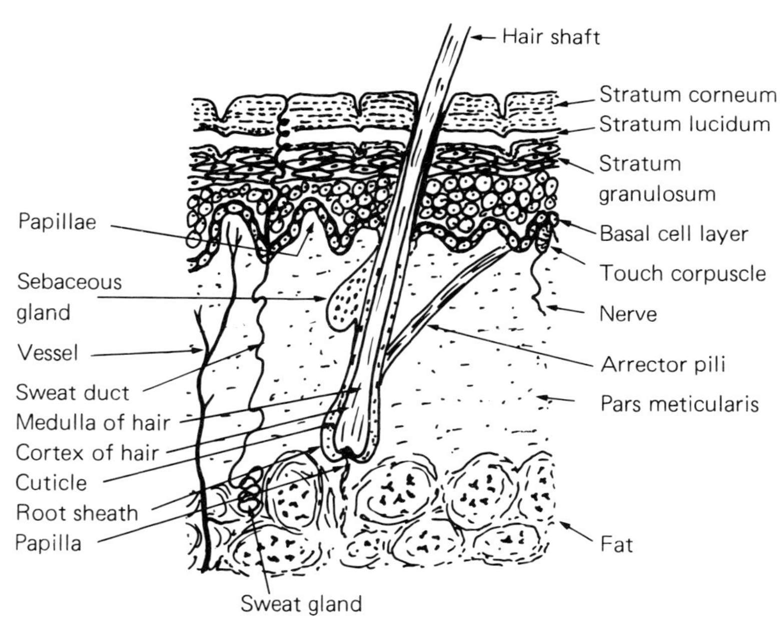


***Figure 6.1*** *A generalized cross-section through skin*

## 6.2 ANATOMY, PHYSIOLOGY AND SPECIALIST TERMINOLOGY

As well as fulfilling its obvious use as a protective covering the skin has several other important functions, being a heat regulator, an organ of the sense of touch, acting as both an excretory and an absorbing organ and being a store of water and chemicals. There are three principal layers; the outer layer or epidermis, the inner layer or dermis (corium) and the subcutaneous tissue. The student should study their structure and functions and those of the sweat glands, the sebaceous glands, the nerve endings and the nails and hair.

The causes of skin changes may be internal or external and may be considered under the following headings. Frequently more than one factor may be present.

(1) Physical causes – Trauma, chemicals, heat, cold, radiation.
(2) Infections – Bacterial, viral, fungal, parasitic.
(3) Internal – Toxic reactions, reflections of metabolic disorders and internal disease in general.
(4) Constitutional disorders and sensitivity disorders.
(5) Tumours – benign and malignant
(6) Congenital disorders.

There is a well defined vocabulary relating to the identification of skin diseases.

*Macules* – Flat circumscribed lesions of altered colour varying in shape and size, not elevated.
*Papules* – Raised and firm lesions up to a centimetre in size, pointed, round or flat.
*Wheals* – Elevated areas caused by oedema of the dermis due to toxins, trauma or allergy. They can be tiny or large.
*Nodules* – Similar to papules but more deeply seated and larger. Also in the sub cutaneous tissue.
*Tumours* – Larger than nodules – may be deeply seated or elevated.
*Vesicles* – Blisters less than 0.5 cm in diameter containing clear fluid.
*Bullae* – As for vesicles but greater than 0.5 cm in diameter.
*Pustules* – As for vesicles but containing pus.
*Plaques* – Raised flat lesions in which the area is large in relation to the elevation. Often formed by a confluence of papules.
*Scales* – Dead and peeling tissue from the horny layer. They may be dry and silvery or greasy and yellowish.
*Crusts* – Masses of dried exudate. May be soft and friable or dry and hard.
*Ulcers* – Irregularly shaped excavations as the result of loss of dermis and epidermis. The shape, floor, base edge and secretion are of importance.
*Excoriations* – Superficial excavations due to scratching.
*Erythematous* – Reddened skin lesion.
*Ecchymosis* – A bruise caused by escape of blood from injured vessels.
*Exudate* – Leaking tissue fluid.
*Discrete* – Separate, discontinuous.
*Exfoliative* – Scaling.
*Desquamatous* – Scaling.
*Lichenification* – Skin appears thickened with accentuated markings rather resembling tree bark.
*Linear* – Arranged in a straight line.
*Discoid or Nummular* – Coin shaped.
*Annular* – Circular with a clear centre.

## 6.3 THE PATIENT

The attitude of photographic staff towards skin patients is important. Patients, particularly those with acute diseases, are sometimes very embarrassed at being photographed. These need tact and reassurance.

Skin conditions are rarely infectious and those that are (if we disregard the skin manifestations of the common childhood infections such as measles and chicken pox) are only transmitted by physical contact, i.e. they are contagious. The following is a list of examples:

Bacterial infections – Impetigo, Syphilis
Viral infections – Viral warts, herpes simplex
Fungal infections – Tinea (ringworm), Candida
Infestations – Scabies, Lice

It is also fair to say that close contact over a relatively long period is necessary for most of these to be transmitted. The simple precaution of washing hands after dealing with each patient will give adequate protection. This point needs to be stressed as it is contrary to popular belief.

People with psoriasis or eczema, for example, are quite used to being treated by the general public with, to say the least, reserve. The dermatologist will have spent considerable time trying to reassure such patients and he does not want his work undermined by the photographer treating them like lepers. (Not that leprosy is highly infectious either.) It is also well to remember that the lesion being photographed may be the skin manifestation of a deeper underlying cause.

Patients with skin disorders presenting for photography are often undergoing treatment and hence their lesions may be obscured by creams, ointments and powders. Before an adequate pictorial record can be made it is essential to clean the skin in a manner which is not injurious to the patient. Often all that is necessary is simple soap and water but sometimes a mixture of 5% medicinal paraffin in ether will be needed. *Never* attempt to clean raw weeping areas – return the patient to the ward or clinic for cleansing of the appropriate areas. Clinical photographs which include dressings or medications are untidy and often useless.

## 6.4 PHOTOGRAPHY – GENERAL TECHNIQUE

### 6.4.1 Materials

Since colour is an important feature in the identification of a skin lesion it is necessary routinely to record patients on colour film. In consequence black-and-white reproductions, usually for publication in books and journals, have often to be made from colour film stock, either negative or reversal. The general requirements of skin photographs are best served by a colour reversal material. Colour negatives are inconvenient for the preparation of transparencies and colour prints of suitable quality are expensive, Colour reversal is ideal for teaching and provides an inexpensive, high quality record for the patient's notes. It is also a good stock from which to prepare colour or black-and-white prints. The emulsion or choice has high resolution good accurate colour rendition particularly in the reds, constant colour balance and speed, and good processing facilities in terms of service, cleanliness and reliability.

### 6.4.2 Positioning and scale

The views chosen will obviously depend on the disease to be photographed. Usually it is necessary to take more than one view. One or more views are required to demonstrate *distribution* or location as well as one or more to show *detail* of lesions. A diffuse erythroderma may gain little by a close up view, there being little change in skin detail, only in colour. However, as a general rule close-up views are valuable. The most common criticism of medical photography by dermatologists is that the views are not close enough. A reproduction ratio on a 35 mm transparency of 1:1 is often required or desirable. However, due to the depth of some small lesions such as a cutaneous horn, sometimes a compromise has to be made. It is important that a raised lesion is sharp throughout its depth and this may not be possible at 1:1.

In general full-length views are to be avoided. The information gained from such views is minimal. A reproduction ratio on 35 mm of not greater than 1:20, i.e. a half-length, should be employed to demonstrate distribution: if necessary take two half-lengths.

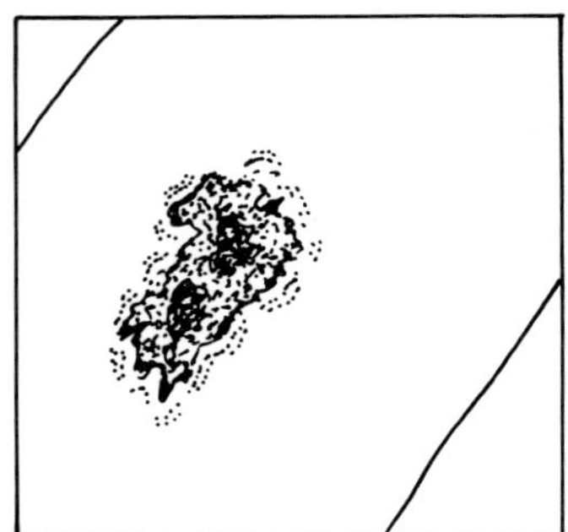

***Figure 6.2*** *The 'ambiguous' lesion – insufficient information is given to enable the viewer to orientate the photograph – is it on the arm or leg?*

### 6.4.3 Background and lighting

The background best suited to skin photography is black, for the following reasons:

(1) The colour in the skin retains maximum saturation – a black background does not produce flare.
(2) There is no chance of a colour cast which can be a problem with large areas of coloured background.
(3) The background remains a constant tone throughout views.
(4) The background does not distract.

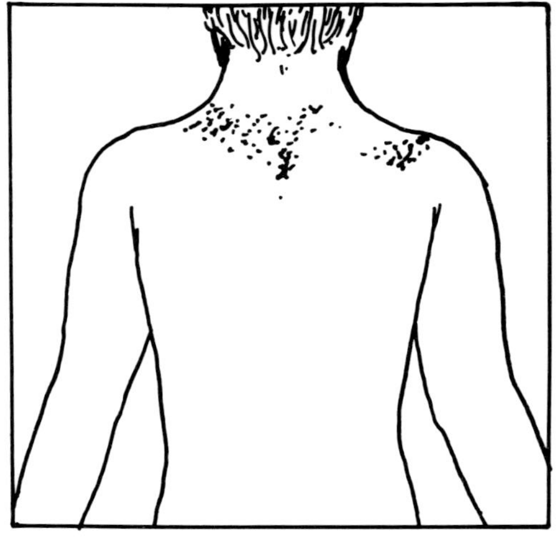

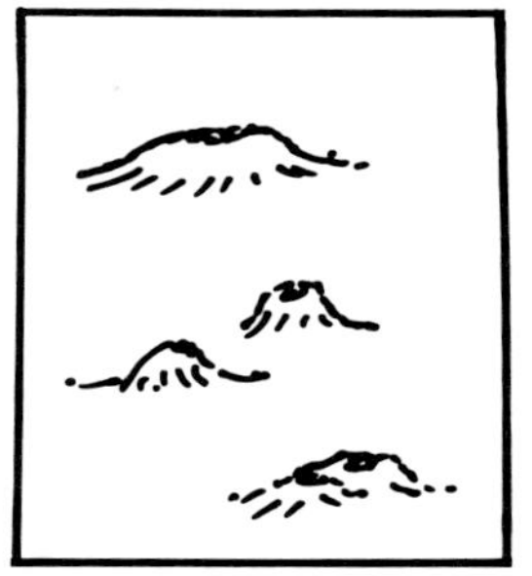

***Figure 6.3 and 6.4*** *The classic pair of dermatological photographs. The general view shows the distribution of the condition whilst the close-up shows the detailed nature of the individual lesions*

The detail that interests the dermatologist includes:

#### *Size*

It is necessary either by reference to a general view or by a 'landmark' to locate the lesion and to give an impression of its size. Recording the scale of reproduction will also help in assessing lesion size and, as a last resort, a centimetre scale may be included in the field of view. This last alternative is on the whole not very satisfactory, in a close up as it obscures a large area, it is difficult to position and retain in sharp focus and is generally rather messy.

#### *Shape*

In at least one view the whole lesion should be included to demonstrate its outline and it is important to provide a comparison with normal adjacent skin.

#### *Colour*

This is dependent upon the choice of film and background as already discussed.

#### *Texture*

The demonstration of texture relies upon the shadows cast by directional lighting. However, this can be overstressed. For colour transparency material the overall lighting must be even – there must not be too high a lighting contrast. When a black background is being used it is *imperative* to 'lift' the subject from the background by the use of lamps at either side of the subject. This then leaves the main light, i.e. the modelling lamp, to provide the necessary lighting contrast. There are exceptional circumstances in which the subtle texture can only be shown by the lamp being brought well off the camera axis, but in most cases the lamp will give sufficient relief to the surface texture without creating unacceptable unevenness when placed just 20° or 30° off axis. This, for close-up work means that due to the size of the relector, the flash-head will be close to the camera.

***Edge configuration*** (i.e. the characteristics of the lesion's margin)

Whether the margin is, for instance, depressed or raised can be highly significant in the diagnosis of a skin lesion and deserves the photographer's attention. Lighting considerations are very similar to those for texture.

### 6.4.4 Monochrome prints

Much of the technique described in this section has been based on the assumption that the record will be made in colour. Some mention, however, needs to be made of the preparation, usually for publication purposes, of monochrome prints. This can either be a further step after the original photograph has been produced as a colour transparency or it can be prepared from a monochrome negative.

***Preparation of monochrome prints from colour transparencies***

The transparencies produced employing a black background and edge lighting as described above lend themselves particularly to black-and-white printing. The even shadowless background and low overall contrast within the subject makes possible the production of very satisfactory prints for publication. It is also possible in the preparation of the monochrome interneg to alter the colour contrast by means of filters.

***Monochrome negatives***

It needs to be categorically stated that if *large* high quality monochrome prints of skin lesions are required these can best be produced on large format (5"×4") orthochromatic film. Unfortunately orthochromatic emulsions are not produced in 35 mm format and panchromatic films do not give the colour contrast. The use of a cyan filter gives a satisfactory result. The lighting for monochrome can afford to leave a higher contrast ratio, but the type of lighting will depend on the subject and background.

## 6.5 DISEASES AND CONDITIONS

To attempt to describe a worthwhile number of skin diseases is beyond the scope of this study guide; they are too numerous and their appearances far too varied. The medical photographer should refer to a standard textbook on skin diseases before photographing any condition with which he is unfamiliar, and if he keeps in mind the basic considerations given in this section under the sub-headings of 'specialist terminology' and 'positioning and scale' he should be able to make a rapid selection of the important visual signs which need to be shown.

There will in many cases be one or two features of such major interest as to form fairly dominant characteristics of the disease. This may for instance be the manner or extent of distribution, as in these examples:

Herpes zoster – A usually well-defined unilateral distribution ceasing at the midline, following a peripheral nerve.
Dermatitis artefacta – Areas within easy

reach of the hands.
Contact dermatitis – The distribution often gives a clue to the causative agent when that is clothing or industrial contact.
Rosacea – Attacks the 'flush' area of the face.

In others the colour changes may be of paramount importance.

Lichen planus – The lilac coloured hue is specific.
Psoriasis – Progress is marked by changes of colour.
Addison's disease – Pigmentary changes are significant.

Shape, texture and configuration are of particular interest in, for example:

Lichen planus – Shiny flat topped, slightly scaly lesions.
Basal cell carcinoma – Rodent ulcers have a characteristic rolled edge appearance.

It is rarely possible and seldom necessary to depict *all* the features of a skin lesion and the medical photographer will learn by study and experience to be selective, taking into account not only the characteristics of the disease but also the purpose of the photographs and the particular aspects that he may know are required by the patient's doctor.

## 6.6 INVISIBLE RADIATION PHOTOGRAPHY

There are a few skin conditions which can be illustrated more vividly by the use of ultraviolet and infrared photography. Such photographs must always be well labelled as having been taken by a particular technique and should be accompanied by a 'control' photograph taken in 'visible' light.

The student is strongly advised to read the two sections on infrared and ultraviolet photography so as to be familiar with the techniques and principles involved.

Normal skin pigment (melanin) absorbs ultraviolet while unpigmented epidermis reflects ultraviolet strongly. Wherever skin changes are faintly observable, or when they are sub-clinical but suspected (as in incipient scleroderma) direct ultraviolet photography can enhance the visualization considerably. Examples of applications are: vitiligo, pigmentary naevi, moles, freckles and keratin plugs, chloasma and Addison's disease the healed lesions of lupus erythematosus, lymphosarcomatosis and related dermatoses, differentiation of verruca vulgaris from molluscum contagiosum, leucoplakia and other pre-cancerous lesions, keloid scars and any hypo-or hyper-pigmentary disturbance.

The shorter the wavelength the less that light penetrates the skin; so ultraviolet radiation is very useful in showing clearly the surface texture of the skin. Clarity of fine detail is possible in, for example, xerodermia, ichthyosis, psoriasis or any condition with desquamation or lichenification.

Ultraviolet fluorescence techniques are also useful in dermatology because a number of conditions, particularly fungal infections, fluoresce under ultraviolet excitation. Examples are tinea capitas which fluoresces a brilliant yellow-green pityriasis versicolor which fluoresces gold or buff-colour, erythrasma which fluoresces coral red and favus which fluoresces grey-green. Some epidermoid carcinomas of the skin demonstrate a red 'live coal' fluorescence under ultraviolet radiation, thought to be due either to bacterial infection associated with the advanced tumour or altered porphyrin metabolism. Other neoplasms, though longstanding and necrotic, do not fluoresce; for example, basal cell carcinoma and haemangioma.

Infrared radiation having a wavelength longer than visible light penetrates the surface of the skin to reveal underlying blood vessels. In general photographic practice it can be assumed that infrared radiation between 700 and 900 nm penetrates to a depth of approximately 3 mm. Venous blood absorbs infrared whilst arterial blood reflects it – so infrared techniques are useful for delineating any abnormality in the superficial venous system. Varicose veins for example can be shown clearly beneath the surface eczema which masks them from the naked eye, whilst the scab covering an area of lupus erythematosus can be made transparent to reveal the condition of the underlying skin. Although fat is transparent to very long wavelengths it reflects infrared well in the 700–900nm region, so xanthomatous plaques are clealy delineated. Hair absorbs infrared so combined with the 3 mm penetration this effect enables accurate records to be made of alopecia even in the beard area which has been clean shaven. Surprisingly, negroid skin does not record any lighter than caucasian skin under infrared illumination – it is probably due to the complex reflectance/transmission characteristics of melanin. Tattoo patterns which have been obliterated to visual examination can often be revealed again by the use of infrared. False colour infrared photography has also been reported as being useful in differentiating between lesions such as pigmented naevi of the fingernail and splinter haemorrhage in the nail bed. In treating burns it is important to be able to assess the depth of the burn and therefore the likely healing rate very early so that skin grafting would be successful should it be necessary. Normally it is several weeks before the eschar has become thin enough to see the healing tissue beneath. Infrared photography penetrates the eschar and enables an early and accurate diagnosis of burn depth. The grey pigmentation of argyria is better differentiated against normal skin by using the false colour infrared film. Similarly, the mottled pattern of congenital phlebectasia or faint lesions of scleroderma are enhanced by false colour infrared film. Deep haemorrhages in haemophilia or in forensic applications are enhanced by the penetrative effect of infrared.

## 6.7 PHOTOMACROGRAPHY OF THE SKIN

Dermatologists are often concerned with the microtopography of the skin surface and will request genuine photomacrography of the epidermis – this may be for research into exfoliation, epidermal ridges or hirsutism, for example. Full details of the optical and photographic considerations are to be found in *Section 16* but mention should be made here of techniques particularly applicable to dermatology.

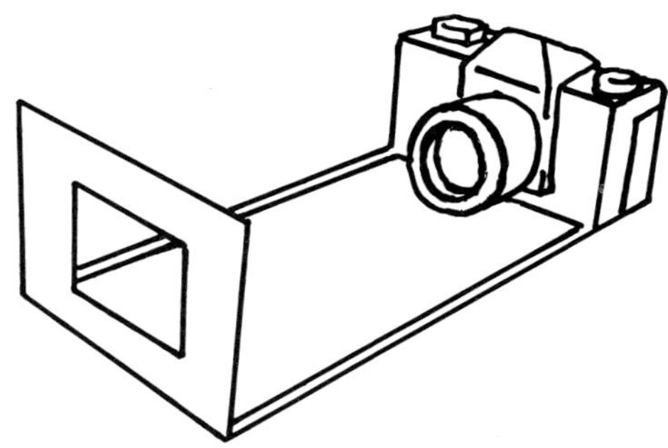

***Figure 6.5*** *A simple frame can be attached to the camera to facilitate easy positioning and automatic focussing when undertaking photomacrography of skin lesions*

The principal difficulty is that the skin surface is semi-translucent, so obtaining adequate sharpness and contrast is very difficult. Various authors have discussed the problem and reported several ways of overcoming it. The three main techniques are:

### *(1) Ultraviolet radiation*

As discussed above the shorter wavelengths do not penetrate the surface of the skin so reflection ultraviolet photography can be used to render better surface detail. There is, however, a problem with this particular technique – accurate focussing. One is often working at wide apertures and depth of field in the macro-ranges is severly limited. Precise focussing of the image is difficult because lenses have unpredictable changes in focal length for shorter wavelengths which are quite significant in close-up photography, and because the filter used is opaque to visible light it is necessary to focus first then cover the lens with the filter prior to exposure. One way of overcoming the latter difficulty is to use a focussing frame attached to the camera which is pre-set to the correct object distance and delineates the area covered by the lens at that magnification. The filter can then be left over the lens permanently.

### *(2) Carbonized creams*

It is possible to apply a cream containing carbon powder or a similar dye to the skin to increase the contrast and prevent light-scatter in the epidermis. This technique works quite well if one is attempting to record the pattern of the epidermal ridges which may be of importance in a number of inherited disorders such as Down's syndrome.

### *(3) Replication*

One of the best ways of obtaining satisfactory photomacrographs is to make a 'plastic' replica of the skin surface which can then be photographed without the attendant problems of 'real' live skin. The skin is coated with a liquid rubber solution which cools to form a rubbery replica of quite remarkable accuracy which is gradually peeled off the skin then photographed.

## References

Aldis, A. and Marshall, R. (1963). Metastatic melanoma, detection by infrared recording. *Med. Biol. Illustr.*, **13**, 2-3

Anselmo, V. and Zawacki, B. (1973). Infrared photography as a diagnostic tool for the burn wound. *Proc. SPIE Seminar II*, **40**, 181-188

Bean, W. (1958). *Vascular Spiders and Related Lesions of the Skin.* (Springfield, Ill: Charles C. Thomas)

Benson, R. and Vogel, M. (1955). The principles of identification and measurement of vulvar fluorescence. *J. Clin. Endocrinol.*, **15**, 784-800

Bluefarb, S. (1977). *Dermatology.* (USA: Upjohn)

Buckley, W. (1963). Localised argyria. *A.M.A. Arch. Dermatol.*, **88**, 531-539

Burgess, C. and Edwards, R. (1978). Hirsutography. *Br. J. Photogr.*, **125**, 770-772

Callender, R. (1974). The optical texture of human skin. *Med. Biol. Illustr.*, **24**, 171-173

Cherrill, F. (1950). Finger prints and disease. *Nature* (London), **166**, 581

Cook, C., Center, R. and Michaels, S. (1979). An acne grading method using photographic standards. *Arch. Dermatol.*, **115**, 571-575

Costello, M. and Lutenberger, L. (1944). Fluorescence with the Wood's filter as an aid in dermatologic diagnosis. *NY J. Med.*, **42**, 1778-1784

Crooks, H. (1953). Photography of epidermal ridges and superficial blood capillaries of the finger. *Med. Biol. Illustr.*, **2**, 198-205

Dorrington, J. (1972). Macrophotography of the skin. *Med. Biol. Illustr.*, **22**, 154-156

Engel, C. (1956). Photomacrography of the skin. *J. Photogr. Sci.*, **4**, 40-43

Figge, F. (1944). Fluorescence studies on cancer. *Cancer Res.*, **4**, 465-471

Fry, L. (1978). *Dermatology – an Illustrated Guide.* (London: Update)

Gibson, H., Buckley, W. and Whitmore, K. (1965). New vistas in infrared photography. *J. Biol. Photogr. Assoc.*, **33**, 1-33

Haxthausen, N. (1933). Infrared photography of subcutaneous veins: demonstration of concealed varices in ulcer and eczema of the leg. *Br. J. Dermatol.*, **45**, 506-510

Kikuchi, I. *et al.* (1979) Reflection ultraviolet photography in dermatology. (Part 1: equipment.). *J. Dermatol. (Tokyo)*, **6**, 81-85

Kikuchi, I. *et al.* (1979). Reflection ultraviolet photography in dermatology. (Part 2: photography of skin lesions.). *J. Dermatol. (Tokyo)*, **6**, 87-93

Levene, G. and Calnan, C. (1983). *A Colour Atlas of Dermatology.* (London: Wolfe Medical Publications)

Lunnon, R. (1959). Direct ultraviolet photography of the skin. *Med. Biol. Illustr.*, **9**, 150-154

Lunnon, R. (1961). Some observations on the photography of the diseased skin. *Med. Biol. Illustr.*, **11**, 98-103

Marshall, R. (1981). Infrared and ultraviolet reflectance measurements as an aid to the diagnosis of pigmented lesions of the skin. *J. Audiovis. Media Med.*, **4**, 11-14

Marshall, R. (1981). Ultraviolet photography in detecting 'latent' halos of pigmented lesions. *J. Audiovis. Media Med.*, **4**, 127-129

Naylor, J.R. (1984). Applications of the skin surface replica technique to dermatology. *J. Audiovis. Media Med.*, **7**, 21–26

Phillips, R. (1976). Photography as an aid to dermatology. *Med. Biol. Illustr.*, **26**, 161-166

Ronchese, F. (1953). The fluorescence of ulcerated epidermoid carcinoma under the Wood's light. *Med. Radiogr. Photogr.*, **29**, 6-8

Sarkany, I. and Phillips, R. (1965). Microtopography of the skin. *Med. Biol. Illustr.*, **15**, (2 Suppl.), 57-61

Schoenfield, W. (1965). The technique, application and evaluation of the dermatogram. *Med. Biol. Illustr.*, **6**, 77-85

Stevenson, J. (1981). Penetration of eschar by infrared photography. *J. Audiovis. Media Med.*, **4**, 141–143

Tredinnick, W.D. (1961). Further advances in fluorescence colour photography. *Med. Biol. Illustr.*, **11**, 16-21

Verbov, J. (1969). Epidermal ridges in diagnostic medicine. *Med. Biol. Illustr.*, **19**, 46-51

Wilkin, J. *et al.* (1980). Infrared photographic studies of rosacea. *Arch. Dermatol.*, **116**, 676-678

## *Practical projects*

(1) Successful dermatological photography demands a knowledge of the disease you are trying to photograph. As a *minimum* requirement the student should look up *all* the following conditions in a good text on dermatology and make short notes on the visual appearances: Acanthosis, Acne rosacea and vulgaris, Actinomycosis, Adenoma sebaceum, Albinism, Alopecia, Atopic dermatitis, Cheilitis angularis, Chloasma, Clavus, Contact dermatitis, Cutaneous horn, Cysts, Dermatitis artefacta, Dermoid cyst, Dermatitis herpetiformis, Dermatographia, Dermatomyositis, Eczema (all types), Epithelioma, Epiloia, Erysipelas, Erythrasma, Erythema (*ab igne*, bullous, induratum, multiforme, nodosum, palmar), Erythematosus (chronic discoid and systemic lupus), Exfoliative dermatitis, Favus, Fibromata, Folliculitis barbae, Gonorrhoea, Granuloma annulare, Granuloma inguinale, Hydradenitis suppurativa, Hyperkeratosis, Hypertrichosis, Ichthyosis, Impetigo, Intertrigo, Keratosis, Koilonychia, Lentigo maligna, Leukoderma, Leukonychia, Leukoplakia, Lichen planus, Lupus, Lymphangioma, Molluscum contagiosum and sebaceum, Mycosis fungoides, Naevi (all types), Onychogryphosis, Pediculosis, Pemphigus, Perleche, Perniosis, Petechia, Pityriasis (capitas and rosea), Polyarteritis nodosa, Pompholyx, Porphyria, Prurigo, Psoriasis, Purpura, Raynaud's disease, Rhinophyma, Rosacea, Sarcoidosis, Scabies, Scleroderma, Seborrhea, Striae, Syphilis, Telangiectasia, Tinea

(all types), Urticaria, Varicella, Vasculitis, Verrucae, Vitiligo, Von Recklinghausen's disease, Warts (all types), Xanthelasma, Xerodermia.

(2) Photograph both forearms at 1:4 magnification against a black background taking care that the outline is clearly visible. Repeat the photographs against a white background. Compare the results.

(3) Photograph an area of skin such as the dorsum of the hand at 1:1 magnification using (*a*) two lights, (*b*) one light with a large reflector, and (*c*) with a single small light source. Make enlargements and compare the results.

(4) Produce a series of colour transparencies to illustrate any dermatological condition with which you are familiar.

(5) Choose three different types of skin lesion and photograph them
(*a*) with reflected ultraviolet rays (*b*) with panchromatic film (*c*) with orthochromatic (or panchromatic plus appropriate filter), (*d*) with infrared film. Produce sets of comparable prints and make detailed notes on your results and observations.

(6) Photograph the tongue of a living subject to demonstrate texture, shape and colour. Produce in a medium of your choice. Note the magnification on the mount.

(7) Produce a mounted set of black-and-white or colour prints suitable for teaching a small group of students the visual manifestations of any skin disease which you choose. (Be sure to include both orientation and close-up views.)

(8) Photograph the fingertip of a colleague at 1 : 1 and 3 : 1 magnification to demonstrate the epidermal ridges. Make notes on any difficulties you encounter and how you overcame them.

## *Examination questions*

Q.1 Describe the visual appearance and photographs that you would take to illustrate:
(*a*) Ichthyosis,
(*b*) Xanthelasma,
(*c*) Psoriasis, and
(*d*) Porphyria

Q.2 Write a short essay on the use of ultraviolet photography in dermatology illustrating your answer by reference to specific applications.

Q.3 Discuss the management and photography of a patient with:
(*a*) A penile syphilitic chancre,
(*b*) Contact dermatitis,
(*c*) Impetigo, and
(*d*) Carcinoma of the breast.

Q.4 List the main visual signs, the lighting you would adopt, and the views you would take for:
(*a*) Leukoplakia,
(*b*) Basal cell carcinoma,
(*c*) Urticaria,
(*d*) Herpes zoster,
(*e*) Molluscum sebaceum, and
(*f*) Keloid scars.

Q.5 Describe briefly the following conditions and the photographs you would take to illustrate them effectively:
(*a*) Alopecia,
(*b*) Scabies,
(*c*) Dermatitis artefacta, and
(*d*) Koilonychia.

Q.6 Describe the ultraviolet fluorescence photography technique and its specific application to dermatological conditions.

Q.7 Discuss the advantages/disadvantages of photography as a method of recording skin texture, as compared with the techniques of dermatograms and plastic replication.

*Multiple choice questions* (any of the statements may be true or false).

Q.8 A doctor requests full length anterior and posterior black-and-white photographs of a male negroid patient:
(*a*) The use of a red filter with panchromatic film would enhance the skin detail.
(*b*) You should obtain the patient's written consent first.
(*c*) Extra exposure would improve the skin detail.
(*d*) The use of a wide angle lens is essential.
(*e*) The patient should be placed in the standardized supine position.

Q.9 Flat, diffuse lighting is particularly suitable for:
(*a*) Neurofibromata,
(*b*) Vitiligo,
(*c*) Infrared photographs of venous congestion,
(*d*) Spider naevi,
(*e*) Psoriasis.

Q.10 Von Recklinghausen's disease may be characterized by:
(*a*) Neurofibroma,
(*b*) Linear striae,
(*c*) Pedunculated tumours,
(*d*) Multiple desquamating patches,
(*e*) Pigmented patches.

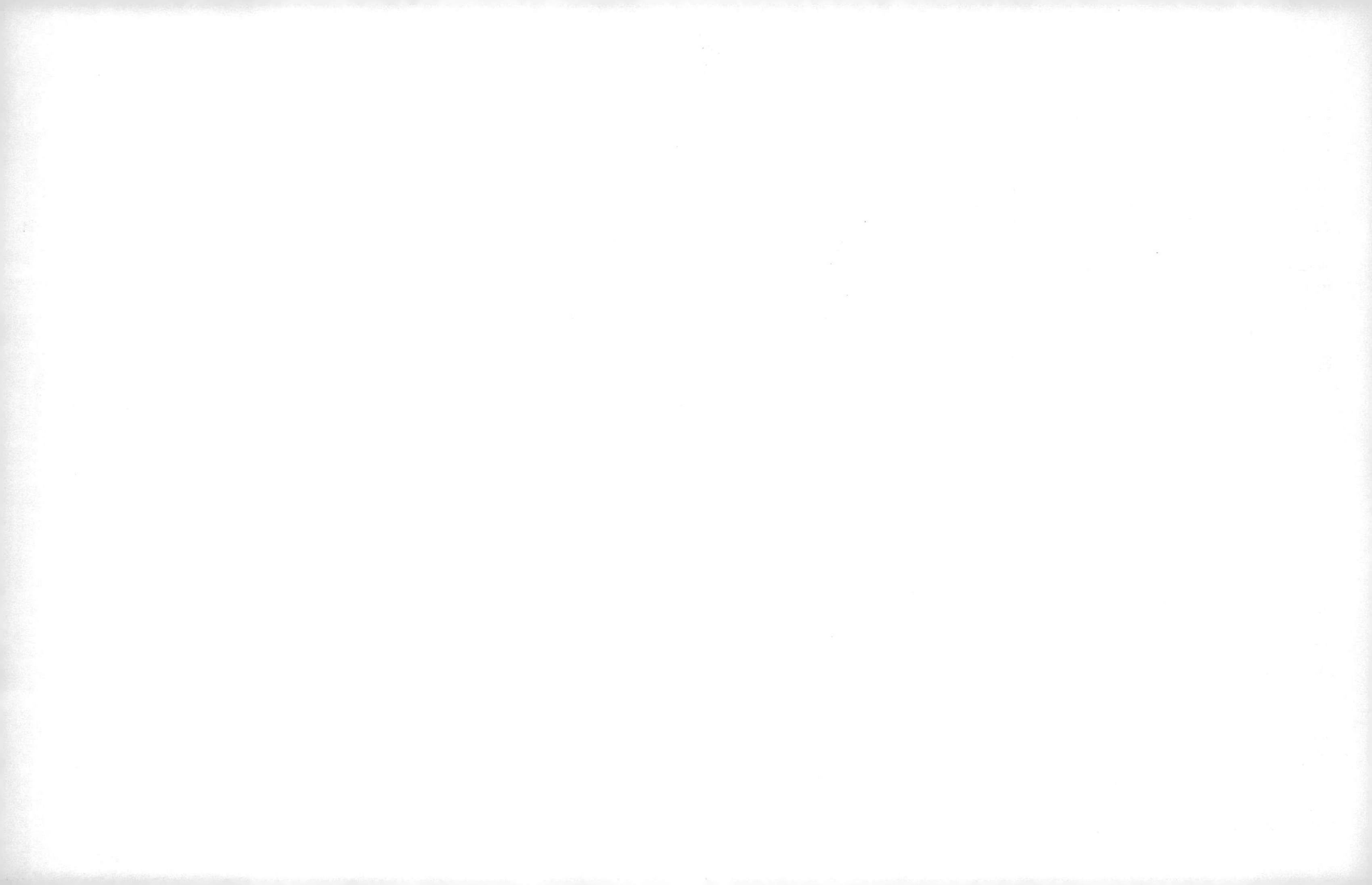

# Section 7
# Photography of endocrine and metabolic disorders

**R.J. Lunnon**, MPhil, FBIPP, FRPS, AIMBI, SBStJ.
Director of Medical Illustration
Institute of Child Health and Hospitals for Sick Children, London

## 7.1 INTRODUCTION

The endocrine or ductless glands consist of the pituitary gland, thyroid, parathyroid, adrenals and gonads. They pass their secretions, which are known as hormones, directly into the bloodstream through which they are distributed to all parts of the body. Among other effects, hormones frequently influence the metabolism or chemistry of the body, and at the same time, hormones may also act on other endocrine glands so that any one disorder may produce signs which are also common to others. Metabolic disturbances are concerned with biochemical abnormalities and disease resulting from deficiency of vitamins and other essential requirements of the body.

The results of endocrine disturbances tend to affect the body as a whole, particularly with regard to growth, distribution of fat, colouration of the skin, etc. As these effects are difficult to describe with precision, photography is much used to record these appearances and their changes in response to treatment or progression of the disease (*see also Section 28.13*).

## 7.2 PHOTOGRAPHY

As well as close-up views of special features, full-length pictures are needed of all these conditions. AP, and one lateral view are essential, but PA and the other lateral views may also be required.

*Standardization is vital* as repeat pictures will be needed over periods of months, years and even decades. The same constant reduction scale must be used for pictures of all patients, whether children or large adults. On the 35 mm format 1:60 (as opposed to the Westminster scale of 1:50) is required to accommodate a patient with gigantism. This technique must be adhered to when making colour transparencies, since the camera image cannot be subsequently modified in the print ing process. Positioning must be accurate and a vertical scale always included in the picture. Camera height should be constant at half the patient's height and the same distance from the patient must always be maintained. Lighting must be symmetrical and capable of standardization. The patient's outline must always be clearly distinguished from the background, which may usefully have a grid ruled upon it.

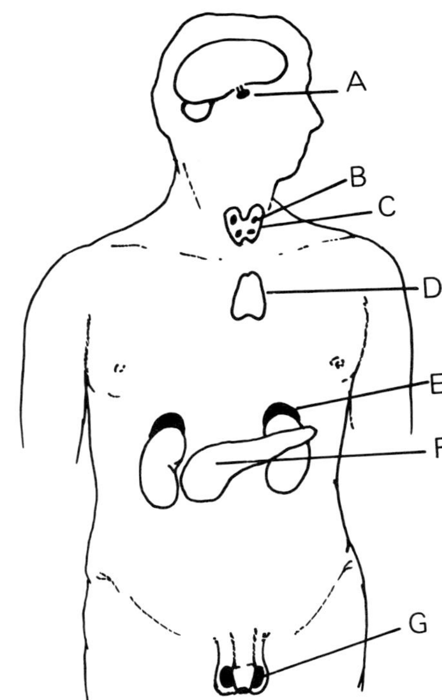


***Figure 7.1*** *The endocrine system: A – the pituitary, B – the parathyroids, C – the thyroid, D – the thymus, E – the adrenals, F – the pancreas, G – the gonads (testes or ovaries)*

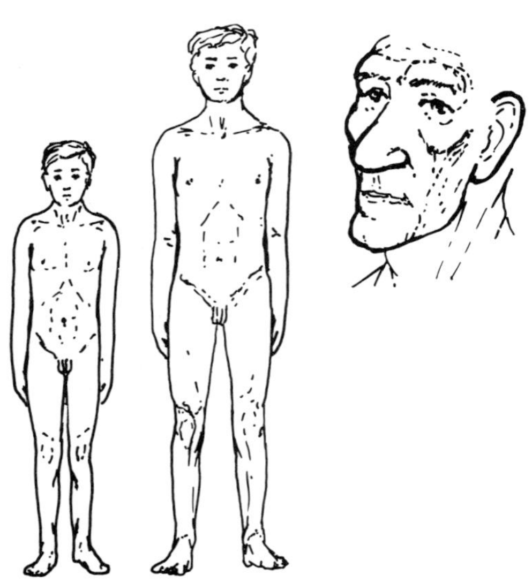

***Figure 7.2*** *Excessive secretion of the thyroid gland causes gigantism in childhood (the drawing shows a normal 12-year-old boy by the side of a child suffering from hyperpituitarism) and acromegaly in the adult (shown in the inset)*

The above views are frequently supplemented by AP and lateral pictures of the head and neck. The same principles apply, but the scale needs to be rather small to accommodate the head of a large man in the lateral position (1:15 is suitable).

When records are required of the female genitalia (*section 12.0*) it is essential that the labia are retracted so that the clitoris is well demonstrated.

## 7.3 THE PATIENT

Since photographs of the patient must be taken at full length in the nude, they should be previously informed of this by the ward or outpatient sister. The studio temperature should be warm, and all photographic preliminaries checked before the patient is asked to pose. It is advisable to take the least embarrassing pictures first, leaving the full length AP until last when confidence is more likely to have been established. Some patients suffering from endocrine disorders may be intolerant of heat or cold, and these special considerations are covered below in relation to the specific disorders.

## 7.4 THE COMMONLY PHOTOGRAPHED ENDOCRINE DISEASES

### 7.4.1 The pituitary gland

The pituitary gland is situated in the pituitary fossa or sella turcica in the sphenoid bone. The pituitary fossa shows well on a lateral X-ray of the skull and may be enlarged in pituitary tumours.

It produces at least eight hormones of major importance, many of which control other endocrine glands, particularly the thyroid, the adrenals and the gonads. Through the medium of the hypothalamus, it is sensitive to blood levels of hormones produced by other glands which induce a 'feed-back' system. Disturbances of the pituitary can thus cause many and complex effects. Tumours (generally adenomas) may cause signs of overactivity or signs of hypofunction, depending on their nature and on the stage of the disease.

*Gigantism* results from excess growth hormone in childhood. The growth pattern is normal but excessive. Later a goitre may appear.

*Acromegaly* results from excessive growth hormone in adults after the epiphyses have closed. Growth in height does not take place, but the bones thicken as well as the soft tissues. The onset of the disease is insidious, so that comparison with old photographs of the patient is of great diagnostic importance. The nose, lips, ears, tongue and lower jaw are enlarged. The teeth become separated due to enlargement of the mandible which also protrudes forward of the maxilla. Frontal bossing or swelling is common due to enlargement of the frontal sinuses. The skin is greasy and thick, the scalp wrinkled and the hair coarse. The hands and feet are large and the fingers thickened. There may also be a kyphosis and a goitre. The voice is hoarse from laryngeal hypertrophy. Photography is of great importance in following the course of this disease. Apart from routine full length pictures, the head and neck should be shown in AP, and lateral views and with the lips retracted to show teeth separation. Individual views of the hands and feet should be taken with a scale and a normal control. Sometimes photogrammetric studies are undertaken of such patients (*Section 22.0*).

*Hypopituitarism* results in *pituitary dwarfism* when occurring in childhood. Growth is simply retarded but if *hypogonadism* with sexual underdevelopment also occurs, it is known as *pituitary infantilism*. The full length pictures should always include a scale with percentile marks on it for the appropriate age. In the adult, panhypopituitarism is known as *Simmonds' disease*, and is most commonly seen in women after a severe post partum haemorrhage causing pituitary necrosis (*Sheehan's syndrome*). It causes premature ageing with loss of pubic and axillary hair, a waxy pallor, emaciation, lethargy, cold intolerance and genital atrophy.

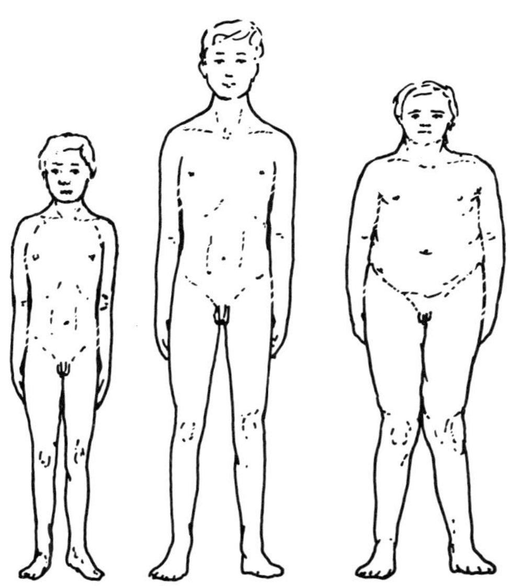

***Figure 7.3*** *Underactivity of the pituitary causes dwarfism. A normal child age 12 (centre) is compared to the Lorain dwarf (left) and the Frohlich's dwarf (right). The Lorain dwarf results from underproduction of somatotrophin alone, whereas the Frohlich's dwarf is the result of deficiency of all trophic hormones*

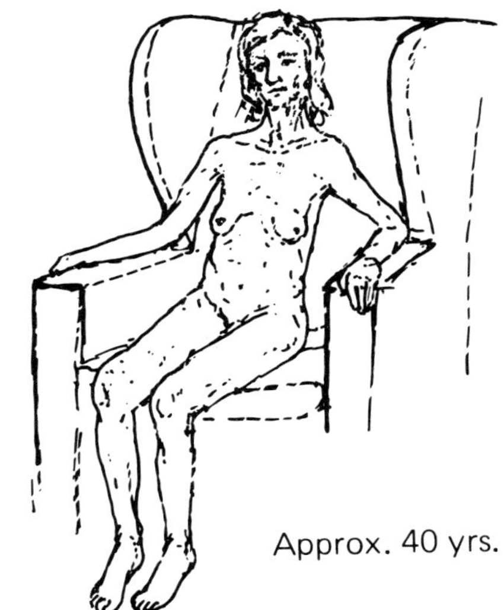


***Figure 7.4*** *The appearance of premature ageing seen in Simmonds' disease*

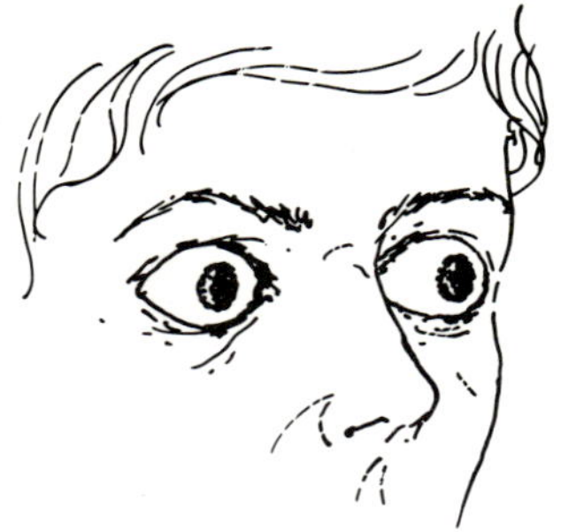

***Figure 7.5*** *Proptosis – protrusion of the eyeballs in exophthalmos*

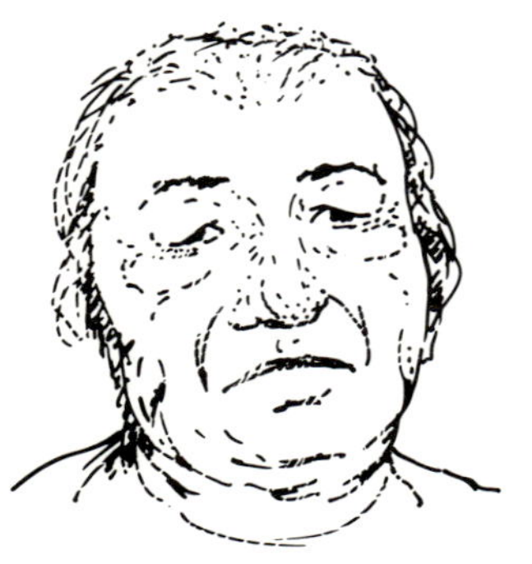

***Figure 7.6*** *The coarse bloated facies of myxoedema*

### 7.4.2 The thyroid gland

Enlargement of the thyroid gland shows as a midline swelling of the neck and should be recorded by an AP and lateral view of the head and neck to below the clavicles. When the lower pole of the gland is enlarged, it will extend behind the sternum and may press on the superior vena cava causing obstruction. This may result in dilatation of the veins over the front of the chest and will show on infrared photography.

*Adenoma of the thyroid* is a nodular swelling which may be non-toxic or toxic when it produces the signs described under Graves's disease.

*Colloid goitre* is a large diffuse non-toxic swelling, also called a struma.

*Thyroglossal cyst* (arises from the thyroglossal duct). This midline swelling of the neck moves up and down with protrusion and retraction of the tongue. Lateral views with or without superimposition will be needed to demonstrate this feature.

*Hyperthyroidism* (Graves's disease). Also known as Basedow's disease, exophthalmic goitre, toxic goitre or thyrotoxicosis. Hypersecretion of the gland. Characterized by an enlarged thyroid gland; exophthalmos (pop eyes): nervous symptoms (over-anxious, excitability); emaciation, tremor of the outstretched hands and sweating. Classically described as a 'startled hare'. Intolerant of heat.

*Pretibial myxoedema* consists of plaques of thickened and possibly rough skin over the shins and dorsum of the feet. It is a rare feature of hyperthyroidism and is not to be confused with generalized myxoedema (*see below*).

*Hashimoto's disease* is a diffuse enlargement of the thyroid due to infiltration by lymphocytes and increase of fibrous-tissue. Tends to produce myxoedema.

*Hypothyroidism* myxoedema. Subfunction of the gland *in adults*. In advanced cases, the face is coarse and even bloated from deposits of a mucin like substance which also shows markedly on the dorsum of the hands and in the supraclavicular fossae. There may be a violaceous hue of the lips and also dilated capillaries in the malar region. The hair is coarse, straight and scanty. The outer third of the eyebrows is often lost. The skin is thickened, dry and often rough on the dorsum of the hands. In addition there may be a slow, hoarse voice, sluggish movements and sometimes mental dullness. These patients are intolerant of cold. In mild cases the changes can only be seen in relation to previous photographs of the patient or in comparison with those taken after treatment. *In children* thyroid inadequacy produces cretinism with stunted growth, arrested mental development, swollen and protruding tongue, distended abdomen and apathy.

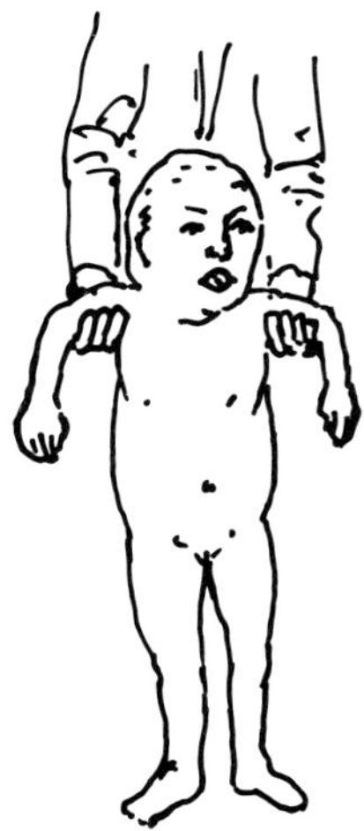

***Figure 7.7*** *Cretinism – the result of hypothyroidism in the child*

### 7.4.3 The suprarenal or adrenal glands

These lie on the upper pole of the kidney. They contain two layers each with a separate function. The inner layer or medulla secretes adrenaline and is concerned with the control of blood pressure. The outer layer or cortex secretes various corticoid and steroid hormones, some of which are concerned with the fundamental chemistry of the body and the androgens and oestrogens which affect gonadal activity.

*Addison's disease* is the result of lack of hormone. The outstanding visual sign is a dusky brown pigmentation of the skin and mucous membranes of the mouth and tongue. It is most marked on the flexures, palmar creases, extension surfaces of the fingers and on old scars. Due to pigmentation of the nail bed, the lunula appears brighter by contrast. A tired expession on the face is due to muscular weakness.

*Cushing's disease* is the result of an excessive production of glucocorticoid hormones, generally from an adrenal tumour, but sometimes secondary to a pituitary tumour. There is a characteristic central adiposity which spares the limbs, with a characteristic 'Buffalo hump' of fat at the back of the neck. The face is plethoric, skin dusky red, greasy and often

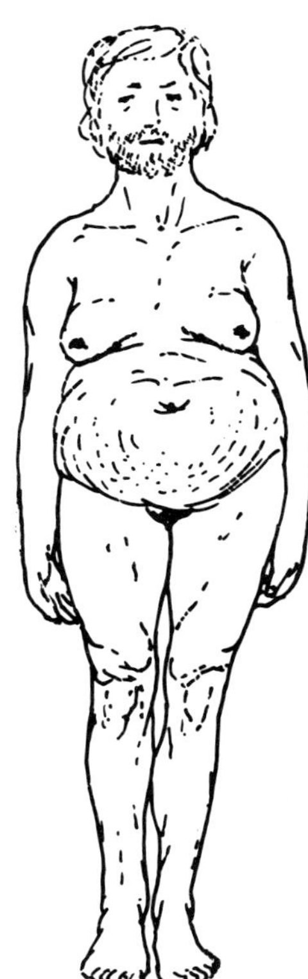

***Figure 7.8*** *Cushing's disease*

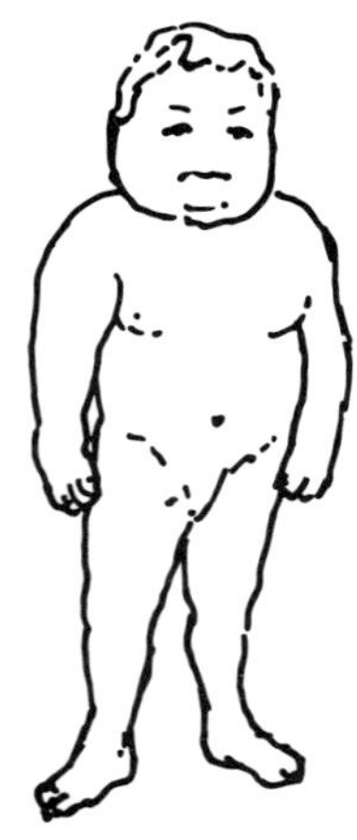

***Figure 7.9*** *The 'infant Hercules', caused by excessive adrenal androgens in childhood*

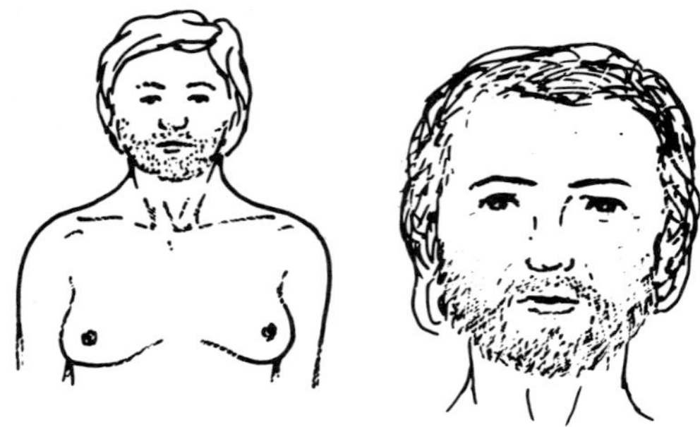

***Figure 7.10*** *Excessive androgens in the female adult result in masculinization and hirsutism.*

mottled, the classic 'moon face'. Purple striae are seen on the abdomen, thighs and shoulders. A downy hirsuties affects the face, trunk and upper arms. Scalp baldness may occur in men. Muscular wasting with weakness and osteoporosis causing collapse of the vertebral bodies may show as deformities.

*The effects of steroid therapy* may produce the signs of Cushing's disease. Serial records of these patients are of importance in the control of long term therapy.

*Adrenogenital syndrome* is caused by excessive adrenal androgens. In children there is excessive sexual development in males resulting in the *'infant Hercules'* picture. In females there is masculinization with developmental abnormalities of the genitals often called pseudohermaphroditism. Hirsutism is common. In adults the female shows regression of the breasts and hirsutism. It is very rare in the male.

### 7.4.4 The gonads

Gonadal dysfunction is frequently secondary to adrenal or pituitary disorders and has been mentioned. There are, however, two important congenital disorders which may present for photography.

*Turner's syndrome* shows hypogonadism in the female. Other signs may be webbing of the neck, low hair at the back of the head, increased carrying angle at the elbows, bent little finger, widely separated nipples and little or no pubic and axillary hair.

*Klinefelter's syndrome* produces testicular atrophy in the male. Genitals are small, hairline female in character, gynaecomastia, sole-to-pubis measurement exceeds crown-to-pubis.

*Gynaecomastia* or enlargement of the male breast occurs in many of the above conditions but may be seen as an apparently isolated and temporary occurrence. A 45° view may be useful.

## 7.5 THE METABOLIC DISORDERS

The metabolic disorders are akin to endocrine disorders in that they tend to affect the body as a whole. The following present aspects of photographic interest.

*Oedema* or the accumulation of excess fluid in the tissue spaces may occur in many varied conditions. It is sometimes localized, such as around an area of inflammation, and sometimes generalized, as in the nephrotic syndrome. To demonstrate oedema, a pit can be produced by pressing on the skin with a finger for 10–15 seconds. The result should be photographed using oblique lighting.

*Diabetes mellitus* is a disorder in which there is a raised blood sugar level due to a failure of the pancreas to produce insulin which is essential for the metabolism of sugar. It occurs most frequently in the obese middle aged female and may be associated with other endocrine disorders. Excess sugar in the urine may show as sugar spots on the clothes or shoes, but the main visual aspects of the disease arise from the patient's susceptibility to infection and from vascular complications. These are: septic spots, boils, rashes and eczema, gingivitis and a large red tongue, ulcers and gangrene of the feet, cataracts and diabetic retinopathy in the ocular fundus. Xanthomas (*see* below) occur on the eyelids and are called xanthelasma in this site. Necrobiosis lipoidica diabeticorum occurs on the shins and shows as waxy yellowish plaques with dilated blood vessels seen through the thin skin.

*Lipidosis or xanthomatosis* is due to an increased blood cholesterol (hypercholesterolaemia). It occurs in many conditions and shows as yellowish plaques or nodules in the skin. Common sites are the elbows, knees, buttocks, hands and eyelids. The extents of the lesions are well revealed by infrared photography, though of course the results bear little relationship to the visual appearance so a panchromatic control picture must always be taken.

*Scurvy* is due to ascorbic acid (vitamin C) deficiency. The gums, which are swollen and congested, bleed readily, and in advanced cases the teeth may become loosened. Petechial rashes occur, particu larly on the legs, possibly with larger ecchymoses as well. Bleeding into muscles may cause brawny swellings.

*Rickets* is usually due to vitamin D deficiency and affects children. The child is often fat and flabby with a distended abdomen. The limbs show swellings at the epiphyses, particularly marked at the wrists and ankles. There may be deformities of the forearms, angulation of the tibia and genu valgum or varum. The skull shows frontal bossing. The thorax may be deformed with a 'rickety rosary' due to bending at the costo-chondral junctions and a transverse groove (Harrison's sulcus) at the insertion of the diaphragm. Vitamin D is manufactured in the skin by UV radiation so children of Asian or negro parents brought up in temperate climates tend to suffer from rickets.

*Chronic anaemia* is the result of a variety of causes, including lack of iron. There is a pallor of skin and conjunctiva and a general weakness. Cutaneous and mucosal haemorrhages occur. Enlarged swollen tongue with papillary atrophy. Koilonychia (spoon shaped nails, demonstrated most effectively by a drop of water which is held in the 'spoon').

*Chloasma gravidarum* also known as melasma. Brown patches of pigmentation especially on the face are caused by hormonal changes of pregnancy or oral contraceptives.

*Argyria* shows as diffuse blue-black pigmentation of skin, mucous membranes and nail beds, occurs in silver and other heavy metal poisonings.

*Icterus* (neonatorum 'of the newborn'), Gilbert's disease or jaundice. Has a variety of causes but is essentially due to a disturbance of bilirubin metabolism in the liver. Patients present with yellow/olive green skin and sclera. Slight variations in the colour of skin are difficult to show convincingly in the absence of a normal control; so it may be helpful to include a healthy hand for example. There may be demonstrable hepato- or splenomegaly.

*Portal cirrhosis* is a chronic structural disease of the liver which may alter all liver metabolism. Gives rise to: bright red shiny lips, 'beefy' red tongue, palmar erythema, finger clubbing and spider naevi. The latter disappear on pressure with a glass microscope slide – this effect needs to be recorded 'before' and 'after' pressure.

*Acanthosis nigricans* characterized by

dark coloured skin folds similar to those seen in Addison's disease; appears as a result of metabolic changes due to malignant tumours of internal organs especially the GI tract.

*Cyanosis* is caused by a lack of oxygen supply to the tissues due to any reason. The patient has a puffy face, magenta coloured nose and lips, cold blue fingers and toes. Chronic cases are accompanied by finger clubbing. Commonly seen in heart/lung diseases.

*Carcinoid syndrome* results in excessive circulating serotonin. Shows as redness and swelling of face, chest and upper arms with telangiectasia.

*Ascites* is a marked accumulation of serous fluid (which glows on transillumination) in the abdominal cavity – due to various causes.

*Gout* is a metabolic disorder marked by an excess of uric acid in the bloodstream. Characterized by deposition of nodules of sodium biurate about joints and cartilaginous areas (tophi), e.g. big toe and pinna of ear.

*Beau's lines.* Major disturbances of metabolism are often reflected in the nail bed and transverse white lines across the nail correspond to major episodes of illness.

*Porphyria* is a disorder of blood pigment metabolism giving rise to brown/yellow pigmentation of the skin in exposed areas with bullous formation following exposure to sunlight. A urine sample fluoresces red under an ultraviolet lamp.

*Pellagra* is a metabolic deficiency of nicotinic acid giving rise to dermatitis, dementia and diarrhoea. Areas of skin exposed to light develop a sharply demarked area of dusky red erythema. The tongue is beefy and swollen.

*Obesity* caused by excessive subcutaneous fat deposits due to endocrine disorders, metabolic disorders, or simply over-eating. Patients are often very sensitive about their size. Standardized full length records will be required to show the distribution of adiposity. Breech obesity (lower-half obesity) means fat distributed around the hips, buttocks and thighs. Silhouette photographs can be very useful for comparative measurement of obesity.

## References


Bloom, A. and Ireland. J. (1980). *A Colour Atlas of Diabetes.* (London: Wolfe Medical Publications)

Briggs, J. (1958). Myxoedema. *Med. Biol. Illustr.* **8**, 196-201

Briggs, J. and Zampa, G. (1960). Cushing's syndrome. *Med. Biol. Illustr.*, **10**, 226-229

Gilson, C. and Summerfield, J. (1981). Clinical photography in liver disease. *J. Audiovis. Media Med.*, **4**, 91-93

Hall, R. *et al.* (1979). *A Colour Atlas of Endocrinology.* (London: Wolfe Medical Publications)

Jones, A. (1951). Acromegaly. *Med. Biol. Illustr.*, **1**, 2-3

Lewis, J. (1973). *The Endocrine System.* (Harmondsworth: Penguin Education (Nursing))

Mason, E. (1964). Some aspects of positioning and standardization in endocrinology. *Med. Biol. Illustr.*, **14**, 8-12

## Practical projects

(1) Produce a mounted set of matching prints to demonstrate the visual features of acromegaly or Cushing's syndrome to a small group of students.

(2) Ask your dematologist to refer a case of koilonychia to you. Take colour transparancies of both a normal control and the Koilonychia (a) with conventional lighting, (*b*) with 'imaginative' lighting to show the spoon shape, and (*c*) as (*b*) with a drop of water placed into the 'spoon'.

(3) Produce a short (approx 5 min) audio – visual programme on the visual signs of any endocrine disease with which you are familiar, designed to teach other medical photographers about the condition.

(4) Prepare a composite teaching transparancy (½ frame) of (*a*) A typical gouty nodule, and (*b*) polarizing microscopy of the sodium biurate crystals from the nodule.

(5) Take full length, AP and both lateral photographs of a colleague in 'silhouette' against a white background. Note any difficulties and the value of the technique for assessing physical build, e.g. obesity.

## Examination questions

Q.1 (*a*) Draw a diagram showing the location of all the endocrine glands.
(*b*) Discuss the activity of the growth hormone, and the results of over and under activity, before and after epiphyseal fusion.

Q.2 Give brief descriptions of the following conditions with special emphasis on the visual signs and symptoms:
(*a*) Hyperthyroidism,
(*b*) Hypothyroidism,
(*c*) Hyperpituitarism,
(*d*) Hypopituitarism,
(*e*) Hyperparathyroidism, and
(*f*) Hypoparathyroidism.

Q.3 Describe the menstrual cycle and the related fluctuations in female hormones.

Q.4 Write short notes on the photography of patients with:
(*a*) Graves's disease,
(*b*) Simmonds' disease,
(*c*) Cushing's syndrome,
(*d*) Klinefelter's syndrome, and
(*e*) Addison's disease.

Q.5 Describe fully the photographs you would take to illustrate:
(*a*) Iron deficiency anaemia,
(*b*) Diabetes mellitus,
(*c*) Osteitis deformans,
(*d*) Icterus,
(*e*) Gout, and
(*f*) Portal cirrhosis.

Q.6 Tabulate the visible effects of hypo- and hyper-secretion of the:
(*a*) Pituitary,
(*b*) Thyroid,
(*c*) Parathyroid,
(*d*) Adrenals, and
(*e*) Gonads.

Q.7 Give a brief description of the following conditions and outline the photographs you would take to illustrate them:
(*a*) Pellagra,
(*b*) Porphyria,
(*c*) Xanthelasma,
(*d*) Cretinism, and
(*e*) Chloasma gravidarum.

Q.8 Write a short essay on 'the importance of standardization in the photographic recording of endocrine disorders'. Illustrate your answer by reference to diseases with which you are familiar.

*Multiple choice (any of the statements may be true or false)*

Q.9 These are features of acromegaly:
(*a*) A micrognathic jaw,
(*b*) Enlargement of the sella turcica,
(*c*) Hypertrophic malar bones,
(*d*) Proptosis,
(*e*) Enlarged hands.

Q.10 A patient is sent for photography with a diagnosis of Graves's disease. You would:
(*a*) Be particularly careful that the studio is warm.
(*b*) Take a lateral picture of the head to

show ptosis.
(*c*) Take a close up of the eyes to show thinning of the eyebrows.
(*d*) Take a picture of the back of the hands to show dry skin.
(*e*) Expect to find striae.

Q.11 You would expect to record the following when photographing a case of Cushing's syndrome:
(*a*) Buffalo hump of fat on the back of the neck,
(*b*) Purple stria on the abdomen,
(*c*) A 'moon face',
(*d*) Muscular wasting of the limbs.
(*e*) Brown pigmentation of the skin folds.

Q.12 You might photograph the hands to show some aspect of:
(*a*) Addison's disease,
(*b*) Turner's syndrome,
(*c*) Porphyria,
(*d*) Pellagra,
(*e*) Ascites.

# Section 8
# Photography in ophthalmology

**R.T. Fletcher**, AIMBI
Formerly Head of Medical Photography
Institute of Ophthalmology and Moorfields Eye Hospital, London

## 8.1 INTRODUCTION

Ophthalmology is concerned with the study and treatment of diseases of the eye and its functional disorders. Such pathology may be only the ocular manifestation of a more general medical condition. The ophthalmologist is a combined physician and surgeon, and works alongside opticians who prescribe and supply corrective lenses and orthoptists who assess and treat abnormalities of eye musculature.

All medical photographers are called upon to take ophthalmic photographs even if only of the external appearance of the eye. The more specialized techniques require very specialized and expensive equipment so tend to be confined to the large department or ophthalmic unit.

Ophthalmic photography, which is mainly photomacrography, is concerned with accurate recording of the following areas:

(1) General views of head and shoulders, to show head posture, etc.,
(2) Close-up external views of one or both eyes, squint sets, etc.,
(3) Translucent and transparent structures and sectional views of the anterior segment,
(4) Angulated views of anterior segment.
(5) The ocular fundus,

and these will be covered in some depth below.

## 8.2 ANATOMY AND PHYSIOLOGY

The detailed anatomy and physiology of the eye should be understood, as should the functional aspects of the visual system. The student should note well the information on the eye in Section 28 and be able to refer to the more advanced works by Duke-Elder and Trevor Roper. An invaluable illustrated volume is Perkins and Hansell's *Atlas of Diseases of the Eye*, which is profusely illustrated with examples of the relevant pathology.

In addition to the gross anatomy of the globe it is necessary to know the terms relating to structures around the eye, e.g. the palpebral fissure, the inner and outer canthus, the caruncle, the superior and inferior fornix, the limbus, the punctum lacrimale and the plica semilunaris. The student must also be conversant with the musculature of the eye, know the names of the six muscles and the effect of paralysis of the nerve supply. The physiology of vision must be understood in terms of binocular vision, refraction and accom-

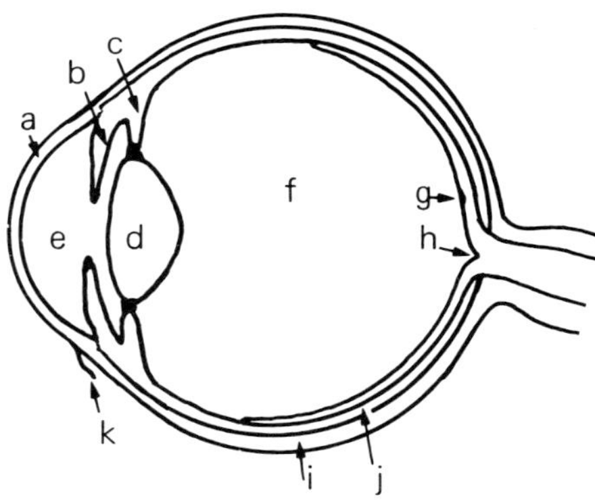


a Cornea
b Iris
c Ciliary body
d Lens
e Anterior chamber
f Vitreous
g Fovea centralis
h Optic nerve head (disc)
i Sclera
j Choroid
k Conjunctiva

***Figure 8.1*** *A sagittal section through the eye*

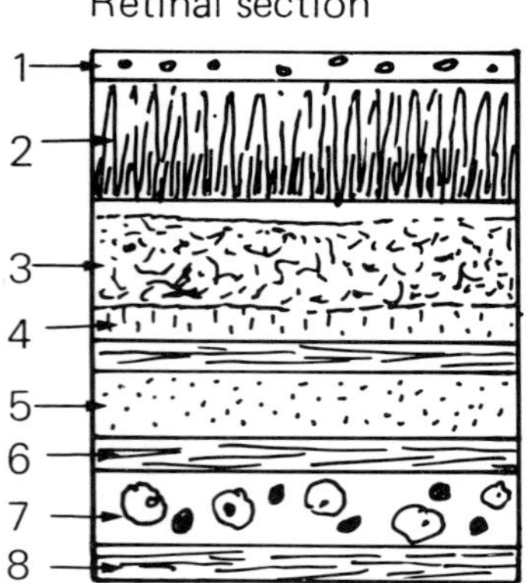


1 Pigment epithelium
2 Layer of rods & cones
3 Outer nuclear layer
4 Outer plexiform layer
5 Bipolar cells
6 Inner plexiform layer
7 Ganglion cell layer
8 Nerve fibre layer

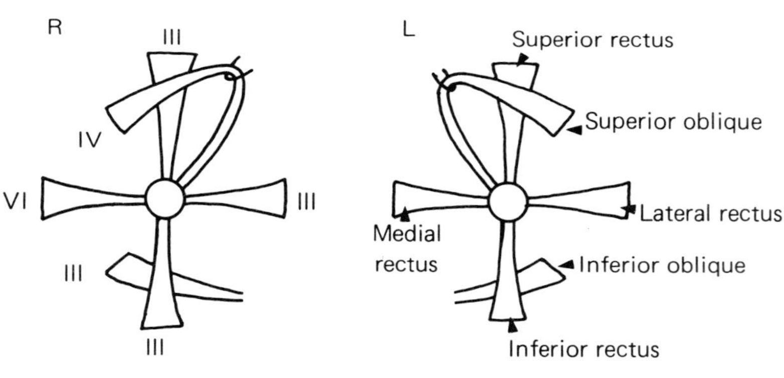


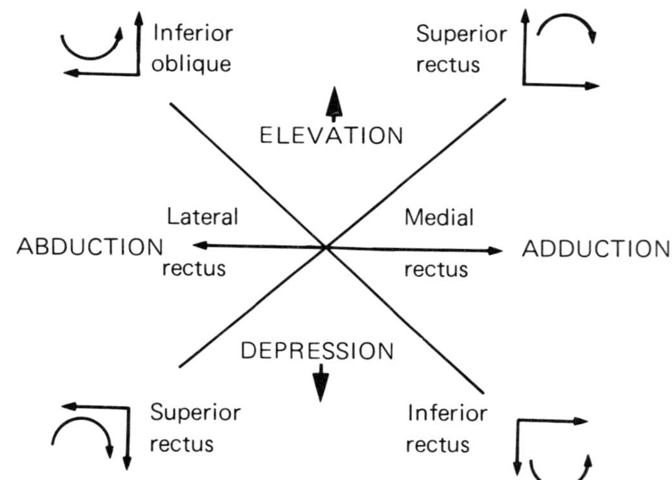


***Figure 8.2*** *(above) The layers of the retina*

***Figure 8.3*** *(right) The muscles used to move the eye, their nerve innervation and a simplified diagram of how they operate in combination*

modation, photosensitivity, colour vision and nutritional supply to the various components of the eye.

The student must be able to compare the eye with a camera in detail, and should have prepared a specification of the eye in photographic terms, i.e. *f* number, focal length, angle of view, relative sensitivity, focussing range, etc. For example, the student must know that the cornea plays a significant role in refraction and that the crystalline lens changes its radius of curvature and hence its focal length during accommodation – it does not focus by changing the image distance as would a camera lens. Again the student should understand, in optical terms, the common disorders of refraction such as astigmatism, aphakia, hypermetropia, keratoconus, myopia, and presbyopia.

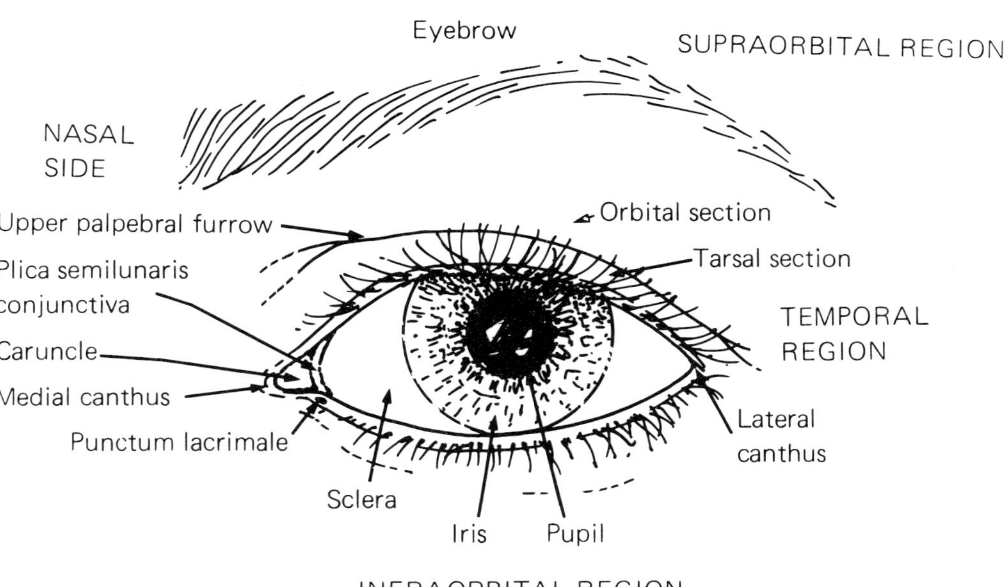


***Figure 8.4*** *The external appearance of the eye and surrounding anatomy*

## 8.3 THE PATIENT

In health the human is dependent on the visual system for most of its information, so when this system starts to fail the patient naturally becomes very apprehensive. They will not only be concerned at an implied threat to their visual system, but in disease the eye itself may become unnaturally sensitive to bright light or physical contact. An easy, confident and reassuring manner on the part of the photographer, combined with clear technical competence, will help to put the patient at ease. If the patient's visualfield or acuity is impaired (as is most likely) they may need physical guidance around camera stands, lighting booms, head rests and even floor cables.

## 8.4 PHOTOGRAPHIC TECHNIQUE

To the photographer the anterior segment of the eye presents a moist, highly reflective, motile, convex, transparent surface with underlying structures. The posterior chamber may be compared to a submarine cave in which the far walls must be studied through a narrow entrance and from above the water surface! Good ophthalmic photography is not

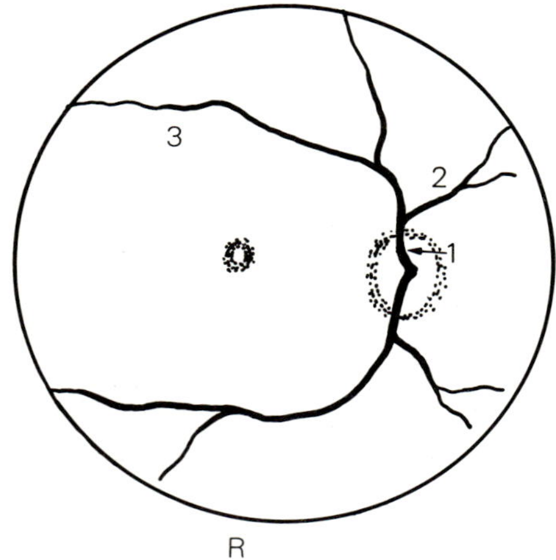


1 Superior papillary artery
2 Superior nasal branch
3 Superior temporal branch

L

1 Inferior papillary artery
2 Inferior nasal branch
3 Inferior temporal branch

***Figure 8.5*** *The patient's right and left retinae as seen by a fundus camera*

easy.

Comfortable, firm, secure positioning of the patient is essential for successful photography. An ophthalmic headrest in conjunction with an adjustable chair is the ideal support. Failing this, much can be done by arranging a chair so that the back of the patient's head is resting firmly against a wall. This will help to prevent the subject from drifting slowly out of focus. For young children a parental lap is often the most secure place, and a few words of explanation to the parent usually leads to the desired result. Both everting lids and instilling ophthalmic drops are best performed by ophthalmic department staff, but if there is a frequent need for such manipulations the photographer should obtain suitably qualified instruction in such techniques, as well as in any contra-indications for the various drugs used. Cycloplegic drugs are used to dilate the pupil and paralyse the ciliary muscle, e.g. cyclopentolate. Mydriatic drugs are used to dilate the pupil but do not paralyse the ciliary muscle, e.g. phenylephrine. Miotic drugs are used to constrict the pupil after ophthalmic examination, e.g. pilocarpine.

### 8.4.1 The external eye

For convenience the regions commonly required to be photographed may be considered as:

(1) Head and shoulders at 1:10 scale (on 35 mm), to demonstrate posture for example, as in the case of a squint which may be consequent upon a torticollis.
(2) Two eyes at 1:6 scale including the bridge of the nose and eyebrows, to demonstrate eye movements for example, as in the nine positions of gaze.
(3) The single eye with accessory structures at 1:2 scale to demonstrate say blepharitis.
(4) Close-up views of the single eye, at 1:1 scale, to show conjunctivis, iris defects, limbal vessels, etc.

Although almost any professional camera could be used for this photography the versatility and ease of use of the 35 mm single lens reflex makes it the camera of choice for all ophthalmic work. A lens of around 100 mm focal length gives a comfortably large working distance, and unless this is of the 'macro' type extension tubes or bellows will be required for the closer views. A solid camera stand with coarse and fine adjustments for movement in X, Y, and Z planes is highly desirable as is an ophthalmic headrest with chin support and forehead location. A desk lamp with dimmer control is needed for viewing and focussing and a single electronic flash unit with a small reflector and computerized thyristor control for exposing. The flash unit should preferably be attached to a swivel arm which can be rotated around the lens, and ideally should have a small light source attached to it to enable the photographer to assess where the light reflex will fall. It is also helpful if a small adjustable light can be positioned anywhere in the range of the patient's vision in order to fix the direction of his gaze – this is called a fixation light. A table to hold both the camera stand and the ophthalmic headrest on a common platform is very useful; this complete apparatus is sometimes called an anterior segment camera,

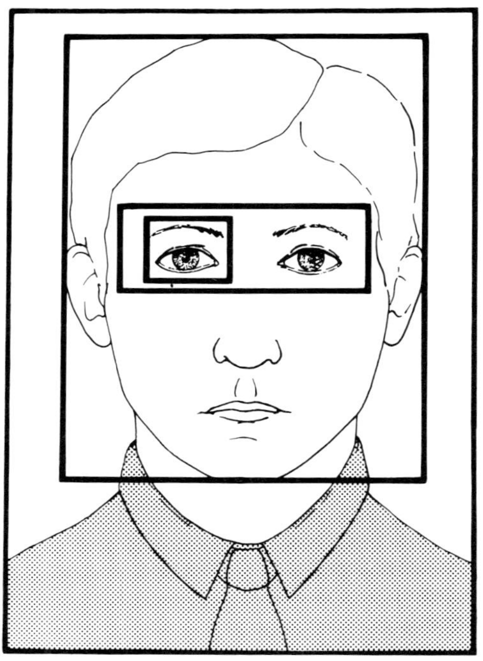

***Figure 8.6*** *The standard representational views for photography of the external eye*

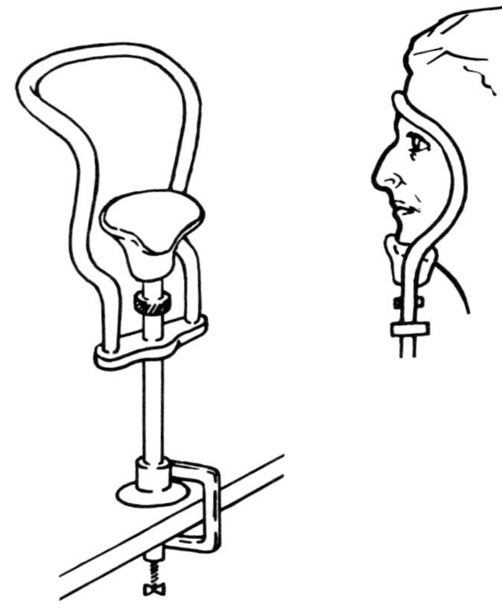

***Figure 8.7*** *An ophthalmic headrest is an invaluable accessory for all anterior-segment photography*

and purpose built ones have been described in the literature.

It is good practice to determine fixed bellows extensions (or tube lengths) and apertures for the scales of 1:10, 1:6, 1:2 and 1:1 and to focus by moving the camera bodily to-and-fro. Rigid adherence to set bellows extensions will ensure comparable reproduction ratios.

Ophthalmic subjects can display much similarity from patient to patient so strict records should be kept of the photographs taken on each film; a loose leaf pocket book with 36 entries per page is the most convenient method. Many departments photograph patients' names onto the film prior to each sequence of photographs.

Lighting from the single flash should be arranged so that the corneal reflex is small and does not obscure relevant detail – for this reason a ringflash is totally unsuited for ophthalmic photography.

The requirements for photography of the external eye might be summarized as:

(1) Subject fixed.
(2) Camera fixed.
(3) Known reproduction ratio.
(4) Known exposure.
(5) Small light source as far away as possible positioned so as not to obscure relevant detail.
(6) Retraction of lids if necessary.

### 8.4.2 The squint set

To adequately record strabismus (or squint) a set of highly standardized photographs is needed. The usual set comprises nine positions of gaze – the so called 'cardinal' positions – in three groups *viz.*

- –primary (or straight ahead)
- –secondary (or up, down, left and right)
- –tertiary (up left, up right, down left, down right)

Commonly, one head and shoulders view is included to show any compensatory head posture.

The head must be immobilized, especially in young children, as any head movement will negate the full range of eye movement being shown. With more bizarre forms of squint it may not be evident from the photographs in which direction the patient is looking. All squint photographs should thus be taken in a known sequence. Perhaps the least ambiguous sequence is clockwise, as seen from the camera, always starting at 12.00 o'clock, with views at 1.30, 3.00, 4.30, and so on, finishing with the primary position.

Some object should be provided for the patient to fixate on and in the three downward gaze positions it is usually necessary to apply slight retraction to the upper lids to prevent them obscuring the iris (this is because the orbicularis oculi muscle automatically lowers the upper lid when the inferior rectus/superior oblique muscles pull the eye downwards) – the ophthalmologist may however ask for this not to be done, as when the lids are asymmetrical. Some departments advocate placing a small arrow on the forehead between the eyebrows to indicate the direction of gaze.

The nine mounted prints, made at life size and masked down to include only the orbital margins, should be arranged in the logical sequence with the primary position in the centre of the mount. Nine positions fit comfortably on the back of an A4 mount, the head and shoulders view for convenience being mounted on the front with all the relevant file data.

### 8.4.3 The anterior segment

Translucent/transparent structures and sectional views of the anterior segment require the use of a photo-slit-lamp. The slit-lamp is a biomicroscope giving magnifications up to about ×40. It has special lighting systems designed to show up anomalies and discontinuities in the translucent/transparent media of the eye. This instrument may also be used to examine

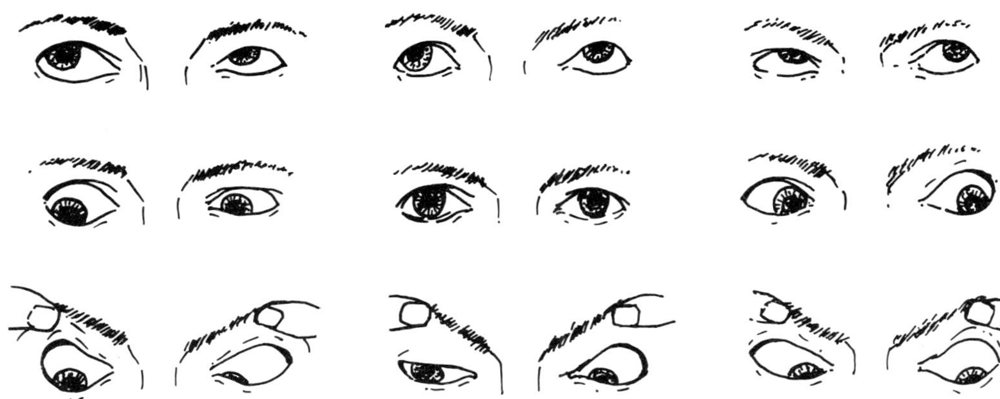

***Figure 8.8*** *The nine 'cardinal' positions of gaze used to record squints and other abnormalities of musculature*

opaque structures.

Slit-lamp illumination can be compared to a car headlamp beam in fog, when viewed from one side. Varying density of the fog can be seen due to the attenuation and refraction of the beam; similarly on a much smaller scale the slit-lamp's focussed beam shows up density changes in the ocular media. Incorporating a camera in the viewing system and a flashtube parfocal with the viewing lamp, enables photographs to be taken which are of high educational value and often of considerable beauty. Several different lighting techniques are possible with the photo-slit-lamp:

**(1)** ***Diffuse illumination*** – a soft general illumination obtained by using a broad slit with or without a ground glass diffuser over the reflecting mirror or prism.

**(2)** ***Direct illumination*** – a narrow beam of light is aimed at the anterior segment at an angle to the viewing axis focussed onto the camera or lens. The image obtained is a 'light-section' of the cornea or lens – a brightly lit parallelepiped. The sections are best seen if the beam angle lies between 45° and 90°. This is the most commonly used form of illumination, and is useful for showing opacities and irregularities in the cornea or lens, detecting foreign bodies, etc.

**(3)** ***Retroillumination*** – a beam of light is directed anteriorly into the eye and focussed onto a reflecting surface such as the retina or a cataract whilst the camera is focussed onto nearer tissue. This type of transillumination shows up clearly such things as changes in the transparency of the lens, precipitates and irregularities in the cornea.

**(4)** ***Specular reflection*** – the light is focussed onto the anterior surface of the cornea to give a brilliant mirror-like reflection. This technique reveals minute details in the surface of the cornea but does have to be adjusted perfectly.

**(5)** ***Indirect illumination*** – a narrow beam of light is focussed close to but not actually on the point of interest and observed at a very steep angle. Translucent deposits and foreign bodies appear dark against a light field.

**(6)** ***Scleral scatter*** – a narrow slit is focussed directly onto the limbus which then acts as an illuminator clearly delineating the various pathological 'rings' which may be seen, such as arcus senilis, or the Kayser–Fleischer ring. Care must

Diffuse illumination
Ground glass
screen
Wide slit

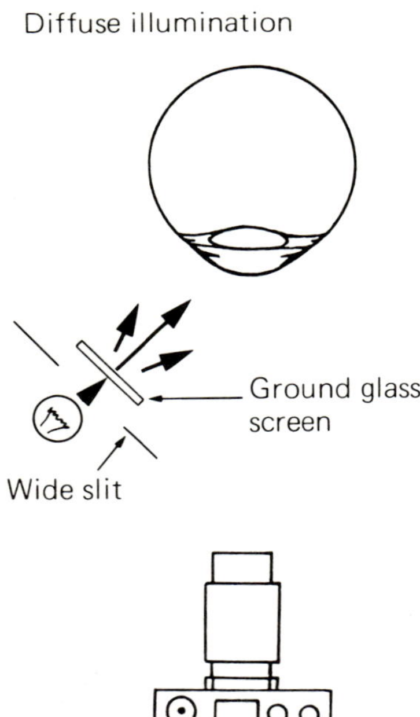

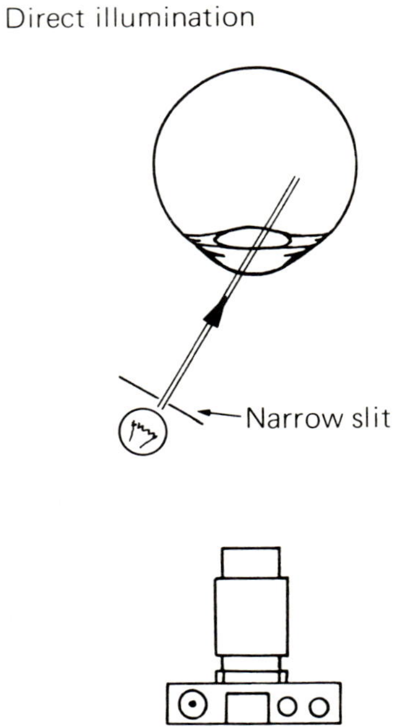

Direct illumination
Narrow slit

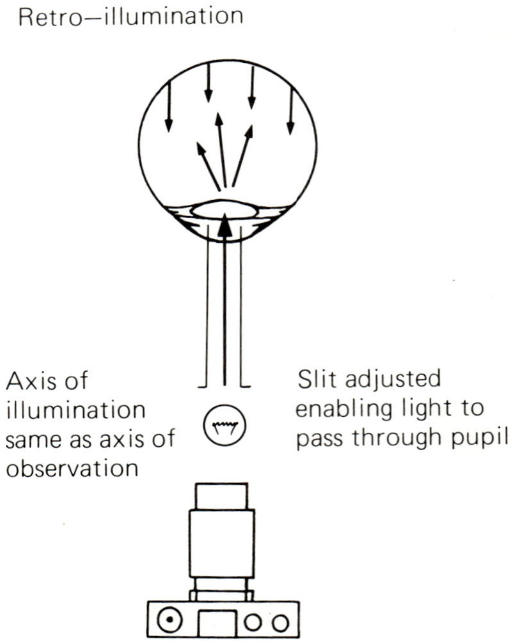

Retro–illumination
Axis of
illumination
same as axis of
observation
Slit adjusted
enabling light to
pass through pupil

***Figure 8.9*** *Six of the lighting techniques which may be employed on the photo-slit-lamp*

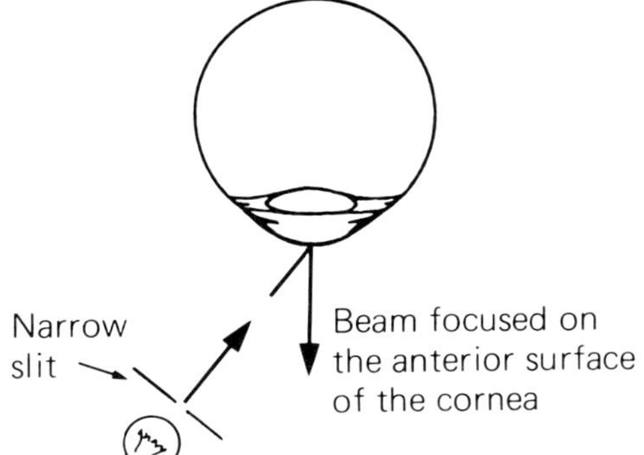
Specular reflection
Narrow slit
Beam focused on the anterior surface of the cornea

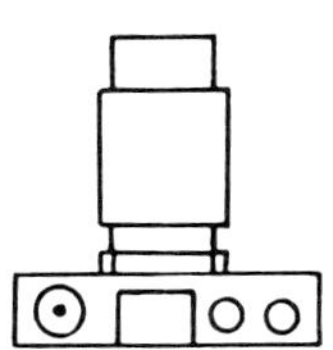

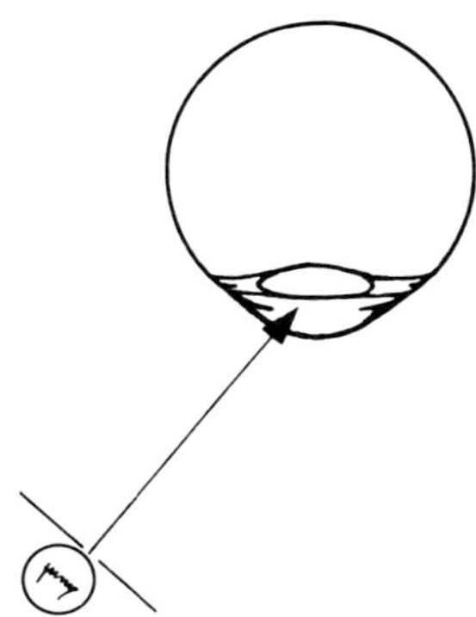
Indirect illumination
Beam focused near to but not actually on subject

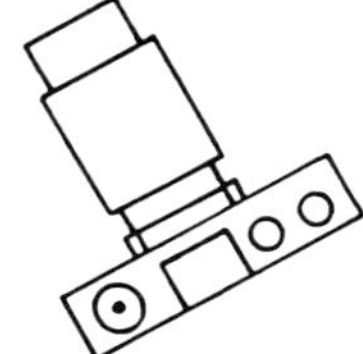

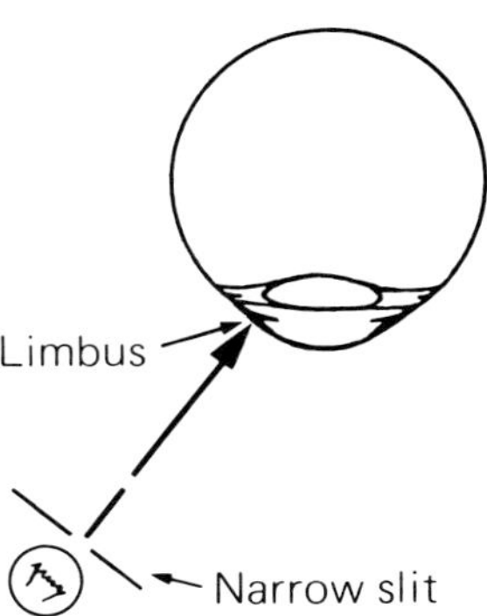
Scleral scatter
Limbus
Narrow slit

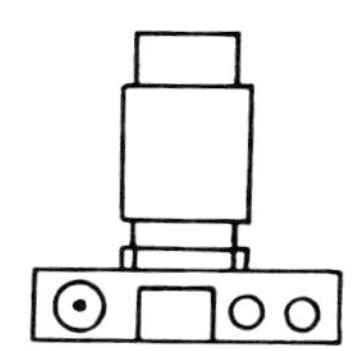

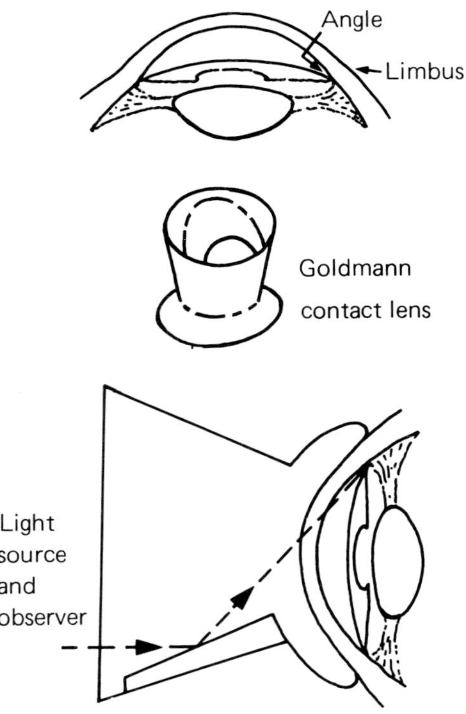


***Figure 8.10*** *Gonioscopy utilizes a Goldmann contact lens to enable the observer to see into the angle of the cornea which is normally hidden by the limbus*

be taken to avoid flare.

The low lighting level obtained with the instrument, combined with its inherently contrasty nature demand a high speed, low contrast colour film of around 200 ASA. Apart from special projects, use of monochrome film on the photo-slit-lamp is negligible. However, the instrument is expensive (at least 30 times the cost of a top quality SLR) and unlikely to be encountered other than in specialist departments.

### 8.4.4 Gonioscopy

Angulated views of the anterior segment are needed in the documentation, particularly of glaucoma, and require the use of a gonioscopic lens (a Goldmann contact lens). This is a contact lens with small mirrors, usually three or five, built into the periphery so as to provide a view across the surface of the iris to where iris, cornea and sclera meet. It is not possible to view this area anteriorly because the limbus overlaps the angle. Topical anaesthetic and a lubricant must be administered to the eye before use of the gonioscopic lens.

The photo-slit-lamp may be used to photograph the anterior segment using the gonioscope, as can the retinal camera, but the enormous depth of field in such views presents considerable problems – the best gonioscopic illustrations are drawn by the ophthalmic artist!

### 8.4.5 Assessment of the cornea

Unless the transparency of the cornea is impaired photography of this structure is difficult. When information about the surface and contour of the cornea is required such records are made with a photo-keratoscope.

In photo-keratography a disc with alternate black and white concentric rings is presented to the eye (a Placido's disc). The spacing and thickness of the rings is calculated so that when reflected in a convex surface of regular curvature, the spacing of the reflected rings is equidistant. This reflection of the disc in the cornea may be photographed via a hole in the centre of the disc. Any discontinuity of the corneal surface breaks up the ring pattern. The technique is used to assess corneal grafts and treatment of keratoconus and other distortions of the cornea. By relating the size and distance of the target to the dimensions of the reflected image measurements of corneal curvature can be made. Monochrome film is of course adequate.

In recording keratoconus it may be sufficient to take standardized anterior and

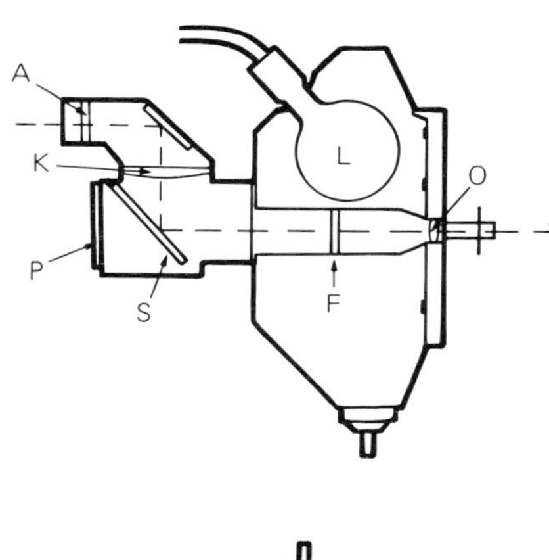


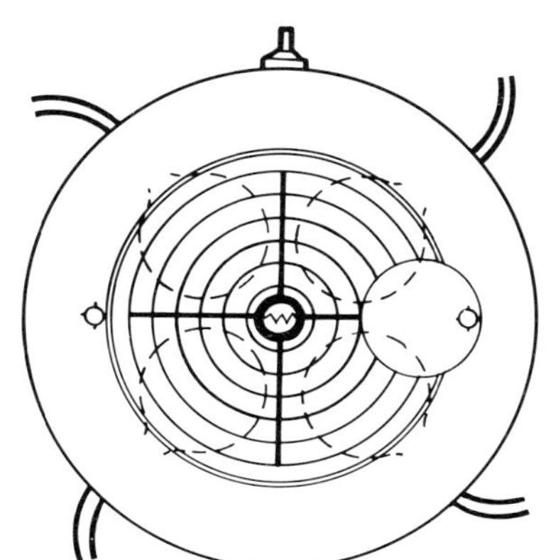

***Figure 8.11*** *The photo-keratoscope (after Amsler) reflects concentric rings of light onto the cornea*

lateral views of the single eye. In the lateral view it may be helpful to place a transparent scale alongside the central axis of the eye. The same technique is used in the assessment of proptosis in exophthalmos where a specially made Perspex rule fits into the outer bony angle of the orbit and enables measurements to be made from the photograph of the exact extent of protrusion. This instrument is called an exophthalmometer.

### 8.4.6 The ocular fundus

The retina is commonly photographed with a 'retinal' or 'fundus' camera, although a photo-slit-lamp with Hruby lens attachment may also be used. Fundus cameras are made by several manufacturers and come in a variety of angles of view – 30° being the standard – with an image magnification of approximately ×2.5. The fundus camera, more common than the photo-slit-lamp, is essentially an endoscope. That is, illuminating and image-forming rays traverse the same optical system. There is a tungsten light source for viewing and electronic flash for photography. The fundus camera is designed assuming a total refractive power in the eye of 58 dioptres, although adjustment of supplementary lenses allows for correction of myopia or aphakia.

Once mastered the fundus camera is a relatively easy instrument to use but much practice is needed to become adept at retinal photography. Good results require:

(1) Good mydriasis of patient (pupilliary diameter of between 5 and 7 mm).
(2) Viewing adjusted to operator's refraction, so that eyepiece and camera are parfocal.
(3) Subject and camera firmly fixed.
(4) Clear ocular media (aqueous and vitreous).
(5) A knowledge of retinal features and diseases.
(6) An accurate fixation system for the patient.

Very briefly the procedure is as follows:

(1) Adjust relative heights of patient's and photographer's stools and the height of the camera to suit.
(2) Check:
    (a) Patient's eye(s) is fully dilated.
    (b) Eyepiece correction set correctly.
    (c) Camera loaded with correct film and mounted properly, with all connections secure.

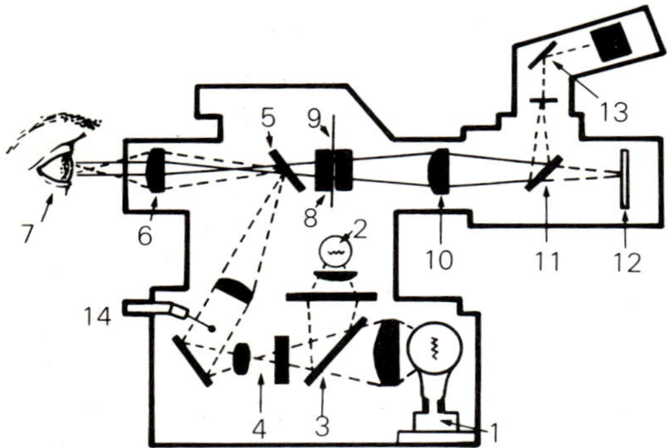


***Figure 8.12*** *The Zeiss–Nordensen fundus camera. Tungsten and flash sources (1 and 2) are aimed into the eye (7) via a series of mirrors and lenses (3, 4, 5, 6). The film (12) and the observer (13) see the image via the beam-splitter. A fixation device (14) is included in the light path*

(d) Flash output selector and recycle time set correctly.
(e) Power on.

(3) Wipe chin/headrest, adjust height of chinrest so that eye is approximately 1" below headrest bar (light axis should hit cornea when camera is in the middle of its elevation/depression range).

(4) Place patient in position, instruct them to breathe through the nose and keep forehead flat against the bar.

(5) Direct the light beam at the cornea of eye to be photographed whilst asking patient to look at fixation light.

(6) Position camera so that the crescent shaped coils of the focussing light are rendered sharply on the cornea at the centre of the pupil.

(7) Now look through the eyepiece and focus the image (apply any astigmatic or dioptre corrections necessary).

(8) Make minor adjustments to illumination using height/joystick controls. Look for even illumination with deepest colour and no 'fringing'. Expose the film. Look out for photographic artefacts:
(a) Orange crescents mean the light beam is hitting the edge of the iris.
(b) Bluish/white highlights within the scene mean the camera-subject distance is too short.
(c) Blue grey veil, particularly peripheral, means the camera to subject distance is too long (this often occurs because the patient gradually moves away from the forehead bar).
(d) Bright flares or streaks caused by patient's eyelashes.
(e) Diffuse bright spots caused by dust on the front of the camera lens.

Frequently in diabetic retinopathy a standard series of views is taken of the retina; with a 30° angle of view – this is normally a series of seven photographs, as defined by the International Diabetic Retinopathy survey.

For a full description of the technique the student is recommended to consult the specialist texts cited in the references.

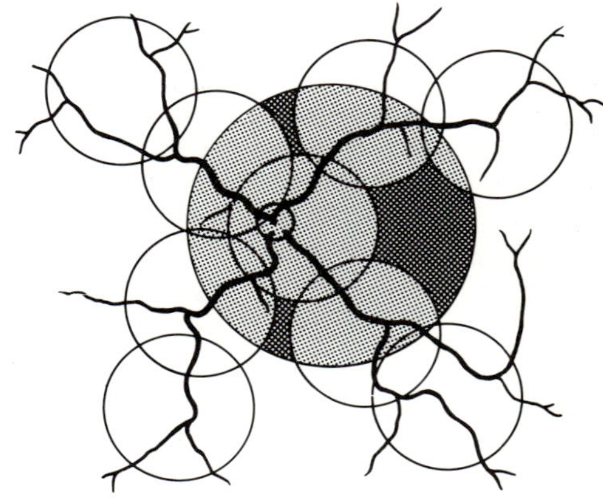

***Figure 8.13*** *A standard series of retinal views*

### 8.4.7 Fluorescence angiography

Fluorescence angiography uses a retinal camera with motorized film transport to make time-lapse studies of the passage of a dye (sodium fluorescein) through the retinal circulation. This is truly a diagnostic application of medical photography.

The fluorescence is of the blue/green variety, i.e. the green (520 nm) fluorescence is excited by blue light (460 nm) not by ultraviolet. The dye is introduced into the circulation by intravenous injection into the antecubital vein, often via a catheter to maintain an undilute bolus of dye for as long as possible. For this reason, the injection is always given by medical staff; instances have occurred of anaphylactic shock and cardiac arrest. It is essential to have an emergency kit or resuscitation trolley at hand for this eventuality – *read* and *learn* Section 4 'First aid'.

Illumination of the fundus camera is modified with exciter and barrier filters, the exciter filter being of the interference type, e.g. Baird atomic B4 to maintain high actinic efficiency and the flash is uprated. Fairly fast monochromatic film of around 125 ASA is preferred, and development is extended by about 50% to maintain speed and increase contrast.

The average arm-to-retina circulation time is of the order of 10–12 seconds, so that it is important to start photography within 5 seconds of the bolus injection. Photographs are then taken every second for approximately 30 seconds from the choroidal flush and filling of the central retinal artery to the full venous phase. It is essential to obtain good control and late venous phase records in addition to the main series.

It is important to describe to the patient just what is going to happen, and to tell him that he may feel slightly nauseous, and that his skin and urine will be yellow for some hours after the injection.

The photographic procedure in angiography is exactly the same as with white light except that the camera needs to be adjusted prior to injection and placing of the blue exciter filter in the light beam. The patient will need to be told to stay very still throughout the procedure.

Colour fluorescence angiography, where a certain amount of red light is passed by the exciter filter, has proved to be of little value apart from the more esoteric research programmes, but it does allow the results to be processed by any colour laboratory should this be desirable.

### 8.4.8 Other techniques

**(1)** ***Cinematography*** – For this work the camera should be capable of at least filling the frame with a single eye. Especially in surgery the camera will often be mounted on an operating microscope. Here, particular care must be taken to ensure that surgeon's and camera's optics are parfocal. In the studio simple lighting, using only one lamp, will avoid confusing double reflexes in the cornea. Lighting contrast can be reduced by a reflector for preference. Occasionally, filming at higher than 16 or 24 fps will be required, for instance with cases of nystagmus and pendular nystagmus.

**(2)** ***Stereophotography*** – Stereo fundus photography is particularly useful in assessing the topographic changes in the optic nerve head, e.g. 'cupping' in glaucoma. Two views of the posterior pole are taken in rapid succession with a parallax difference introduced between the two. It is possible to do this by swinging the camera but much more common is the use of the Allen stereo-separator. This device is simply a parallel sided glass block placed in front of the camera lens. The glass block is angled to the left for one view and to the right for the other view. This artificially introduced parallax gives very acceptable stereo perception. The Allen stereo-separator can be motorized and activated electronically. Various specialized stereo cameras have been devised to photograph the external eye and anterior chamber in stereo – the most notable of these is the Donaldson stereo camera.

**(3) *Dye staining*** – Where the corneal surface has been damaged, e.g. in corneal abrasions or ulceration, the surface becomes porous and absorbent. Visualizing this kind of traumatic damage is very difficult with visible light so either sodium fluorescein (green) or Rose Bengal (pink) drops are instilled into the eye. The porous abrasion absorbs the dye and becomes well delineated against the intact and unstained cornea. A similar technique is used to demonstrate the fit of contact lenses.

**(4) *Various other highly specialized techniques*** – Such as indocyanine fluorescence, infrared photography, adaptation of Scheimpflug's principle to assessing cataracts, iris angiography and pupillary aqueous flow measurement have been described. The advanced student would do well to read the appropriate references.

## References

Aan De Kerk, A., Verhallen, J. and Vijvinkel, G. (1973). A new portable photokeratoscope. *Med. Biol. Illustr.*, **23**, 206-209

Aan De Kerk, A. and Steenbergen, G. (1981). Wide angle retinal photography using contact lenses. *J. Audiovis. Media Med.*, **4**, 139-140

Allen, L. (1971). Stereoscopic fluorescein angiography of the ocular fundus. *J. Biol. Photogr. Assoc.*, **39**, 89-93

Allen, L. and Frazier, O. (1976). Photography with corneal contact fundus cameras. *Doc. Ophthal. Proc. Serv.*, **9**, 1-7

Brown, N. (1973). Slit image photography and measurement of the eye. *Med. Biol. Illustr.*, **23**, 192-203

Bruun-Jensen, J. (1969). Fluorescein angiography of the anterior segment. *Am. J. Ophthalmol.*, **67**, 842-845

Craandijk, A. and Aan De Kerk, A. (1970). Fluoresence angiography of the iris. *Br. J. Ophthalmol.*, **54**, 229-232

Cubberly, M. (1976). Infrared photography as a diagnostic tool in ophthalmology. *J. Biol. Photogr. Assoc.*, **44**, 80-85

Dallow, R. (1974). Colour infrared photography of the ocular fundus. *Arch. Ophthalmol.*, **92**, 254-258

Donaldson, D. (1955). A stereocamera for medical photography. *Med. Biol. Illustr.*, **5**, 209-216

Donaldson, D. (1976). Stereophotographic systems. *Int. Ophthalmol. Clin.*, **16**, 109-131

Drachenko, K., Shaer, E. and Starodubtseva, E. (1979). Fluorescence angiography of the anterior segment of the eye. *J. Audiovis. Media Med.*, **2**, 49-53

Duke-Elder, S. (ed.). (1958). *A System of Ophthalmology* (15 volumes). (London: Henry Kimpton)

El-Hage, S. (1971). Suggested new methods for photokeratoscopy – a comparison for their validities. *Am. J. Optom.*, **48**, 897-912

Fincham, E. (1953). The photokeratoscope. *Med. Biol. Illustr.*, **3**, 87-93

Hansell, P. (1957). *A System of Ophthalmic Illustration.* (Illinois and Oxford: Charles C. Thomas)

Hansell, P. (1967). Retinal camera review. *Med. Biol. Illustr.*, **17**, 81–89

Kottler, M., Drance, S. and Schulzer, M. (1975). Simultaneous stereophotography: its value in clinical assessment of the topography of the optic disc. *Can. J. Ophthalmol.*, **10**, 453-457

Kulwant, S. (1982). Red-free photography of the retina. *J. Audiovis. Media Med.*, **5**, 142-144

Matsui, M., *et al* (1969). Fluorescein fundus angiography in colour. *Acta Soc. Ophthalmol. Jpn.*, **73**, 653-658

McIntyre, D. (1967). The stimulation of fluorescein in external ophthalmic photography. *J. Biol. Photogr. Assoc.*, **35**, 155-157

Mikuni, M. *et al.* (1969). Stereo-gonioscopy by means of the Kowa fundus camera. *Jpn. J. Clin. Ophthalmol.*, **23**, 765-772

Ollerenshaw, R., Kilshaw, P. and Dervin, E. (1978). An optical bench for anterior photography of the eye. *J. Audiovis. Media Med.*, **1**. 137-139

Parr, J., *et al.* (1972). Grading of diabetic retinopathy by point-counting on a standardized photographic sample of the retina. *Am. J. Ophthalmol.*, **74**, 459-465

Parry, D. (1975). A technique for high magnification photography of the ocular fundus and for accurate fixation. *Med. Biol. Illustr.*, **25**, 25-27

Pearce, N. (1974); Slit-lamp photography of the eye. *Med. Biol. Illustr.*, **24**, 21-27

Perkins, E. and Hansell, P. (1971). *An Atlas of Diseases of the Eye.* (Edinburgh and London: Churchill Livingstone)

Rosen, E. (1979). *Fluorescence Photography of the Eye.* (London: Butterworths)

Rosen, E. and Young, E. (1976). Five years experience with automatic processing of fluorescein angiograms. *Med. Biol. Illustr.*, **26**, 227-230

Rutherford, A. (1973). Ultraviolet fluorescence photography in ophthalmology. *Med. Biol. Illustr.*, **23**, 204–205

Ruben, M. (1982). *A Colour Atlas of Contact Lenses.* (London: Wolfe Medical Publications)

Sheehan, B. (1980). The use of the photographic slit lamp. *Br. J. Photogr.*, **127**, 863-865

Siertsema, J., *et al.* (1982). Automatic development of retinal fluorescein angiograms. *J. Audiovis. Media Med.*, **5**, 17-19

Stenstrom, W. (1978). Guidelines for external eye photography. *J. Biol. Photogr. Assoc.*, **46**, 155-158

Trevor-Roper, P. (1980). *Lecture Notes in Ophthalmology.* (6th ed.). (London: Blackwell Scientific Publications)

Turk, A. (1978). Clinical indocyanine green fluorescence angiography of the choroidal circulation. *J. Audiovis. Media Med.*, **1**, 133-135

Wong, D. (1976). Fundus photography and fluorescein angiography. (Part 1: Photography in ophthalmology and the apparatus). *J. Biol. Photogr. Assoc.*, **44**, 105-115

Wong, D. (1976). Fundus photography and fluorescein angiography. (Part 2: Anatomy). *J. Biol. Photogr. Assoc.*, **44**, 148-153

Wong, D. (1977). Fundus photography and fluorescein angiography. (Part 3: The photographic procedure). *J. Biol. Photogr. Assoc.*, **45**, 26-30

Wong, D. (1977). Fundus photography and fluorescein angiography. (Part 4 : Photography of the external eye, photographic artifacts, patients). *J. Biol. Photogr. Assoc.*, **45**, 69-77

Wong, D. (1977). Fundus photography and fluorescein angiography. (Part 5 : Fluorescein angiography). *J. Biol. Photogr. Assoc.*, **45**, 104-114

Wong, D. (1980). *Techniques of Fundus Photography.* (Kodak publication M3-718). (Rochester, NY: Eastman Kodak)

### ***Practical projects***

(1) Good ophthalmic photography demands that you know what you are looking at. Look up the following terms in a good dictionary or illustrated textbook of ophthalmology and write short notes on the visual appearance of each:
Achromatopsia, Albino, Amaurosis, Amblyopia, Aphakia, Astigmatism, Blepharitis, Bulbar conjunctivitis, Buphthalmos, Cataract, Chalazion, Chemosis, Cyclitis, Dacryoadenitis, Dacryocystitis, Diplopia, Ectropion, Entropion, Enucleation, Epiphora, Evisceration, Exophthalmos, Glaucoma, Hemianopia, Hordeolum, Hypermetropia, Hyphaema, Hypopyon, Iridectomy, Iridocyclitis, Iris bombe, Iritis, Keratitis, Keratic precipitates (KP), Keratoplasty, Keratoconus, Meibomian cyst, Myopia, Nystagmus, Ophthalmia neonatorum, Panophthalmitis, Papilloedema, Photophobia, Presbyopia, Proptosis, Pterygium, Ptosis, Retinal dialysis, Retinoblastoma, Scotoma, Strabismus, Symblepharon, Synechia, Tarsorrhaphy, Trichiasis, Uveitis.

(2) Prepare a composite of the nine cardinal eye positions of gaze, preferably of a patient with strabismus. Produce black-and-white matched prints mounted on an A4 mount.

(3) Demonstrate the standard series of views for a diabetic survey of the fundus by producing a series of colour slides.

(4) Produce a fluorescein angiography series of the macula as a black-and-white contact proof sheet with an indication of timing sequence. Make enlargements of four frames from the series with notes on your observations.

(5) Produce a slit-lamp photograph(s) of a tumour, vascular change, or corneal lesion in a medium of your choice. Draw a diagram of the type of lighting used.

(6) Photograph a single eye with (*a*) ring-flash, (*b*) studio type electronic flash, and (*c*) portable electronic flash. Mount the series of prints together and provide observations on your results.

(7) By moving either the camera or the subject take a stereopair of photographs of (*a*) the external eye and, (*b*) the optic disc. Produce slides mounted for viewing in a standard stereo mount.

### *Examination questions*

Q.1 A patient suffering from a tumour of the brain shows abnormal eye movements and a marked nystagmus. How would you set about recording this case with a view to the execution of a follow-up sequence after operation?

Q.2 Write short notes on squints and ocular palsies. State in detail the methods you might employ to record and present such cases.

Q.3 You are asked to record on cine film the reaction of the pupil of the eye to light. Describe the procedure.

Q.4 Describe in detail the procedure for retinal photography.

Q.5 Write short notes on three of the following:
(*a*) Fluorescein angiography of the optic fundus,
(*b*) Gonioscopy,
(*c*) Indocyanine dye photography,
(*d*) Stereo-photography of the optic nerve head,
(*e*) The photography of corneal abrasions.

Q.6 With the aid of simple diagrams describe at least three distinct lighting methods that can be employed on the photo-slit-lamp. Give examples of the types of condition best suited to each technique.

Q.7 Discuss the technical requirements for the range of standard representational photography of the external eye. Briefly describe specific problems of dealing with patients suffering from eye conditions.

Q.8 Describe fully the technique of photokeratography and the ophthalmic conditions that it may be applied to.

*Multiple choice questions (any of the statements may be true or false).*

Q.9 You may need to photograph the eyes to show some aspect of:
(*a*) Opisthotonus,
(*b*) Osteogenesis imperfecta,
(*c*) Abducent nerve palsy,
(*d*) Nystagmus,
(*e*) Icterus neonatorum.

Q.10) In the technique of fluorescein angiography of the optic fundus:
(*a*) The patient's pupil should be dilated to not less than 5 mm.
(*b*) Ultraviolet light is used to stimulate the fluorescence,
(*c*) The fluorescence has a wavelength of 520 nm,
(*d*) The photographs should be taken every 10 seconds,
(*e*) A late phase picture should be taken to show the choroidal flush.

# Section 9
# Photography in orthopaedics

**K.P. Duguid**, FBIPP, FRPS, AIMBI
Head of Medical Illustration
Westminster Hospital and Medical School, London

## 9.1 INTRODUCTION

The word 'orthopaedic' is derived from two Greek words: *'orthos'* meaning straight, and *'paedion'* meaning a child, and was originally applied to the art of correcting deformities in children. Modern orthopaedics is however, concerned with all age groups and is not confined to bones and joints but covers many diseases of the associated muscles, tendons, ligaments, nerves and blood vessels. Injuries to the skull and the jaws are, however, considered to be the specialities of the neurosurgeon and dental surgeon, respectively. Thus there is bound to be considerable overlap with these and other specialities, such as endocrine, vascular and plastic surgery.

In orthopaedic photography there is particular emphasis on demonstrating by suitable lighting techniques external abnormalities resulting from skeletal deformities, and on the recording and measuring of normal or limited joint movement by either still, cinephotography or television.

Deformities are defects causing the formation of an abnormal convexity or concavity in the normal peripheral shape of the body. The causes of deformities are:

(1) Congenital (born with) e.g. syndactyly, Sprengel's shoulder, torticollis, etc., including deformation of growth, e.g. scoliosis, hallux valgus, kyphosis, Marfan's syndrome.
(2) Traumatic (injury). Fractures of all types, dislocations, burns, Volkmann's contracture, etc.
(3) Pathological, e.g. osteitis deformans, all neoplasms, osteogenesis imperfecta, etc.

## 9.2 ANATOMY AND PHYSIOLOGY

While it is not necessary to know in detail all the two hundred bones in the body, it is essential to have a sound knowledge of the majority of them, their shapes, purposes and formation, and the terminology used to describe them, e.g. articulation, condyle, crest, facet, foramen, fossa, border, process, tubercle, trochanter, tuberosity. Of similar importance will be a familiarity with the clinical methods and vocabulary used in examining joints and their movements. Adduction and abduction, extension and flexion, pronation and supination, and rotation are all terms much used by medical staff when requesting photography of orthopaedic patients – the student must be fully familiar with them.

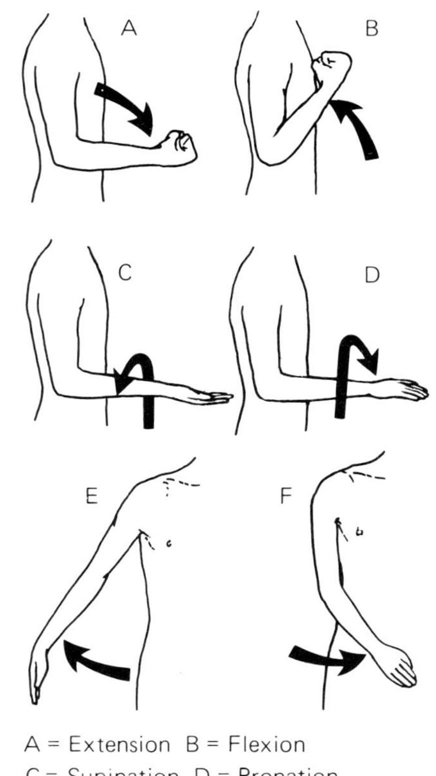


***Figure 9.1*** *The terms used in orthopaedics to describe the movements of joints and limbs*

The Institute of Orthopaedics *Photographic Standardisation Chart* is often useful for accurate communication between clinician and medical photographer which, in orthopaedics, is perhaps more difficult than usual. A good knowledge of standard clinical examination practice is of the greatest value and the medical photographer should take every opportunity to attend some practical demonstrations.

## 9.3 THE PATIENT

When applying the general principles and practice given in the Section 2 (*Care of the Patient*) it should also be remembered that many orthopaedic patients will have long term or 'chronic' conditions; their mobility or lack of it may not be obvious from their general appearance, and their attitude towards their disease may well be different to that of patients with 'acute' conditions.

Orthopaedic patients are often sent for photography after surgical operation. If the occasion is their first time out of bed and they are asked to stand they may be unsteady; this is not only dangerous but will also make the photographs of doubtful value as records of any improvement. It is best to advise a later appointment.

Where patients' mobility is restricted there is often the temptation to photograph them on the ward – resist this – good orthopaedic records require good lighting and backgrounds and full-length views, all of which are difficult to achieve on the ward. Have the patient brought to the studio in a wheelchair and use an assistant to help them stand. The patients will often appreciate and welcome this 'trip out' away from the confines of the ward.

## 9.4 PHOTOGRAPHY – GENERAL TECHNIQUE

No specialized apparatus or sensitive materials are necessary, other than those used in general photography of patients. **Standardization** is the key to all orthopaedic photography, the only variant should be the current condition of the patient – this is sometimes very difficult when 'creative' lighting may be needed to show the condition properly. Because of the considerable time factor, the negative and print filing system assumes great importance in orthopaedics, where matched prints may be required over many months or years.

Preparation and positioning of the patient is most important in orthopaedic cases in order to establish the best viewpoint; both for observation of the condition and also so that the subject is correctly placed in regard to its natural function. This is particularly important when joint movements are being recorded, and where there is likely to be a long delay until future comparable records are requested. Where the stance of the patient is of interest, care must be taken to ensure that he assumes his 'natural' position and does not over- or undercompensate in the mistaken belief that this is what is required of him.

As much of orthopaedics is concerned with normal or abnormal growth the scaling of photographs is often essential. Metric scales are preferred for measurement, and should be placed in the plane of principal focus. The inclusion of a 'normal' control patient within the photograph for immediate comparison can be of particular value for teaching. The 'Westminster' reproduction ratios are particularly recommended.

The superimposition of a squared grid or a protractor image at the printing stage can help assessment of joint movement. Some difficulty may be found in placing the centre of the protractor over the axis of the joint since not even all anatomists will agree as to its exact position. Either of these methods combined with a double exposure technique can give a very clear picture of the range of movement of a joint.

In many orthopaedic patients the only visual sign of deformity is that the normal contours of the body are either lacking, misplaced or increased. The wrong choice of lighting during photography can easily diminish or exaggerate these changes so that they are presented inaccurately as either too gross or too mild. The right balance of light and shade must be obtained while still maintaining an uncomplicated lighting arrangement which can be matched in subsequent serial photographs. Correct choice of background in conjunction with effective lighting should ensure that the body or limb outlines are never 'lost' – black backgrounds with rim-lighting are much favoured in this area of photography. This is of course a general criterion for all patient photography but perhaps above all in orthopaedics where the outline is of such importance.

## 9.5 SPECIAL TECHNIQUES

***(1) A double exposure*** *(or multiple exposure) technique* can be effectively used to demonstrate a range of movement of either a single joint or of the spinal column in the cervical or lumbar regions. Separate exposures are made, usually at the two extremes of movement, against a black background. No exposure variation is necessary but great care must be taken with the positioning of the subject so that the axis of the joint remains stationary. This may be relatively easy, in for instance the case of a wrist joint where it can if necessary be anchored while still allowing full range of movement of the hand; it may be far more difficult in the case of the spinal column when trying to record the patient's ability to bend forwards and back while preventing the pelvis from moving.

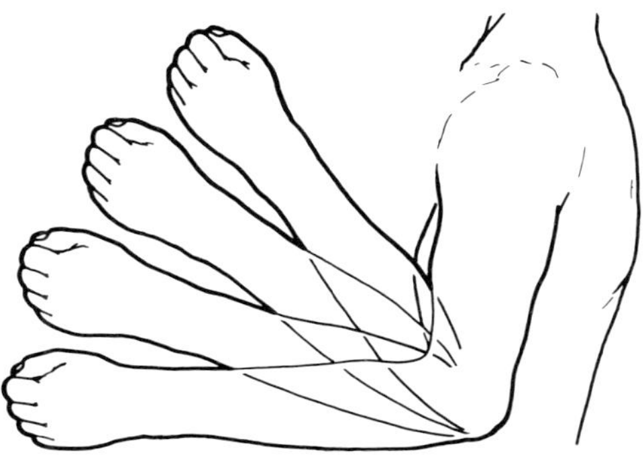

***Figure 9.2*** *Multiple exposure records are very useful in assessing joint movement. Care must be taken to ensure that only one part of the joint is allowed to move*

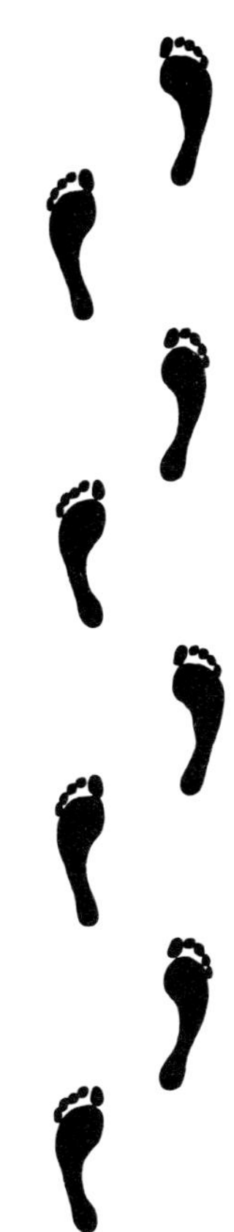

***Figure 9.3*** *'Footprints' such as these may be obtained in a variety of ways, as explained in the text. They are useful for assessing many types of deformity*

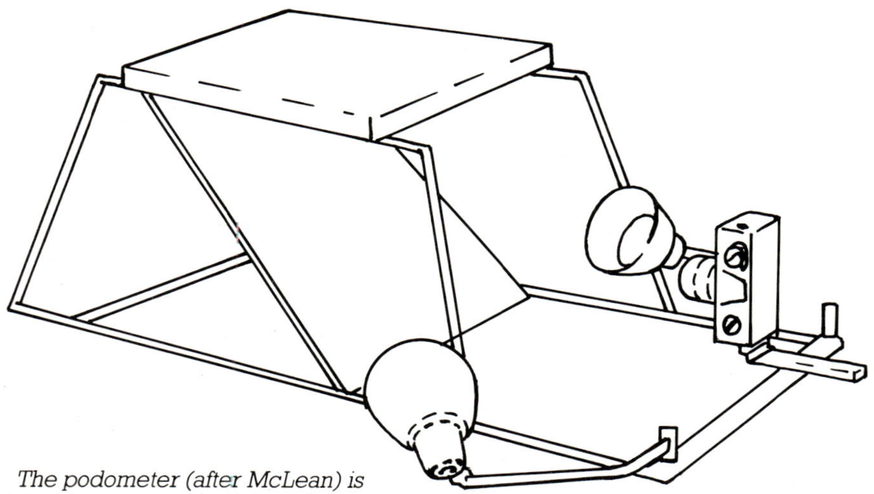

**Figure 9.4** *The podometer (after McLean) is used to obtain clear records of the plantar surface of the foot whilst weight-bearing*

***(2) Theatre photography*** in orthopaedics only presents two differences from normal practice. Firstly, the whole surgical team will be doubly careful about sterility, secondly the operative field will frequently be made bloodless by the application of a tourniquet so care must be taken when judging exposure.

***(3) Recording the plantar surface of the foot***. Several techniques have been used to record the weight-bearing pattern of the plantar surface. These include wiping the sole of the foot with ink and asking the patient to impress his footmark on a white paper, or wiping the sole with Vaseline and impressing an image of the foot onto bromide paper which is then fogged and processed. The Vaseline prevents development of the print, and a white image remains on a black ground. The best technique, however, is to get the patient to stand on a sheet of armour plate glass and by using a 45° mirror beneath it record photographically the pressure areas. Special instruments with lighting arranged to demonstrate the pressure effectively have been described, and can be used conveniently even for mass screening of patients.

## 9.6 ORTHOPAEDIC CONDITIONS

Some of the more common diseases and conditions which may be referred for photography are:

***(1) Scoliosis***. This is described as lateral curvature of the spine. It is usually a primary curve with secondary compensating curves, one above and one below the main curve which may be lumbar, thoraco–lumbar or thoracic. Subclassified as congenital, idiopathic or myopathic.

Photographs to show both posture and the deformity are required from anterior, posterior and lateral viewpoints. An additional posterior view with the patient bending down as though to touch the toes will help to show the associated 'rib hump' deformity. Marking out the individual spinal processes with a skin marker is a helpful technique. Such marking must be done with the patient already in the intended position for photography, otherwise a movement such as bending down will alter the positions of the marks. When photographing scoliosis, it is important to show the whole patient including the head and feet. Scoliosis may well either cause or be the result of other bodily abnormalities – which should also be recorded. Photogrammetry is much used for the recording and early detection of this condition (*see Section 22*).

***(2) Kyphosis and lordosis.*** Kyphosis is an exaggeration of the normal dorsal curve (hunchback) and lordosis is an exaggeration of the normal curve in the lumbar region, with anterior protrusion of the lower abdomen. Full length lateral views are required. It is often necessary to get the patient to flex the arms at the elbow so that the arms do not hang down and obscure the lumbar curvature. Do not get them to put their hands behind the head – this will alter the spinal configuration.

***(3) Hallux valgus.*** Lateral deviation of the big toe. This often involves both feet and can give rise to a bunion caused by rubbing on the shoes. Additional deformities occur in advanced cases. Accurate serial photographs are required for evaluation during treatment which is usually surgical. A viewpoint from above should be chosen and the whole of both feet included.

***(4) Talipes equinovarus*** (congenital club foot). The foot is turned so that the sole is facing inwards. There is adduction of the toes relative to the hindfoot and also plantar flexion. As this is a congenital condition early and prolonged treatment is essential, serial pictures will be needed over a lengthy period. With very young children some care will need to be exercised to ensure that the child adopts the abnormal stance – one technique is to get the parent to hold the child vertically and then lower him until his feet just touch the floor. Both feet should be shown and also the legs up to and including the patellae so as to record the relative positions and angles. Both anterior and posterior views are essential. It is important to be able to see the surface on which the child is standing – completely white shadowless backgrounds are useless to the orthopaedic surgeon in recording these conditions.

***(5) Congenital dislocation of the hip.*** In this condition, the head of the femur is displaced out of the acetabulum in an upwards direction. It is a spontaneous dislocation, present at birth. It is usually diagnosed at the post-natal examination and special views may then be required. At a later stage, an abnormal gait, a delay in learning to walk and restricted abduction of the affected limb (which may also show extra skin folds) are all characteristics which may be filmed or photographed. Photographs of the patient demonstrating Trendelenburg's manoevre may also be required. This involves posterior views of the trunk and lower limbs; first with the patient standing at rest and then with the weight on the affected limb while raising the other foot just off the ground. Normally this would raise the pelvis on the lifted side, but in CDH the opposite will occur and it will drop. In order to see this tilt of the pelvis, it may be advisable to mark the right and left posterior iliac crests.

***(6) Arthritis.*** This is an inclusive term covering both inflammatory and degenerative conditions in joints. There are many types, including rheumatoid arthritis, tubercular arthritis, osteo-arthritis and ankylosing spondylitis. Restricted joint movements, local swellings and characteristic deformities, particularly in the hands, wrists and feet are the features which will concern the medical photographer most often.

***(7) Ankylosing spondylitis.*** This is a progressive condition of the spine, mostly affecting young men. The main feature is the poker like rigidity of the spine and consequent loss of its mobility. A lateral view using a double or triple exposure technique is often preferred to separate photographs for recording this limitation of movement.

***(8) Paget's disease*** (osteitis deformans). A progressive condition which affects the pelvis, the vertebrae, the femur, the tibia and the skull. In well-established cases, softening of the bones leads to the patient having a characteristic posture and appearance with marked bowing of the legs, a shortened trunk and an enlarged skull (the patient finds as the years go by that he needs larger and larger hats).

***(9) Achondroplasia*** (chondrodystrophy). This is dwarfism characterized by short limbs, which are caused by a defect of long bone growth but with a normal sized head. Adult achondroplastics are usually less than 4 feet (1.2 m) in height and the hands are short and broad.

***(10) Infantile torticollis* (wry neck)**. The head is tilted to one side by contracture of the sternomastoid muscle. There may also be facial asymmetry. Photographs should show both of these facets, and also, if possible, the tightly contracted muscle which contrasts with the normal muscle on the other side of the neck. The view must include both clavicles. There may also be a squint which will need recording in the nine positions of gaze (*see Section 8.4.2,*).

***(11)* Dupuytren's contracture**. A condition of the hand in which there is a typical flexion of one or more fingers caused by a thickening of the palmar fascia. The first sign, before any flexion occurs, is a thickened nodule in the middle of the palm. The hand should be photographed in full extension from both the palmar and the ulnar aspects. The ulnar view is best taken from *slightly* above rather than from on a level with the palm. Serial pictures are certain to be required during treatment or follow up.

***(12) Chest deformities***. Among the chest deformities to be demonstrated are the long chest, the flat chest, the barrel chest, the pigeon chest (pectus carinatum) and the hollow chest (pectus excavatum). For these it is important to show the line of the ribs and of the spinal column and the outline of the sternum. It may be helpful to inscribe anatomical points on the patient with a skin pencil. The body section and contours may be accurately demonstrated and measured by photogrammetry.

***(13) Foot deformities***. Pes planus (flat foot) and pes cavus (claw foot) which are characterized by flattened or raised longitudinal arches respectively, are best recorded with both a medial view with the patient lying supine at rest, then another with the patient standing (weight bearing). Standardized views for the documentation of foot deformities have been reviewed in the literature.

***(14) Knee deformities***. Genu valgum (knock knee) and genu varum (bow legs) need anterior and posterior views of both lower legs from mid-thigh to floor then anterior and lateral close-ups of both knees to demonstrate the deformity in detail. Views for foot attitude and general body habitat may also be useful.

***(15) Gait abnormalities***. Several diseases are characterized by particular styles of walking, e.g. the lame gait of pes planus, the 'heather-step' gait of alcoholic neuritis, the jerky gait of spastic paralysis, the tremulous short-stepped gait of Parkinson's disease, the bizarre jerky gait of Huntington's chorea, the dragged leg of hemiplegia and the waddling gait of congenital dislocation of the hip. The recording of gaits is most commonly carried out by cinematography or television (*see Section 21*) but photogrammetry (*Section 22*), chronocyclography and stroboscopic photography (*Section 23*) are sometimes used. To make an intelligent representation of a gait with still photography calls for considerable patience and a fast motor drive. It is important that the patient has sufficient area in which to walk and that the area is evenly illuminated. Light levels are considerably higher than those required for still photography. The lighting technique is to have sufficient diffuse lighting to cover the area and to augment this with a key light. If indoor facilities are not sufficient the recording of gaits outside is perfectly satisfactory. The orthopaedic surgeon may sometimes request that the walking surface of a patient's shoes be photographed as these often record clearly abnormalities of gait and posture.

## References


Adams, J. (1971). *Outline of Orthopaedics* (Edinburgh: Churchill Livingstone)

Dommasch, H., *et al* (1972). Investigations into techniques of gait analysis. *J. Biol. Photogr. Assoc.*, **40**, 106-116

Duguid, K. and Ollerenshaw, R. (1962). Standardization in records of the foot. *Med. Biol. Illustr.*, **12**, 241-245

Ebrahim, H. and Williams, A.R. (1981). Comprehensive photo-optical gait recording. *Br. J. Photogr.*, **128**, 929-931

Kessel, L. and Boundy, U. (1980). *A Colour Atlas of Clinical Orthopaedics*. (London: Wolfe Medical Publications)

Kilshaw, J. and Ollerenshaw, R. (1954). Assessment of spinal movement. *Med. Biol. Illustr.*, **4**, 166-177

McLean, K. (1977). Photography of the plantar surface of the foot. *Med. Biol. Illustr.*, **27**, 141-144

Murray, E. (1972). Investigations into techniques of gait analysis. *J. Biol. Photogr. Assoc.*, **40**, 106-110

Rutherford, A. (1983). Footprints. *J. Audiovis. Media Med.*, **6**, 80-88

Whitley, R. (1959). Lighting in orthopaedic medicine. *Med. Biol. Illustr.*, **9**, 226-230


## *Practical projects*

(1) Photograph the palmar surface of the hand in the medium of your choice.
(*a*) With frontal bilateral lighting,
(*b*) low angle lighting,
(*c*) rim lighting.

(2) Produce a series of three matched black-and-white prints of the back from neck to iliac crest with:
(*a*) 45° copy lighting,
(*b*) Strong top lighting,
(*c*) Strong side lighting.

(3) Produce a series of not less than eight matched colour transparencies to illustrate some orthopaedic operation, e.g. hip replacement. Pay particular attention to standardization and anatomical orientation.

(4) Use multiple exposure technique to demonstrate the range of movement of either the knee or spine. Supply a 10" × 8" print with a superimposed protractor inserted at the printing stage.

(5) Make a short film-loop of a characteristic gait and write short notes on the disease to accompany the film.

(6) Photograph both hands in a medium of your choice:
(*a*) anteriorly (palmar),
(*b*) posteriorly (dorsal),
(*c*) ulnar side,
(*d*) radial side.

Experiment with different background arrangements until you find a convenient method.

(7) Use any method you choose to demonstrate the 'pressure areas' of the plantar surface of a patient's foot.

(8) Produce a series of black-and-white prints suitable for inclusion in a patient's case notes of a case of idiopathic scoliosis.

## Examination questions

Q.1 (*a*) Draw an annotated cross-sectional diagram of the hip joint, and with the aid of simple diagrams describe the range of movements at the hip.
(*b*) Briefly describe a photographic technique for recording the range of movements of joints.

Q.2 Describe fully two specialized photographic recording techniques that are of use in orthopaedic photography.

Q.3 List the main features of visual interest in the following conditions and state the photographs you would take to demonstrate them:
(*a*) Ankylosing spondylitis,
(*b*) Torticollis,
(*c*) Carpal-tunnel syndrome,
(*d*) Sprengel's shoulder, and
(*e*) Osteogenesis imperfecta.

Q.4 'Creative lighting and standardization are the cornerstones of orthopaedic photography,' discuss this statement fully.

Q.5 Describe the common orthopaedic deformities of the foot and the standardized photography of such conditions.

Q.6 What photographs would you take to fully illustrate:
(*a*) Paget's disease (of bone),
(*b*) Pectus excavatum,
(*c*) Genu valgum,
(*d*) Talipes equino–varus, and
(*e*) Lordosis.

Q.7 Distinguish between:
(*a*) Osteitis deformans and osteogenesis imperfecta,
(*b*) Genu varum and genu valgum,
(*c*) Pott's fracture and Colles's fracture,
(*d*) Pes planus and pes cavus,
(*e*) Talipes equinus and talipes calcaneum.

*Multiple choice questions (any of the statements may be true or false)*

Q.8 When asked to show scoliosis you would:
(*a*) Take a posterior–anterior view of the patient,
(*b*) Use flat lighting,
(*c*) Have to use colour film to make an adequate record,
(*d*) Use a multi-exposure technique,
(*e*) Include the crests of the ilium in the photograph.

Q.9 Multiple exposure techniques are very useful for recording the ranges of limb movements, but:
(*a*) A white background is essential.
(*b*) Long shutter speeds are required.
(*c*) If three exposures are taken each one should receive only ⅓ of the metered exposure.
(*d*) A 5" × 4" view camera is quite suitable.
(*e*) The technique cannot be used to assess spinal column movements.

# Section 10
# Photography in paediatrics

**M.K. Johns**, FIMBI, ARPS
Deputy Director of Medical Illustration
Institute of Child Health and Hospitals for Sick Children, London

## 10.1 INTRODUCTION

Paediatrics is the term applied to the development of children, their care and to the treatment of their diseases. The age range encompassed by paediatrics is normally from birth to 14 or 16 years, although in some paediatric hospitals a small number of older children will sometimes be seen. Paediatrics is only a specialty insofar as all the patients are children: within the specialty will be seen almost all the conditions that are seen in any adult hospital, although some congenital deformities that can be treated early in life will not be seen in their 'gross' state in the adult. Consequently the techniques of medical photography that can be applied to paediatrics are wide-ranging and a careful study of this book will equip the medical photographer for the technical aspects of his work with children.

## 10.2 HANDLING CHILDREN

Successful photography of people – and not children alone – can only be achieved easily if the photographer is prepared to take the necessary time to build a relationship with his subject. People in hospital either as inpatients or visiting as outpatients are always under some form of stress due more often than not to fear (however hard they may try to rationalize this). A hospital is an alien world to the layman and in a strange situation it is little wonder that worry about one's condition or whether the next investigation will be painful or whether there might even have to be an operation all conspire together to change the patient's outlook on life. In the case of children it is probably not so much the prospects of recovery that loom largest in his mind – rather the prospect of another 'needle' that causes the most concern.

The patient in hospital, therefore, needs a little more consideration than would otherwise be necessary and the little extra effort that it takes to build a proper relationship will pay dividends in two ways. In the first place the photographs will be that much easier to obtain simply because the patient will be that much more co-operative. The other benefit, although perhaps not so directly helpful to the photographer, is that the patient will gain that little more confidence in the health care team if he is made to feel that he is a little bit special. This is true of all patients, but particularly true of children.

### 10.2.1 Establishing a relationship

The first and most important thing to remember is that the patient is a person and not a disease. In a busy session it is easy to start thinking of the next 'fluorescein angiogram' or the next 'scoliosis' rather than of 'Peter' or 'Barbara', the children who require these investigations.

From the moment a patient enters the door of the department to the moment he leaves at the end of the session, he should be addressed by name. Very often young patients will be accompanied by their parents, especially if coming from the outpatient department. Despite this, all questions and discussions should be aimed at the child and questions asked of him directly. Should the parent interrupt and answer on the child's behalf, it is likely that the photographer will succeed in his search for a relationship if the child is taken alone to the studio, or with an escorting nurse or secretary asking the parent politely to 'wait here while we go to take the pictures'. In this context it is as well to note that some children will either want their parent to accompany them or not; in these cases this wish should be respected.

Appropriate dress for medical photographers has been mentioned elsewhere in this study guide; superficially it may seem that it would be better to dress casually when dealing with children. This is not the case. Children respond to people more than they respond to dress, but adults tend to make more of first impressions. In the case of the paediatric photographer, therefore, the dress is for the parent and the relationship for the child. It is significant that 'professional dress', clean white coat, collar and tie, and so on, can provide an air of solidity which will give confidence to a worried parent.

A photographer wearing a white coat can in fact help the younger child to realize that not all 'white coats' are automatically going to stick needles into them, and to give him confidence when he sees other members of the health care team.

The child should be collected from the waiting room and taken to the studio by the photographer rather than be summoned by a loudspeaker calling his name. The short walk to the studio will take place on 'neutral ground' and the alert photographer will learn a great deal in these few moments about the behaviour of the child. An exaggerated example is the case where a patient is referred for a film or video recording of gait. While going from the waiting room to the studio the child will be walking naturally because he will feel relaxed on 'neutral ground'. Once in front of the camera he may well, consciously or otherwise, alter his natural walk either to make it look worse or, more likely, to try to make it look better, in which case he will tense up and in fact the gait will seem to be worse! The photographer who has seen the natural gait will be able to ensure that this is what he records in the studio.

### 10.2.2 In the studio

Once in the studio, the patient should be seated comfortably (or, in the case of a baby, held in mother's or nurse's arms) and examined by the photographer. During this time the photographer must work out what he is going to do for the patient – how many views, what equipment, what lights need to be on and so on. All the time a conversation should be carried on so that the actual photographic session seems almost an incidental part of the whole proceedings.

While the patient or parent takes off any clothing and/or dressings that might intrude, the photographer should be preparing his equipment. It is a sensible idea to have a small wheeled trolley for accessories which can 'follow the photographer around' so that everything that will be needed is to hand. To break off in the middle of the session to fetch an extension tube from the other side of the room not only disturbs the relationship with the child but also interrupts the flow of the photography.

The patient who is old enough should be sat on a tall adjustable stool so that his feet do not quite touch the ground. This will naturally limit his ability to move and make it easier to light the subject!

Younger children can be photographed on a couch or on their mother's knee. If a couch is used it is important to appoint someone to take care of the child to stop him falling off – an accident which can happen in a second while the photographer's back is turned.

Traditionally, clothing does not appear in medical photographs and this should largely be the aim in paediatric photography. There will be occasions when the subject will not want to get undressed and in this situation a compromise should be reached. An instance is a child who would strip to the waist from both ends, but not at the same time! A full length equivalent of two half lengths in this particular case was suitable and the request was met in this way! As a general rule, if clothing has to appear in the picture it should be subdued and not detract from the subject.

In cases where regular sets of photographs are taken to illustrate given conditions, it is worthwhile evolving a 'patter' for each set of pictures; not only does this enable the photographer to keep a conversation going through a longer session, it can also help to cue his actions with the cameras and lights and so help to speed up the session.

Some children will naturally be awkward or non-cooperative. If a baby, it may be because he is tired or hungry, and often a brief wait while a feed is given will resolve the problem. A toddler or older child may also be uncooperative. Unless the photographs *must* be taken in this session – because the patient is going to theatre or is an outpatient, for example, (and in which case the best possible result must be obtained) it is probably better to give up gracefully and to arrange a new appointment for earlier in the next day An 'off duty' visit to the ward to see the child and play with him for 5 minutes or so may well break the ice sufficiently to allow a good photographic session – as indeed may just a good night's sleep.

On no account should children be either bribed or rewarded with sweets. They may be on special diets or going to theatre soon, but are unlikely to be able or willing to tell the photographer so.

By the same token, the photographer should never lie to a patient in order to gain his cooperation. Saying something will not hurt and then hurting the patient is almost expected by an adult. But a relationship with a child is built on trust rather than on the sort of code that an adult understands. A reluctant child may well be persuaded to pose by the photographer promising 'not to touch'. If this or any other promise is made, it must be kept. If not, you might get away with it on this visit – but your patient will remember next time and you will have to work all the harder!

Avoid hurting the young patient unnecessarily. When recording cleft lip and palate cases, for example, some photographers advocate pinching the baby to make him cry – thereby obtaining a good view of the palate. This is unnecessary; most often if you hold the baby's head gently on either side, covering both ears and gently tilt the head back, they will oblige by crying loudly. This latter technique does not hurt the child and is just as effective.

At the end of the photographic session, the relationship should be broken as cleanly and gently as possible, and the child should be invited back again to the department next time he comes to the hospital.

The key to success lies in the two words 'time' and 'relationship'. It is worth the time it takes to get the relationship right, if only to make the next visit that bit easier – it is a fact that children provide more photographic repeat visits than adults and the paediatric photographer will get to know many of his patients well as he follows their progress from birth to maturity.

## 10.3 EQUIPMENT AND LIGHTING

Correct posing and viewpoints can be difficult to achieve when photographing children – either through hyperactivity and/or short attention span or physical inability to take up standing or sitting positions.

Consequently the best approach will be to use a handheld single-lens reflex camera system, thus allowing continuous correction of viewpoint to compensate for changes in posing.

Because of the problem of movement, electronic flash will be the lighting method of choice, and for most conditions it is adequate to use fairly flat lighting of a wide subject area, so allowing the patient a range of movement without 'falling out' of the lit area.

Many conditions that involve only small areas of the patient – for example, the mouth, the fingers, an ear, a foot – will often be more than adequately lit using a small portable unit close to the lens and this indeed may be the apparatus of

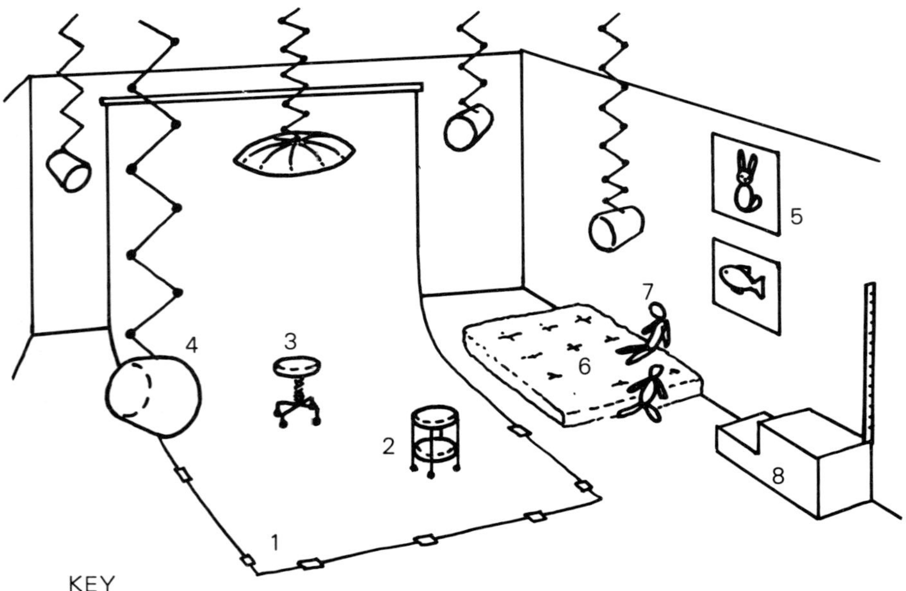


KEY

1 Disposable black background, firmly fixed down
2 Trolley on wheels with ALL necessary equipment
3 Small stool (adjustable for height)
4 Electronic flashes - ceiling mounted
5 Wall pictures to fix child's gaze
6 Floor mattress for babies
7 Assortment of dolls, toys etc to attract attention
8 Stepped box with calibrated height scale

***Figure 10.1*** *The paediatric studio*

choice at other times. If the patient is apprehensive, he can often be photographed whilst sitting on a parent's or nurse's knee. By working in tight close-up, problem backgrounds can be avoided.

The choice between ringflash and point-source flash is one that will be discussed wherever medical photographers gather! One view is that the ringflash is inappropriate for nearly every sort of medical photography, with the exception of very deep cavities (as in photographing a cleft of the soft palate, for example). In all other cases, a small point-source light will provide much better modelling and relief, even in cavities, particularly if used in combination with a mirror.

Ideally all studio lighting should be suspended from the ceiling so that the floor of the studio is a clear as possible; mains cables can easily be tripped over, and can represent a more serious hazard if a patient's young sibling – who may well have accompanied the family to the studio – decides that the cable might be fun to chew at!

Standardization of scale in the photographs can be difficult, due to the change in size of the subject. A 5″ × 7″ print of a newborn baby full length may well require a 20″ × 24″ print to make the full length to the same scale 16 years later!

It is recommended, however, that standard sets of photographs are used, together with a fairly standardized lighting system. In paediatrics more than in any other branch of medicine, it seems, the patients will return to the hospital. A fairly standard approach to the photography of each condition will ensure that, so far as is possible, a series of pictures of each patient taken on different occasions will stand a fair chance of comparability.

In nearly every session, the photographer will want the patient to look away from the camera in a given direction. In order to make the patient look the appropriate way, there should be simple pictures positioned around the studio walls. The use of pictures about 150 mm square, of such subjects as a black-and-white cow, a red chicken, a yellow duck and so on is recommended.

It is easy for the photographer to ask the child simple questions about these pictures, so maintaining the correct posing position (for example, 'can you see a duck over there?', 'What colour is it?', 'Is it still there?').

The very young child will need an audible stimulus or a light stimulus to make him look away from the camera or his parent. Squeaky toys can be useful, as can small torches, but equally effective is a bunch of keys. If such 'attention-getters' are used, care should be taken to keep them out of the picture or to position them in such a way that they can be masked out later.

## 10.4 PAEDIATRIC CONDITIONS

As mentioned above, the very young patient may suffer from any of the diseases described in the specialist sections for adults, but certain conditions are most often seen in the young. Congenital malformations for example, i.e. those present at or before birth regardless of cause, are recorded in the neonatal stage. Disorders of growth and development and the childhood infections, are all photographed.

However, when photographing the salient features of certain diseases, the way in which they present in adult life or in childhood may show a remarkable contrast; the significance of many signs and symptoms can be vastly different at different ages. Many diseases are related to the age of the child, for example:

(1) At birth – Congenital malformations, birth traumas, etc.,
(2) Newborn – Gynaecomastia, haemorrhagic and haemolytic diseases, etc.,
(3) Infancy – Nutritional disorders, spasms, napkin rashes etc.,
(4) School age – Infections, accidents, enuresis etc.,
(5) Puberty – Acne, anorexia, etc.

The student should familiarize himself with the following types of conditions, taking particular care to note the visual appearance.

### *(1) Congenital malformations*

Eg. Down's syndrome, cleft lip and palate, Pierre–Robin syndrome, Klippel–Feil syndrome, club foot, dislocation of the hip, Hurler's syndrome, Hunter–Hurler's syndrome, Fallot's tetralogy. hypospadias, Wilm's tumour, Hutchinson's teeth, Apert's syndrome, Treacher–Collins syndrome, Crouzon's disease, Hirschsprung's disease, Marfan's syndrome, Peutz–Jeghers syndrome, Sprengel's deformity, bat ears, polydactyly, syndactyly, pyloric stenosis and ankyloglossia.

### *(2) Birth injuries*

Eg. facial palsy, brachial plexus palsy, cerebral haemorrhage, forceps marks, compressions and fractures, Erb's palsy.

### *(3) Neonatal pathologies*

Eg. umbilical granuloma, exomphalos, gynaecomastia/mastitis neonatorum, erythema toxicum neonatorum, premature twins, etc.

***(4) Disturbances of growth and metabolism***

Dwarfism, diabetic embryopathy and fetopathy, hypopituitarism, hypothyroidism, goitre, Turner's syndrome, genu valgum, genu varum, cystic fibrosis, coeliac disease, scoliosis, kyphosis, lordosis, osteogenesis imperfecta, adrenogenital syndrome, rickets.

***(5) Dermatoses***

Congenital ichthyosis, Henoch – Schönlein purpura, eczema, haemangioma, urticaria, etc.

***(6) Disorders of the nervous system***

Eg. spina bifida, meningitis, encephalitis, hydrocephalus, spastic hemiplegia, ataxia, athetosis, meningocele, meningomyelocele, microcephaly, encephalocele.

***(7) Infections/infestations***

Eg. scabies, tonsillitis, varicella, epidemic parotitis, tinea, pertusis, etc.

## 10.5 TRANSILLUMINATION OF THE INFANT SKULL

The skull of the young infant is relatively transparent to light and transillumination has been used for many years to visualize gross lesions such as hydrocephalus and hydranencephaly. Whilst new techniques such as computerized axial tomography have certainly improved the recording of such conditions, there is still a place for photographic transillumination, especially where such sophisticated diagnostic imaging facilities are unavailable. Two types of illumination may be distinguished: (1) axial and (2) angular. Axial illumination as its name implies, is carried out with the light source, the patient's head and the camera lying on the same axis, i.e. in a straight line. 'Superficial' lesions cannot be seen, since they will be illuminated only on the blind side of the head from the camera viewpoint. In the case of angular transillumination, however, the camera–patient axis is at an angle to the patient–light source axis. It has been found most effective to use the light source either at the anterior fontanelle or posteriorly at approximately the occipital fontanelle. The occipital fontanelle closes at a few months but the anterior fontanelle remains open to about 18 months. So long as these fontanelles are open and the transilluminating source is placed over them, it has less solid tissue to traverse and consequently more light is available. A further advantage of placing the light at the fontanelles and viewing at an angle is that the light only has to pass through one cerebral hemisphere. Some workers have used very powerful electronic flashguns (300 joules) whilst others have used condenser lenses to focus the light from less powerful flashguns. The use of condenser lenses also helps to sharpen the shadows obtained. Even with good illumination the amount of light available to expose the film is small and exposures are typically in the range f/2.8 – f/5.6 with 200 ASA film.

## 10.6 CONCLUSION

It is possible to carry out nearly all types of medical photography on children of all ages. At one London paediatric hospital even retinal fluorescein angiography is routinely carried out on children as young as 4 years old and techniques have been evolved to provide the medical staff with this test on babies and younger children.

As has been stressed above, it is not what you are doing to a child that will distress him – it is the way you do it. Time, care and respect for your patient will allow you to build up the necessary relationship. With it anything is possible. Without it, nothing.

## References

Allen, G. (1978). Paediatric photography in comparison to adult patient photography. *J. Biol. Photogr. Assoc.*, **46**, 57-67

Dynski-Klein, M. (1975). *A Colour Atlas of Paediatrics*. (London: Wolfe Medical Publications)

Ford, R. (1974). Infrared photography of trans-illuminated infant skulls. *J. Biol. Photogr. Assoc.*, **42**, 94-102

Johns, M. (1979). Retinal photography and angiography of children and babies. *Br. J. Photogr.*, **126**, 889-891

Johns, M. (1979), Transillumination of the infant skull. *J. Audiovis. Media Med.*, **2**, 140-149

Jolly, (1981). *Diseases of Children*. (Oxford and Edinburgh: Blackwell Scientific Publications)

Martin, D. (1961). Some facies in the diseases of childhood. *Med. Biol. Illustr.*, **11**, 76-84

Moll, H. (1976). *Atlas of Paediatric Diseases*. (Philadelphia: W.B. Saunders)

Rogers, G. (1976). Paediatric photography. In Newman, A. (ed.). *Photographic Techniques for Scientific Research*. Vol. 2, (London: Academic Press)

Shurtleff, D. (1964). Transillumination of skull in infants and children. *Am. J. Dis. Childr.*, **107**, 14-19

Vaughan, V. (ed.). (1975). *Nelson's Texbook of Paediatrics* (Philadelphia: W.B. Saunders)

## *Practical projects*

(1) Really study the conditions listed in Section 10.4 and make notes on what you would photograph if asked to record patients with those diagnoses.

(2) Choose any paediatric condition with which you are familiar and produce a series of photographs in a medium of your choice to demonstrate clearly the features of this condition.

(3) Produce a series of at least three black-and-white prints of exhibition quality to show characteristic facies of childhood diseases, e.g. Down's syndrome. Mount the photographs suitably for display along with a short description of each condition.

(4) Produce a series of 35 mm colour transparencies to demonstrate the features of a case of cleft lip and palate (a) before reparative surgery, (b) after surgery. Make notes on the technique used and any difficulties you encountered.

(5) Photograph any orthopaedic malformation in a young infant, such as talipes equinovarus; and produce a series of photographs suitable for inclusion in the patient's notes.

(6) Produce a colour transparency (in vertical format) suitable for publication on the front cover of a brochure describing careers in paediatric nursing. The photograph should show a nurse in uniform and a young patient and attempt to capture the rewards of working with young children. Submit the transparency and also an exhibition quality print from the transparency.

### *Examination questions*

Q.1 Describe fully the photographs you would take to illustrate the following conditions:
(*a*) Hypospadias
(*b*) Down's syndrome
(*c*) Hurler's syndrome
(*d*) Pyloric stenosis.

Q.2 Discuss the difficulties which you might encounter when photographing very young patients and the technique that you would adopt to overcome them.

Q.3 Describe with the aid of diagrams the lighting arrangement you would choose for recording full length pictures of infants (*a*) in the studio (*b*) in the ward.

Q.4 Write a description of the technique you would use for transillumination photographs of the infant skull.

Q.5 What is a syndrome? Describe the features of the following syndromes:
(*a*) Pierre–Robin
(*b*) Klippel–Feil
(*c*) Apert's
(*d*) Treacher–Collins
(*e*) Marfans,
(*f*) Peutz–Jegher's.

Q.6 Describe the equipment and technique you would use to record a case of meningomyelocele which is being barrier-nursed in an incubator.

Q.7 You are asked by your paediatric department to photograph ten pairs of twins, four times a year, from age 2 to age 16 for a research project on child growth. Full length anterior, lateral and posterior photographs will be required to measure from. Discuss fully the factors you would consider when preparing for such a project and describe the technique you would adopt.

Q.8 Describe the equipment and methods you would use to record babies with cleft lip and palate. What is the value of such records?

*Multiple choice questions (any of the statements may be true or false).*

Q.9 The following may be congenital:
(*a*) Poliomyelitis
(*b*) Cataracts
(*c*) Ankyloglossia
(*d*) Pyloric stenosis
(*e*) Variola.

Q.10 A photograph of the face would be particularly beneficial in recording:
(*a*) Exomphalos
(*b*) Sprengel's deformity
(*c*) Trisomy 21
(*d*) Hurler's syndrome
(*e*) Erb's paralysis.

# Section 11
# Photography in plastic surgery

**A.R. Williams**, MPhil, FBIPP, FRPS, FBPA, AIMBI
Head of Medical Illustration and Teaching Services
Charing Cross Hospital and Medical School, London

## 11.1 INTRODUCTION

Plastic or reconstructive surgery is the removal, addition, replacement or manipulation of tissue in order to repair, restore or enhance appearance and/or function. Photography is used for records of the surgical stages, which may be of great number occurring over a period of many years; for teaching and publication purposes; for research; for medico-legal purposes (a) on behalf of patients, where evidence of original injury and subsequent treatment can help substantiate a claim for insurance or compensation, or (b) on behalf of the surgeon, in a case of litigation where the patient is not satisfied with the outcome of his treatment; for boosting morale by encouraging a patient by showing him a first and last photograph of a comparable case or to encourage him during protracted treatment by showing photographs illustrating progress already achieved.

The general anatomical scope of photography for plastic surgery includes those parts of the body which are visible including the palate, the nasal septum and the interior walls of the nose. There is a certain amount of overlap with other surgical specialities such as oral surgery, neurosurgery, orthopaedics and paediatrics.

Plastic surgery is carried out in the following circumstances:

(1) Congenital abnormalities where function and/or appearance is impaired by:
   (a) Total or partial absence (agenesis) of a limb or external organ.
   (b) Excess tissue, such as supernumerary digit, hypertrophy and embryonic remains (naevi).
   (c) Malformation.

(2) Traumatic injuries caused through industrial, traffic and domestic accidents and war. Function and/or appearance is impaired by lacerations, fractures or amputation.

(3) Burns and scalds destroy deeper tissues by flame, hot liquids, chemicals, electricity or radiation. Scarring and contracture during healing may be involved.

(4) Diseases which impair appearance and/or function, or are malignant. (rodent ulcer, lupus vulgaris, Dupuytren's contracture).

(5) Cosmetic treatment to improve appearance. This applies to a certain extent to all the above categories. The term 'cosmetic surgery' usually applies to treatment of patients whose appearance causes them mental suffering (neurosis). Examples include hypertrophy of breasts – mammaplasty; abnormal nose–rhinoplasty; skin blemishes such as keloids, pock marks and slack skin.

## 11.2 ANATOMY AND PHYSIOLOGY

In this field the photographer must familiarize himself with the various anatomical and technical terms which may be found in a textbook on plastic surgery. This will include the various types of operation and methods used. Basically there are only five types of skin graft:

(1) The free graft in which a piece of skin is completely detached from the donor site and embedded on a prepared base of healthy granulation tissue elsewhere in the body. These are subclassified as:
   (a) Split skin (Thiersch, Ollier) where a dermatome or Humby knife is used to excise just the epidermis and part of the dermis, from thigh, arm, abdominal wall, etc.

(b) Full thickness (Wolfe, Krause) where a free excision is made of epidermis and dermis from the back of the pinna, mastoid area or abdominal wall.

(c) Pinch graft, where 1 centimetre discs are excised from upper thigh or arm consisting of epidermis at the edges, with dermis and subcutaneous fat at the centre.

(2) The pedicle graft in which a larger and thicker piece of skin is detached at one end and reattached to a new site. The tissue gains a new blood supply through the transplanted end, and gradually the connection at the donor site is detached. These are again subclassified as:

(a) Flaps, for multiple stage: cross legs at the calf, abdominal wall for hand or forearm.

(b) Tubes, for multiple stage: chest for arm or neck, forehead for face, abdominal wall to forearm, thence to neck and forehead, and finally to nose or face.

All pedicle grafts consist of epidermis, dermis, subcutaneous fat and blood vessels.

The student should also be aware that cartilage and bone grafts are also used in reconstructive surgery. Bone is taken from the crest of the ilium, cartilage is obtained from the front portion of the ribs.

## 11.3 THE PATIENT

In the initial stages the patient may be in considerable pain and unable to move around due to his graft and supporting bandages. In these cases photography will have to be done in the ward and at times when dressings are being changed. Barrier nursing may be in effect on the wards in cases of burns. The patient undergoing cosmetic surgery will usually be particularly anxious about their appearance at all stages of surgery and may ask for the photographer's opinion of changes since the last photographs were taken – never venture to give it. Be encouraging in an unspecific way especially, for example, to parents of a child with cleft lip and palate deformity.

## 11.4 PHOTOGRAPHY – GENERAL TECHNIQUE

Plastic surgeons themselves have frequently commented on the need to standardize all parameters in photography of their patients. Too low a viewpoint before rhinoplasty and too high after will make it appear that the surgeon has slimmed the nose and tucked the nostrils underneath – whereas in fact he may have done nothing of the sort. Strong toplight may make breasts appear large and pendulous whereas softlight angled upwards will make them appear firm and smaller. It has been said that much cosmetic surgery can be performed by lighting alone! The production of comparable and accurate serial records demands meticulous attention to standardization of all the factors.

### *(1) Views*

Views for any particular condition must be established in consultation with the surgeon with a mind to the treatment likely to follow, which varies from patient to patient. Viewpoints must be chosen to minimize perspective distortions (see Section 22.1.2).

### *(2) Scale*

The scale of reproduction must be constant for any given area both at the negative and printing stage. The 'Westminster' reproduction ratios are recommended.

### *(3) Positioning*

Positioning must be exactly the same each time for both patient and camera. Record standard views first and unorthodox views to further illustrate the condition if necessary. Include enough surrounding area for an anatomical identification and to allow recording of subsequent surgical steps e.g. flap formation.

***(4) Lighting***

The lighting must also be in the same position each time. It is most important that the same type of lamp, i.e. directional or diffuse, is used in the same way. If a directional beam shows the lesion well before surgery then use it, but the subject area should be lit in exactly the same manner on follow-up although the lesion itself may have been removed or reduced. Otherwise photographic comparison is impossible – absolute professional integrity is required in lighting pre and post-operatively.

***(5) Backgrounds***

The background should provide a clear outline and must be a constant colour or tone throughout a series of photographs. Colour photography demands a background of a contrasting colour to the subject. It is surprising how much influence background colour exerts over the subjective impression of scars for example.

***(6) Clothing***

As a rule clothing should never appear in clinical photographs – all jewellery, watches, etc., should be removed. The same applies to make-up where the patient may be obscuring facial scars. The only possible exception is at the end of a course of plastic surgery when the surgeon may wish to demonstrate the satisfactory appearance of the patient when clothed; e.g. scar lines may be deliberately placed beneath clothing or under a wig. The same is true of prostheses and implants – it will be necessary to photograph the patient with and without these appliances.

## 11.5 ULTRAVIOLET PHOTOGRAPHY

Direct ultraviolet recording may be used to enhance the image obtained of scar tissue, e.g. keloid scars (*see Section 19 for technique*), but a control panchromatic record must always accompany such a picture.

Fluorescence techniques are used in plastic surgery to examine the blood supply, particularly to pedicle flaps. Sodium fluorescein is injected into an appropriate vessel and blue light from a suitably filtered electronic flash source excites the green fluorescence which is recorded on colour film. When photographing exposed tissues in this way it is important to avoid ultraviolet burns. The Kodak Wratten filter number 47A has been especially designed to provide efficient excitation of sodium fluorescein, but it does transmit some long-wave ultraviolet radiation and this needs to be absorbed by a Kodak Wratten 2B ultraviolet absorbing filter. The excitation filters are placed over the light source; whilst the camera requires a 2E or 2B filter over the lens (it is usually helpful to include some pale yellow and cyan filters to reduce the blue cast and eliminate any red light leaked by the excitation filter). Various workers have described this technique and its application to plastic surgery.

### References


Barron, J. and Saad, M. (eds.). (1980). *Operative Plastic and Reconstructive Surgery.* (In 3 volumes) (Edinburgh: Churchill Livingstone)

Chapple, J. and Stephenson, K. (1970). Photographic misrepresentation. *Plast. Reconstr. Surg.*, **45**, 135-137

Davidson, T. (1979). Photography in facial plastic and reconstructive surgery. *J. Biol. Photogr.*, **47**, 59–67

Davidson, T., Hoffman, H. and Webster, R. (1980). Photographic interpretation of facial plastic and reconstructive surgery. *J. Biol. Photogr.*, **48**, 87-92

Dickason, W. and Hanna, D. (1976). Pitfalls of comparative photography in plastic and reconstructive surgery. *Plast. Reconstr. Surg.*, **58**, 166-171

Erol, O., *et al.* (1981). An improved method for fluorescein dye photography. *Plast. Reconstr. Surg.*, **68**, 120-121

Jemec, B. and Jemec, G. (1981). Suggestions for standardized clinical photography in plastic surgery. *J. Audiovis. Media Med.*, **4**, 99-102

Krugman, M. (1981). Photoanalysis of the rhinoplasty patient. *Ear, Nose, Throat J.*, **60**, 328-330

Krugman, M. *et al* (1979). Facial series of photographs as viewed by the plastic surgeon with special emphasis on the nose. *J. Biol. Photogr.*, **47**, 201-203

McDowell, F. (1976). On the necessity of precision photographic documentation in plastic surgery. *Plast. Reconstr. Surg.*, **58**, 214-218

Morello, D., *et al.* (1977). Making uniform photographic records in plastic surgery. *Plast. Reconstr. Surg.*, **59**, 366-358

Welsh, J. (1982). The photography of fluorescein. *Plast. Reconstr. Surg.*, **69**, 990-994

## *Practical projects*

(1) Borrow a good textbook on plastic surgery such as Barron and Saad (1980) and make short notes on the most common grafts and operative procedures such as blepharoplasty, canthoplasty, cranioplasty, dermabrasion, Kapetansky repair, Le Fort operations, lipectomy, mammaplasty, microsurgery, osteotomy, pharyngoplasty, reconstructions, W-plasty, Z-plasty.

(2) Photograph in black-and-white an area of skin at a magnification of 1:4 on the negative preferably with some fine scar detail.
(*a*) At the correct exposure,
(*b*) One stop underexposure, and
(*c*) Two stops overexposure.
Produce a set of matching prints at life-size and make notes on the effect of exposure on fine skin detail.

(3) (*a*) Photograph a head and shoulder view (anterior and both laterals) and a hand (palmar, dorsal, radial and ulnar views) in colour, and produce a set of matching colour prints suitable for issue to a jury in a court of law.
(*b*) Some weeks later repeat the views without referring to the prints prepared at the time.
(*c*) Compare the results and make notes on any differences between the two sets, or difficulties which you encounter.

(4) Produce a series of three matched black-and-white prints of the female chest and abdomen in anterior aspect with:
(*a*) 45° copy lighting,
(*b*) Strong top lighting, and
(*c*) Strong side lighting.
Make notes on your results.

(5) In a medium of your choice photograph a face anteriorly at a magnification of 1:8 (on 35 mm)
(*a*) With the camera level with the lower orbital margin,
(*b*) With the camera level with the lips, and
(*c*) With the camera level with the eyebrows
Note the spectacular changes in nose shape on the finished photographs induced by these small changes in viewpoint.

(6) Produce a series of colour transparencies of any plastic surgery operation.

### ***Examination questions***

Q.1 It has been said that much plastic surgery can be accomplished with just clever lighting. Discuss this statement fully.

Q.2 Describe fully the applications of ultraviolet photography to plastic surgery.

Q.3 Describe briefly the following conditions and the photographs you would take to illustrate them effectively:
(*a*) Bat ears,
(*b*) Blepharochalasis,
(*c*) Dupuytren's contracture,
(*d*) Keloid scars,
(*e*) Microstomia, and
(*f*) Nasal septal defect.

Q.4 Describe the views you would take, and what special measures you would employ to ensure standardization of results, pre-and post-breast augmentation surgery.

Q.5 Discuss the uses of photography in plastic surgery illustrating your answer with specific applications.

Q.6 Standardization is the cornerstone of all plastic surgery photography; discuss the factors you would consider in attempting to achieve highly accurate and repeatable photographs.

Q.7 'Clothing should always be removed in clinical photography' – discuss this statement in the context of plastic surgery.

Q.8 Describe the principal types of skin graft and the use of photography in assessing flap viability.

*Multiple choice questions (any of the statements may be true or false)*

Q.9 In the photography of patients undergoing treatment by plastic surgery:
(*a*) The patient should remove dentures for intra-oral photography.
(*b*) The main use of photography is for medico–legal purposes.
(*c*) They should always remove clothing prior to photography.
(*d*) In cleft palate cases the ulna head must be shown.
(*e*) The patient should sometimes be shown photographs of similar cases to encourage confidence.

Q.10 The following conditions may be corrected by plastic surgery:
(*a*) Micrognathia,
(*b*) Mastocytogenesis,
(*c*) Achondroplasia,
(*d*) Ulerythema,
(*e*) Lipomatosis.

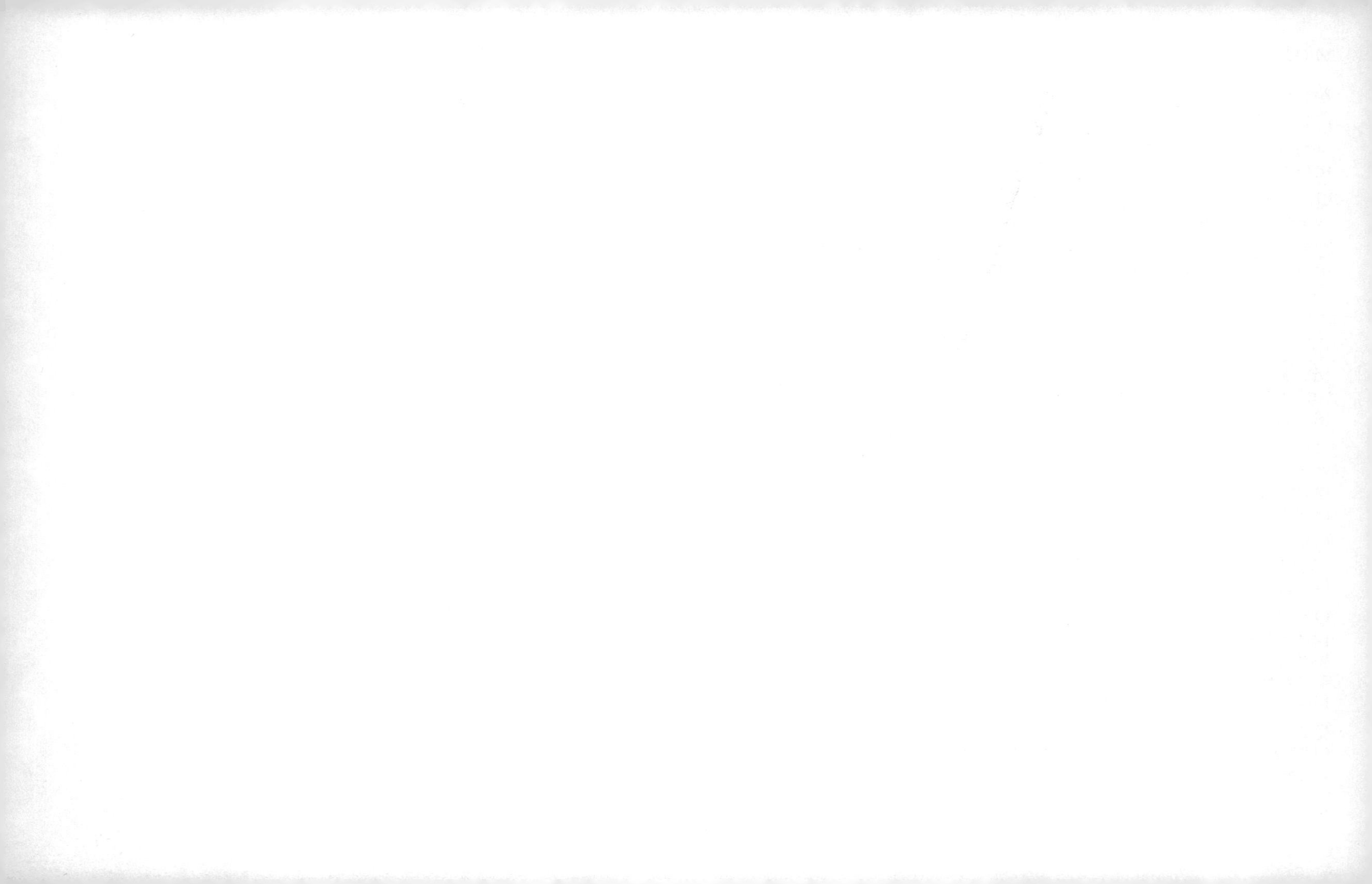

# Section 12
# Photography in genito-urinary medicine and gynaecology

**A.R. Williams**, MPhil, FBIPP, FRPS, FBPA, AIMBI
Head of Medical Illustration and Teaching Services
Charing Cross Hospital and Medical School, London

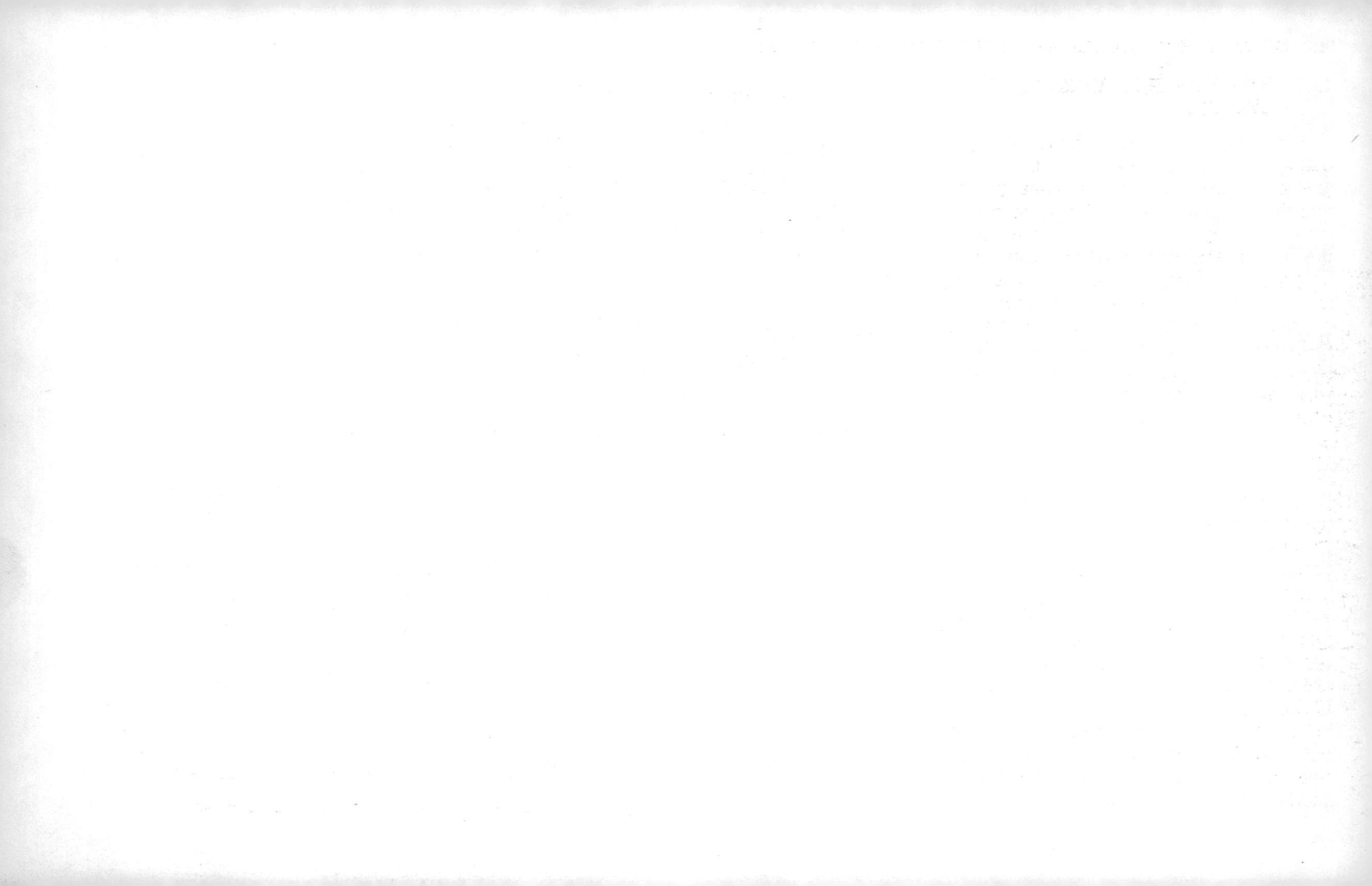

## 12.1 THE FEMALE REPRODUCTIVE SYSTEM

Gynaecological photography is the application of orthodox methods to the photography of the external genitalia (vulva) and the application of cavity photography for recording diseases and conditions of the vagina and cervix uteri. True endoscopic techniques may also be involved, as in culdoscopy where a straight rod endoscope similar to a cystoscope is inserted into the pelvic cavity through the vagina. Photography of the internal reproductive organs may also be required during surgery.

### 12.1.1 Anatomy

It is essential that the photographer is completely familiar with the anatomy and physiology of the female reproductive system – including the physiology of menstruation and pregnancy. The external genitalia consist of the labia majora, mons pubis, clitoris, labia minora, vestibule, hymen, vaginal and urethral orifices and fourchette. The intra-abdominal organs are the ovaries, Fallopian or uterine tubes, and uterus. Their detailed structure, function, position and relationship to other abdominal organs should be clearly understood.

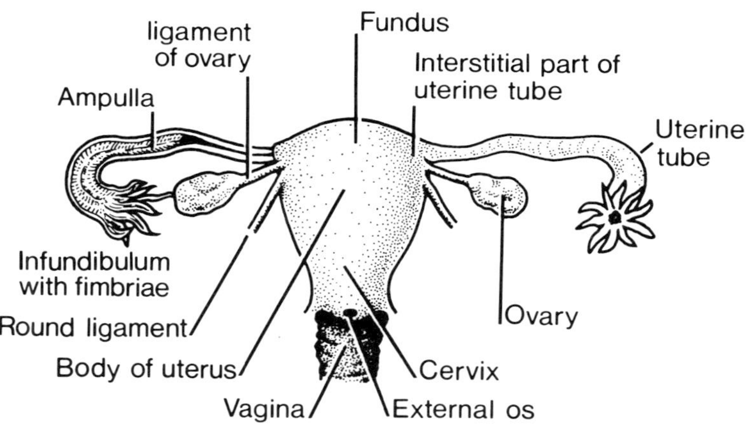


**Figure 12.1** *The intra-abdominal female reproductive organs*

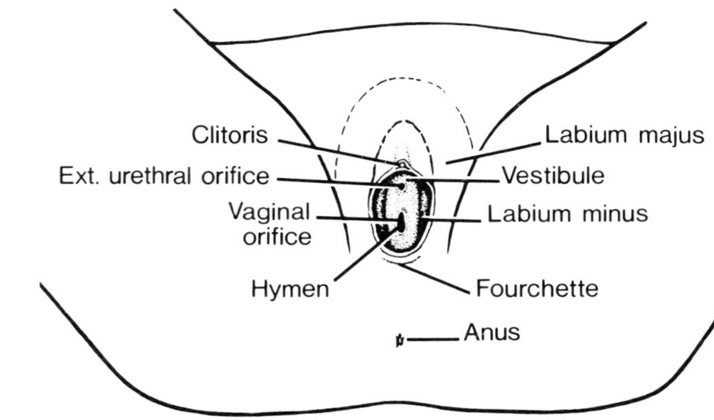


**Figure 12.2** *The female external genitalia*

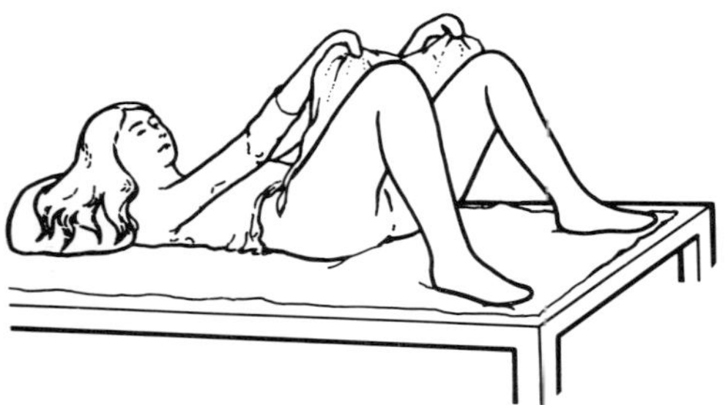

***Figure 12.3*** *The semi-lithotomy position*

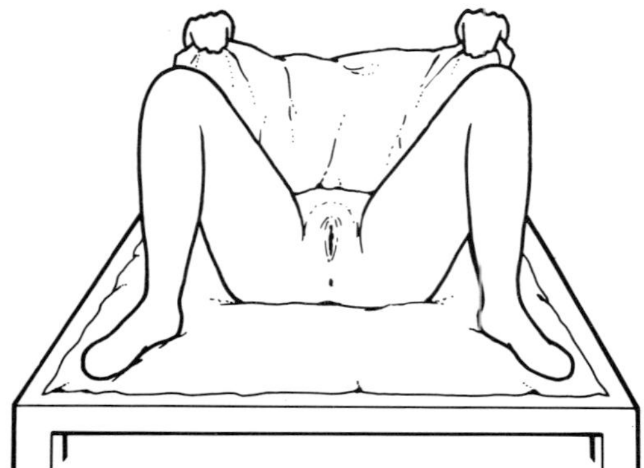

***Figure 12.4*** *A pillow used as a simple background*

### 12.1.2 The patient

Tact and understanding of the patient's natural embarrassment at this type of photography are essential. Detached efficiency is the key to success. If a female photographer is not available, male photographers must always have a chaperone present. Such a person can be either a nurse or female assistant but never a female relative of the patient. (This need not apply in the case of the mother of a female child, but discretion should be used in each individual case.) If no chaperone is available photography should not be undertaken until one can be provided. This is simply to protect the photographer – you have no record of the patient's psychiatric history. The patient should be allowed to undress in privacy and need remove clothing up to the waist only. A clean dressing gown must be provided. Good hygiene is essential – particularly when dealing with cases of venereal disease.

### 12.1.3 Photography of the vulva

The patient should lie on a couch in the semi-lithotomy position, i.e. on the back with thighs and legs flexed and abducted but with the heels flat on the couch. The buttocks should rest on a disposable white background. If the lesion to be photographed extends to the mons pubis, a background such as a pillow or sheet of card may be required and can be held by the patient. Should it be necessary to separate the labia majora in order to demonstrate the lesion more effectively, surgical examination gloves must always be worn. (It is usually best to allow the patient to do this herself.) Sometimes vulval lesions will extend into the vagina in which case it will be necessary to insert a speculum to demonstrate the lesion more clearly, this must be done by a doctor.

The routine view, taken to scale, should include the whole of the vulval area; close-ups of particular lesions may also be required. The whole procedure should be carried out as rapidly and discreetly as possible. If it is known that the patient has to be operated on in the near future, it is often preferable to take the photographs while the patient is under a general anaesthetic.

### 12.1.4 Photography of the vagina and cervix

This is usually carried out in the gynaecological clinic, the ward or the operating theatre. The patient will normally be in one of the standard positions – such as

Sims', knee–elbow or lithotomy. The gynaecologist will insert specula to demonstrate the lesion required and photography according to the principles of cavity photography is carried out (*Section 20*). A black anodized speculum is best for this type of photography. Many clinics are equipped with a colposcope, which is a binocular microscope especially designed for the examination of the cervix uteri. These often have a camera attachment, with built-in electronic flash.

### 12.1.5 Some diseases and conditions

The more common conditions which you may have to photograph are contained in the following list:

Carcinoma of the vulva, vagina or cervix; congenital abnormalities of the genitalia; syphilitic chancre; cervical erosion, Bartholin's cysts; haemangioma; haematoma; leukoplakia; uterine prolapse; moniliasis or thrush; vulvitis; vaginitis and vulval warts.

Sometimes a prolapse of the cervix cannot easily be seen and it will be necessary for the doctor to insert a speculum to demonstrate the condition clearly. It may be necessary to ask the patient to 'produce' the prolapse. This occurs when the patient 'bears down', i.e. contracts her abdominal muscles and pushes down, thereby presenting the prolapse *per vagina*.

## 12.2 THE MALE REPRODUCTIVE SYSTEM

Standard photographic methods are applied to the photography of the male external genitalia. Photographs of the internal reproductive organs may be required during a surgical operation or as pathological specimens.

### 12.2.1 Anatomy

The position and functions of the internal organs, the testes, the prostate, the seminal vessels and the ejaculatory ducts must be understood, and also their relationship to the adjacent structures of the bladder, urethra and perineum. The external organs are the penis and scrotum. The end of the penis is enlarged to form the glans penis which is covered by a fold of skin, the prepuce. (Circumcision is the excision of this fold of skin).

### 12.2.2 The patient

Though the choice of photographer and the need for a chaperone is not so important as in gynaecological photography, it is kinder to the patient and will be appreciated by the female members of staff if a male colleague undertakes the case. Patients with venereal diseases

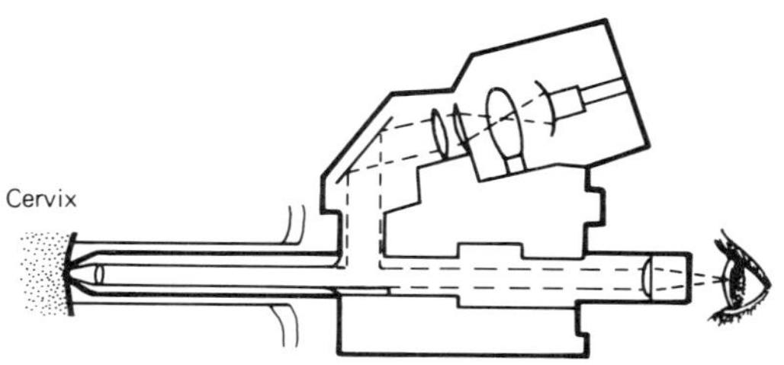


**Figure 12.5** The colpomicroscope

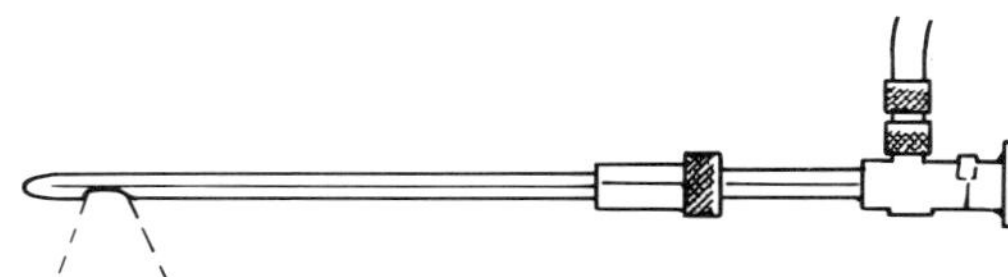

***Figure 12.6*** *A culdoscope*

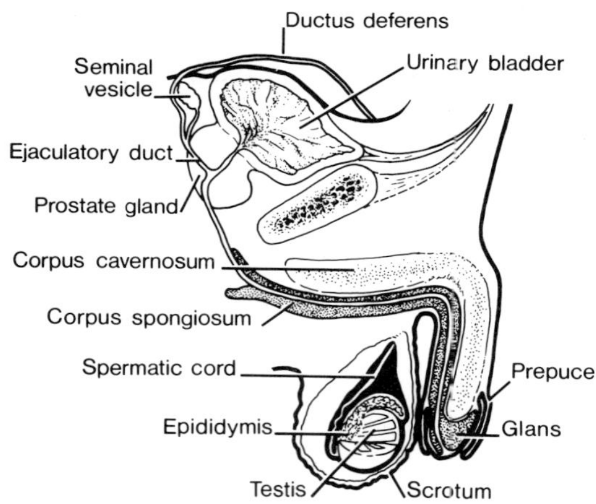


***Figure 12.7*** *The male genitalia*

must be handled with particular care as regards risk of infection. Although it is essential that the photographer is thoroughly familiar with the correct anatomical nomenclature it should be appreciated that the uneducated patient may not understand this terminology.

### 12.2.3 Photography of the external genitalia

Views of the penis and scrotum can be taken with the patient standing, if of course, he is able to do so. Close-up views are best obtained with the patient lying on a low couch. Clothing should never be allowed to appear in the picture area.

Close-up views will usually require the penis to be held so that the lesion can be clearly demonstrated. This is best done by the patient himself or by an assistant – disposable gloves should always be worn. Retraction of the prepuce may be necessary to show the glans properly. When photographing the scrotum, the penis should be held out of the way in order to obtain a suitable picture.

### 12.2.4 Some diseases and conditions

Skin diseases, including the venereal diseases, will form the bulk of cases referred for photography of the external male genitalia (*Section 6*).

When requested to photograph the genitalia of patients with endocrine disorders, it is important that the photograph shows the degree of development in relation to the whole patient, his age, height and other bodily characteristics. Full-length and close-up views will be necessary.

Undescended testicles, hydrocoele, spermatocoele and epididymal cysts can all be successfully demonstrated by using a low power electronic flashgun to transilluminate the scrotum. Conventional views must also be taken as a control.

Other conditions frequently photographed are: orchitis, seminoma, teratoma and hernia. The most common site for a hernia is in the inguinal region. They may be congenital or caused by excessive strain. In some instances it may be necessary to ask the patient to cough to 'bring down' the hernia. Most inguinal hernias disappear when the patient is asked to lie down so bear this in mind.

## 12.3 THE URINARY TRACT

Photography of the urinary tract is mainly confined to views of the kidneys, ureters, bladder and urethra during operative surgery; to endoscopic views of the bladder; and to that portion of the urethra which is visible externally.

### 12.3.1 Anatomy

The student should be familiar with the size and shape, position and function of the kidneys, ureter, bladder and urethra. It is also important that the student should be able to orientate a single kidney (fixed or fresh) in correct anatomical position for photography. (Remember the right kidney is lower, and that the ureters curve downwards.) The external meatus of the female urethra is situated centrally between the folds of the labia minora, anterior to the vaginal orifice. The external meatus of the male urethra is situated centrally at the end of the glans penis.

### 12.3.2 Some diseases and conditions

Hypospadias and epispadias are congenital conditions where the opening of the urethra is formed at some place other than the tip of the penis. A photograph taken during micturition will usually demonstrate this abnormality but in practice this is very difficult to arrange. In order to show an abnormally placed orifice, a probe may need to be inserted by the doctor – this is generally more satisfactory.

The photographer should be familiar with the visual appearance of the commonest renal pathologies such as nephritis, polycystic kidneys, and arterial occlusions. (*see Section 15 for technique*).

## References

Beischer, N. and Mackay, E. (1981). *Colour Atlas of Gynaecology*. (Philadelphia: W.B. Saunders)

Conn, R. *et al.* (1975). A simple inexpensive technique for cystoscopic photography. *J. Urol.*, **114**, 927-928

Kleidon, D. and Singh, K. (1982). Photography through the hysteroscope. *J. Biol. Photogr.*, **50**, 5-6

Lloyd-Davies, R. (1983). *A Colour Atlas of Urology*. (London: Wolfe Medical Publications)

Phillips, J. (1977). Increased mobility with an articulated lens in gynaecological endoscopic photography. *Med. Instrum.*, **11**, 13-16

Stafl, A. (1981). Cervicography – a new approach to cervical cancer detection. *Gynecol. Oncol.*, **12**, 292-301

Tindall, V. (1981). *A Colour Atlas of Clinical Gynaecology*. (London: Wolfe Medical Publications)

Warner, E. and Kleidon, D. (1980). Increasing size in laparoscopic photography. *J. Biol. Photogr.*, **48**, 27-29

Wolnik, L. (1980). Colpophotography with a large format camera. *Am. J. Obstet. Gynecol.*, **137**, 141-143

## *Practical projects*

(1) Make yourself three cylinders of black paper and three of polished aluminium foil (approx. 3 cm in diameter and 3,7,11 cm long). Produce a series of colour photographs of moist skin through these various tubes using (*a*) a single point source of light and (*b*) a ring-flash. Make notes on your results especially in terms of exposure, illumination evenness, flare, etc.

(2) Go to the gynaecology department, explain your course of study and ask if you might be shown:
(*a*) The different vaginal specula, e.g. Simm's, Duck-bill, etc.
(*b*) The culdoscope in action.
(*c*) The colposcope in action.
When observing (*b*) and (*c*) take special note of the internal anatomy and the visual appearance of the disease demonstrated to you.

(3) Look up the references cited and learn the construction of the culdoscope and colposcope. Also read the section on cavity illumination and endoscopy (*Section 20*) and note the relevance to GU and gynaecological photography.

(4) Obtain a good illustrated atlas (e.g. Wolfe) and study the visual appearance of cervical, vaginal and bladder diseases. Make notes as necessary.

## *Examination questions*

Q.1 What considerations are important when photographing:
(*a*) Penile chancre,
(*b*) Vulval warts, and
(*c*) Cervical erosion.

Q.2 Describe the photographic technique and patient handling factors involved in photographing carcinoma of the cervix.

Q.3 Discuss the use of chaperones in medical photography.

Q.4 Write brief notes on the following:
(*a*) Bartholin's cyst,
(*b*) Gonorrhoea,
(*c*) Episiotomy,
(*d*) Priapism,
(*e*) NSU, and
(*f*) WR.

Q.5 Discuss the relative merits of a photo-colposcope versus the Kowa portable fundus camera for photographing lesions of the vagina.

Q.6 Discuss photography of the cervix uteri under the following headings:
(*a*) Care of the patient,
(*b*) Lighting, and
(*c*) Optics.

Q.7 Draw an annotated mid-sagittal section through the female reproductive system. Write brief notes on the principal considerations in gynaecological photography.

Q.8 Describe the photographs you would take and any special precautions necessary for:
(*a*) Balanitis,
(*b*) Spirochaetal condylomata,
(*c*) A prolapsed uterus,
(*d*) An inguinal hernia, and
(*e*) Phimosis.

*Multiple choice questions (any of the statements may be true or false)*

Q.9 Special precautions should be taken to avoid infective dangers in photographing these conditions:
(*a*) Spirochaetal condylomata,
(*b*) A gumma,
(*c*) A primary chancre,
(*d*) Vulval leukoplakia,
(*e*) Balanitis circinata.

Q.10 In gynaecological photography:
(*a*) The colposcope is used for laparoscopic examination of the ovaries.
(*b*) The culdoscope is used to photograph the cervix *per vagina*.
(*c*) Black lined specula are preferable to polished chrome.
(*d*) Simms' position is often used.
(*e*) The semi-lithotomy position is best used for photographing the vulva.

# Section 13
# Photography in neurology and psychiatry

**A.R. Williams**, MPhil, FBIPP, FRPS, FBPA, AIMBI
Head of Medical Illustration and Teaching Services
Charing Cross Hospital and Medical School, London

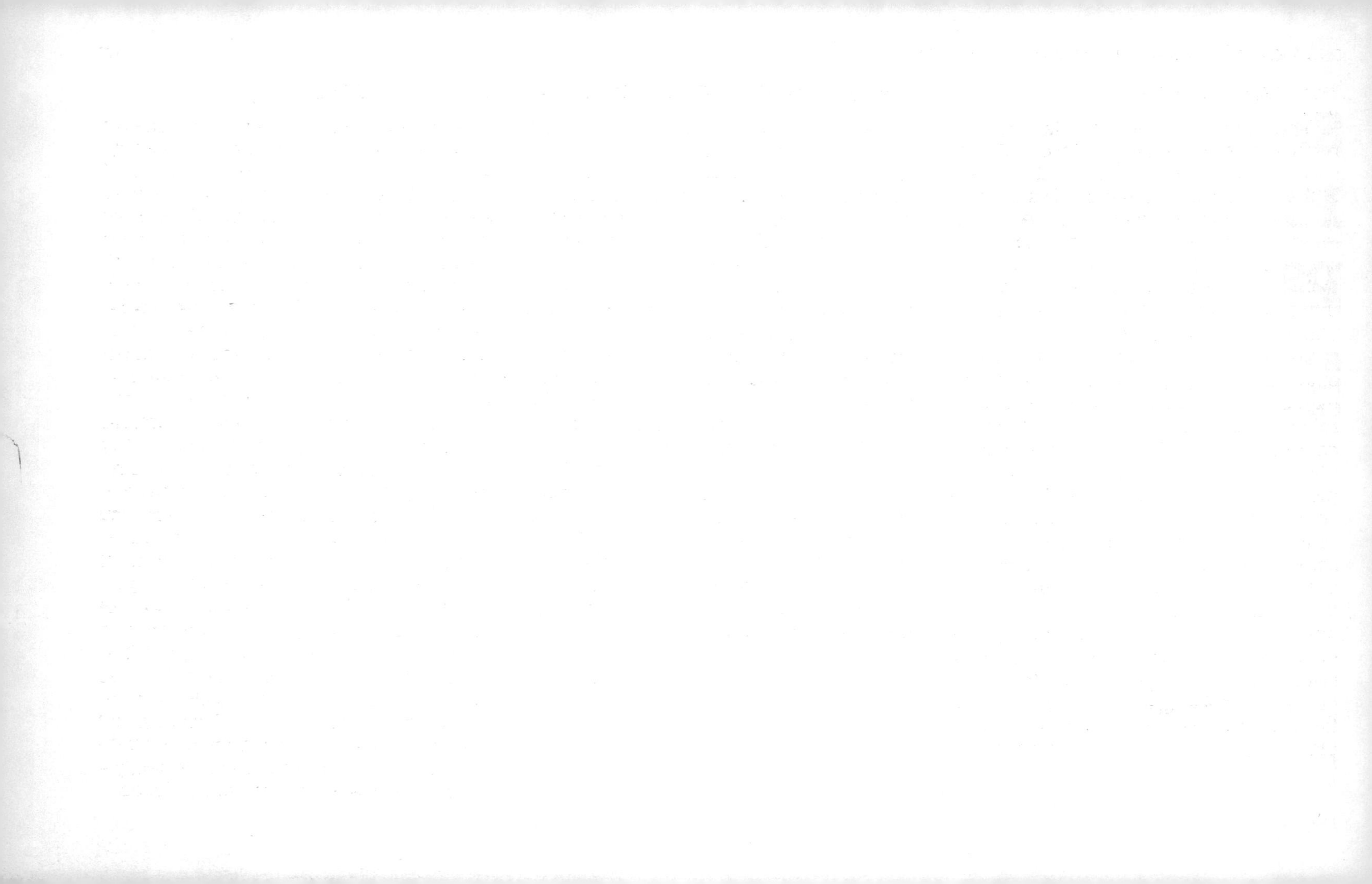

## 13.1 INTRODUCTION

Photography plays an important role in recording the visible evidence of diseases of the nervous system and diseases of the mind. Most often there is a need to record movement, so cine and television techniques are required, but sometimes a single picture or short series of pictures will demonstrate and describe the condition effectively. Photographic prints placed in the case notes are an invaluable aid where the treatment invariably extends over long periods. Deformities may be caused by a whole range of neurological conditions such as meningocoeles, atrophy of muscles due to peripheral nerve lesions, poliomyelitis, paraplegia, etc. and the majority of these are adequately recorded by still photography. As a general rule psychiatrists seldom request still photographs of their patients but occasionally they are of value for monitoring progress, e.g. anorexia nervosa or for use in teaching, e.g. the characteristic posture of a manic depressive. It should be remembered that some of the earliest medical photography was taken in the fields of neurology and psychiatry by Duchenne and Hugh Diamond.

## 13.2 ANATOMY AND PHYSIOLOGY

It is essential that the student is familiar with the general design of the nervous system and its division into the central nervous system and peripheral nervous system and its division into the central sympathetic and parasympathetic nerve pathways. He should understand the structure and function of nerve cells, be able to describe monosynaptic reflex arcs and the chemical/electrical transmission of nerve impulses along neurones and across synapses. The relationship between muscles and nerves and the concept of muscle tone should be learnt. The location and function of the major nerves should be known, as should the major divisions of the brain. It is important to know the effects of paralysis of the various cranial nerves especially III, IV, VI, and VII, and the major functional areas of the cerebrum. The formation, function and circulation of cerebrospinal fluid must be understood.

## 13.3 THE PATIENT

Psychiatric patients need to be treated very carefully when sent for photography. Whether they are suffering from mild mental illness (neuroses) such as anxiety states, phobias and obsessional states or whether they are suffering from the more severe mental illnesses (psychoses) such as melancholia or schizophrenia with delusions and hallucinations, they may be unstable and behave in a very unexpected fashion. The problem of patient consent becomes very difficult with psychiatric patients because they are of 'unsound mind' and therefore incapable of 'informed consent'. Any request/consent form signed by a psychiatric patient is, therefore, worthless in law. They may be suspicious of why you wish to photograph them; sometimes even positively antagonistic. You must remember that the patient is ill – despite the absence of obvious physical signs of disease. Even though the patient may do bizarre things treat him with respect. The neurological patient may have lost the use of limbs, have curious gaits or tremors, or be unable to talk coherently; but always remember that they can probably hear and understand you perfectly – their mental faculties are rarely dulled.

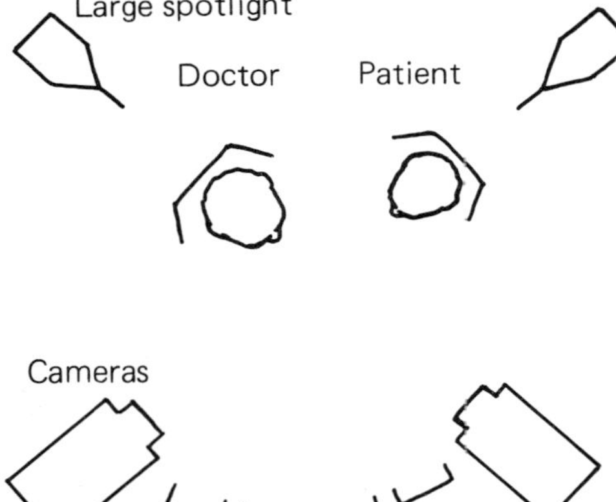


***Figure 13.1*** *A simple psychiatric interview arrangement using two cameras*

## 13.4 GENERAL PHOTOGRAPHIC PRINCIPLES

Still photography in this field of medicine is usually confined to the recording of deformities in neurology and the recording of characteristic attitudes in psychiatry. Both follow the normal principles of good clinical photography outlined in Section 1. Good lighting is the key to photographing the deformities, and the advice given in the section on orthopaedics should be followed.

Most often some record of movement is required and so cine or television must be used (*see Section 21*). This applies to all tremors or involuntary movements such as nystagmus, facial tics, or Parkinsonism; and also to abnormalities of locomotion in, for example, spastic paraplegia or Huntington's chorea. When it can be anticipated that photographs will be required for publication still photographs should also be taken. Still images taken from cine film or television screen are always of poor quality.

A motor drive may be used to advantage to capture a number of key points in a movement cycle, and other ingenious methods can be employed to show movement in a still photograph. The hand tremor of a Parkinson's can be demonstrated by asking the patient to write on a piece of paper and then photographing the shaky result: or alternatively a longish time exposure can be used to demonstrate tremor.

Neurological patients who exhibit voluntary or involuntary movements may require some restraining during photography whilst patients who have paralyses or weaknesses from other causes may require supports. Areas of paraesthesia or anaesthesia will need to be marked with a black skin marker.

Sometimes in psychiatry candid views are required of patients taken through one-way mirrors – there are no special requirements for this, other than that the film usually has to be uprated to cope with the low light levels. Still photographs are also taken of patients' activities in rehabilitation and occupational therapy centres. Often neurologists and psychiatrists will accompany patients when they attend for photography to ensure understanding on the part of both photographer and patient of what is to be recorded.

## 13.5 SOME COMMONLY PHOTOGRAPHED CONDITIONS

*Anorexia nervosa.* A condition marked by great loss of appetite leading to emaciation and metabolic derangement attended by serious neurotic symptoms.

It occurs in predominantly white, middle class, teenage girls. Full length AP, PA and lateral views should be taken to show wasting.

*Alzheimer's disease.* A progressive brain disease occuring between the ages of 40 and 60 years characterized by a generalized atrophy of the brain. Cine or television records of difficulty of locomotion and speech are required.

*Argyll–Robertson pupils.* Small and irregularly shaped pupils which respond to convergence but not to light.

*Bell's palsy.* Benign unilateral facial paralysis, usually caused by a self-limited lesion of the VIIth cranial nerve. There is distortion of the face with the mouth being drawn to one side – this is best demonstrated by asking the patient to smile, blow or whistle. There is absence of eyebrow movement and the inability to completely close the eyelid on the affected side. A series of still photographs of the AP face is needed; they should be annotated, e.g. smiling, whistling, raising eyebrows, at rest, etc.

*Cerebral palsy.* A group of disorders of the motor system, present at birth but perhaps not evident until the child is 1 or 2 years of age. Includes *spastic paraplegia* with paralysis of both legs and the classic 'scissors deformity' caused by spasm of the adductor muscles of the thigh; and *athetosis* characterized by constant, slow, involuntary movements of the hands, fingers and sometimes feet.

*Cerebral vascular accidents* (apoplexy, stroke). There is a variety of vascular accidents which lead to ischaemia and neuronal destruction. There may be hemianaesthesia, hemiplegia, aphasia, vertigo or loss of vision.

*Cretinism.* Severe arrested mental development caused by inadequate production of thyroid hormone in early infancy. There is stunted growth, apathy, distended abdomen and protruding swollen tongue.

*Epilepsy.* Strictly speaking epilepsy is a symptom not a disease; it may be due to congenital neuronal dysfunction, systemic metabolic disorder or structural brain disease. Although common it is rarely photographed. *Grand mal* is characterized by violent convulsive movements of the limbs, incontinence, and the lips and tongue may be bitten. This is followed by a period of unconsciousness with dilated and unresponsive pupils. *Petit mal* consists of brief interruptions of consciousness sometimes accompanied by rhythmical blinking of the eyelids.

*Erb's palsy.* This is due to injury of the brachial plexus during birth, particularly with a breech delivery and gives rise to a flaccid paralysis of the muscles supplied. The arm hangs by the side with the forearm pronated and fingers flexed (the so called 'Policeman's tip' position.

*Facial tics.* Involuntary, brief and recurrent twitching of a group of muscles under the control of specific nerve branches, e.g. *tic douloureux* involving the trigeminal nerve. Some of these tremors are very fine and very fast.

*Habit spasms or cramps.* Liable to occur in individuals of almost any handicraft, e.g. artists, writers, typists, tailors, shoemakers and musicians. In the first instance there is gradually increasing difficulty in conducting the movements required for the work with loss of manual dexterity. Eventually the muscle groups become seized with spasm or cramp. Spasmodic wry-neck also occurs in the same way.

*Herpes zoster.* An infection of the ganglia of the posterior roots of the spinal nerves, or the Vth cranial nerve, by the varicella-zoster virus. Marked by vesicular eruptions running along the cutaneous nerves. Usually unilateral.

*Horner's syndrome.* Constriction of the pupil (meiosis), ptosis, apparent enophthalmos and the cessation of sweating over that side of the face (anhydrosis). Caused by a lesion of the supraspinal sympathetic neurones in the lower brain stem.

*Huntington's chorea.* Inherited progressive dementia with bizarre involuntary movements. Curious springy gait, progressing to a drunken stagger. Facial grimacing is common.

*Meningitis.* Inflammation of the membranous coverings of the brain and spinal cord. Features include headache, neck stiffness, pyrexia and sometimes photophobia and a haemorrhagic rash.

*Munchausen's syndrome.* The fabrication by an itinerent malingerer of a clinically convincing simulation of disease. It may include complex self-induced injuries, signs and symptoms, and there is usually a long history of hospitalization – frequently under many different names. Clinicians may require a photographic record of the signs and symptoms for teaching or simply a facial record for distribution to other hospitals.

*Muscle wasting.* Progressive muscular atrophy occurs whenever muscles are deprived of neurological stimulus for long periods, it may be symptomatic of a generalized motor neurone disease. There is gradual wasting of individual muscles, or groups of muscles, often starting in the thenar eminences spreading to the muscles of the arms, shoulders and trunk.

*Muscular dystrophy.* In the child there is symmetrical weakness and wasting of the muscles of the pelvic girdle and back. This makes the child walk with a 'waddling' gait and an exaggerated lumbar lordosis. It also makes him rise to his feet in a characteristic way by climbing hand over hand up his legs. The degenerative process is steadily and rapidly progressive – within 10 years the patient can seldom walk, and long periods of immobility cause osteoporosis and skeletal deformity.

*Myasthenia gravis.* A chronic disease characterized by variable degrees of muscular weakness leading eventually to paralysis. It begins with the muscles of the eye causing ptosis and diplopia.

*Nystagmus.* A rhythmical oscillatory movement of the eyes resulting from a disorder of co-ordinated eye movement and fixation. Jerky nystagmus is characteristic of cerebellar disease, while pendular nystagmus is due to defects in ocular fixation.

*Parkinsonism* (paralysis agitans). A syndrome characterized by stiffness and slowness of voluntary movement, stooped posture, propulsive gait, rigidity of facial expression (mask like facies) and rhythmic tremor of the limbs.

*Sydenham's chorea* (St. Vitus' dance). A benign disorder of childhood and one of the manifestations of rheumatic fever. In addition to the jerky movements of the limbs the child makes smirking grimaces.

*Syringomyelia.* Progressive cavitation of the grey matter especially in cervical regions. Characterized by dissociated sensory loss, lower motor neurone weakness and trophic changes in the upper limbs and spasticity of the legs. There is occasionally scoliosis of the lumbar spine.

*Tabes dorsalis.* The tertiary stage of syphilis, with sclerosis of the sensory nerve roots. Symptoms are shooting pains, muscular inco-ordination and atrophy and functional disturbance of major organs. There is often erosion and dislocation of joints, optic atrophy and small irregular pupils, which react to convergence but not to light.

*Von Recklinghausen's disease* (neurofibromatosis). Inherited disorder characterized by multiple pedunculated tumours, which follow the course of the peripheral nerves. There are also light brown '*cafe au lait*' spots on the skin.

## 13.6 PHOTOGRAPHY OF NEUROSURGERY

Photographs may be required of any neurosurgical procedure, such as removal of subarachnoid tumours, extradural haematomas, drainage of hydrocephalus or correction of meningomyelocele. Normal photographic principles apply as described in Section

1. Some special techniques have been described in the literature; notably that of fluorescein tracers to establish blood flow to tumours.

## References

Campbell, W. (1953). Medical illustration and psychiatry. *J. Biol. Photogr. Assoc.*, **21**, 28-34

Draper, P. (1980). *Lecture Notes in Neurology* (5th ed.). (Oxford: Blackwell Scientific Publications)

Feindel, W. *et al.* (1967). Intracarotid fluorescein angiography. *Can. Med Assoc. J.*, **96**, 1–7

Garrison, L. (1970). History of illustration in psychiatry. *Br. J. Photogr.*, **117**, 880-884

Hodge, C. *et al.* (1978). Fluorescein angiography of the brain – the Photographic procedure. *J. Biol. Photogr. Assoc.*, **46**, 67–99

Marshall, R. (1979). Infrared recording of neural tube defects. *J. Audiovis. Media Med.*, **2**, 92–94

Parsons, M. (1983). *A Colour Atlas of Clinical Neurology*. (London: Wolfe Medical Publications)

Priest, R. (1978). *Minski's Handbook of Psychiatry for Students and Nurses*. (London: Heinemann Medical Books)

Sclare, A. and Thomson, G. (1968). The uses of closed circuit television in teaching psychiatry to medical students. *Br. J. Med. Educ.*, **2**, 226-228

Wallace, F. (1957). Neuropsychiatric photography. *J. Biol. Photogr. Assoc.*, **25**, 96-97

Wilmer, H. (1968). The undisguised camera in psychiatry. *Visual Sonic Med.*, **3**, 5-9

Yonge, K. (1965). The uses of closed circuit television for the teaching of psychotherapeutic interviewing to medical students. *Can. Med. Assoc. J.*, **92**, 747-749

## *Practical projects*

(1) Produce a series of still pictures to effectively demonstrate Bell's palsy. Annotate the photographs appropriately. Produce in a medium of your choice.

(2) Make a short cine film or videotape to demonstrate some abnormality of movement or locomotion due to a neurological disorder. Write short notes on the condition you have chosen to record.

(3) Produce a 12″ × 10″ exhibition quality print to illustrate some aspect of occupational therapy for stroke patients.

(4) Produce two photographs in a medium of your choice to illustrate effectively two psychiatric conditions, e.g. depression or schizoprenia.

## *Examination questions*

Q.1 Describe how photographic recording is of value in psychiatry; cite specific examples to illustrate your answer.

Q.2 What are the main visual signs, and what photographs would you take to illustrate the following conditions:
(*a*) Anorexia nervosa,
(*b*) Cretinism,
(*c*) Erb's palsy,
(*d*) Horner's syndrome,
(*e*) Parkinsonism.

Q.3 Discuss the relative merits and uses of still and cine photography in recording neurological diseases.

Q.4 What is 'chorea'? Describe fully two examples and discuss the photographic recording of these disorders.

Q.5 Describe the photographs you would take to illustrate the following conditions:
(*a*) Munchausen's syndrome,
(*b*) Muscular dystrophy,
(*c*) Myasthenia gravis,
(*d*) Nystagmus, and
(*e*) Bell's palsy.

Q.6 Describe fully the technique of fluorescein angiography of the brain.

Q.7 Discuss the concept of 'patient consent' in the context of recording psychiatric interviews. Why are such recordings of great value?

Q.8 With the aid of simple diagrams describe the lighting you would arrange for a two camera television recording of psychiatric interviews. What other factors are particularly relevant in recording such an event.

*Multiple choice questions (any of the statements may be true or false)*

Q.9 You would take a photograph of the face to illustrate an aspect of:
(*a*) Munchausen's syndrome,
(*b*) Bell's palsy,
(*c*) Erb's palsy,
(*d*) Parkinsonism,
(*e*) Spastic paraplegia.

Q.10 The following conditions are characterized by peculiar gaits:
(*a*) IIIrd Cranial nerve palsy,
(*b*) Paralysis agitans,
(*c*) Huntington's chorea,
(*d*) Alzheimer's disease,
(*e*) Athetosis.

# Section 14
# Photography of vascular, blood and lymphatic disorders

**A.R. Williams**, MPhil, FBIPP, FRPS, FBPA, AIMBI
Head of Medical Illustration and Teaching Services
Charing Cross Hospital and Medical School, London

## 14.1 INTRODUCTION

This section concerns disorders of the blood its constituents and its transportation. In medical terms this covers a vast range of conditions treated by specialists in general medicine, thoracic and vascular surgery, cardiology, haematology and oncology. In photographic terms this section primarily covers local pathological changes caused by vascular insufficiency, visible changes in the vessels themselves and neoplastic pathology. Patients suffering from such conditions need special care, ranging from avoidance of physical exertion to complete barrier nursing. The photographer should be aware that patients suffering from hypertension or angina pectoris often appear to be in robust health.

## 14.2 ANATOMY AND PHYSIOLOGY

The student must be completely familiar with the major venous and arterial networks, the names of the major vessels and the areas of tissue they supply. The difference in structure between arteries and veins must be understood, as should the nature of emboli, aneurysms and collateral circulation. The common cardiac abnormalities should be learnt (*study carefully Section 28.7*). A knowledge of the components of blood, the mechanisms of blood cell production/destruction and clotting is expected, as is the function and circulation of lymph. Without this fundamental appreciation, the student will find it difficult to illustrate the relevant pathology intelligently.

## 14.3 PHOTOGRAPHIC TECHNIQUE

There is nothing in the recording of such conditions which is of a unique character, but a meticulous and sometimes innovative approach is necessary. Colour fidelity, for example, is particularly important where a slight blue cast from a coloured background might suggest, quite erroneously, cyanosis. Slight overexposure of a colour transparency might suggest pallor and ischaemia where none existed. Good lighting is also important – the surface evidence of an aneurysm might be only a very delicate superficial pulsation which will require expert lighting and cinematography to record it adequately.

The use of invisible radiation photography, especially infrared, is often called for to record abnormalities in vascular pattern. Often the requesting surgeon or physician will not appreciate, or will misunderstand, the use of infrared photography for recording such conditions and the good clinical photographer may well have to take the initiative in such situations. It is particularly important therefore for the student working in this field to study Section 18.

Like every other branch of medical photography standardization is particularly important in following, for example, the progress of leg ulcers which may even require photogrammetric techniques to measure the rate of healing.

## 14.4 SOME COMMONLY PHOTOGRAPHED CONDITIONS

### 14.4.1 Venous changes

All recording of superficial veins is best accomplished with infrared radiation which is able to penetrate the skin and is heavily absorbed by carboxyhaemoglobin. The infrared record should always be accompanied by a visible light photograph to enable to doctor to interpret accurately the results. Varicose veins record well with this technique but great care has to be taken to provide even 'wrap-around' lighting for the legs or detail will be lost in dark edges. Collateral venous channels appear as either a pale blue, diaphanous vascular net, or as large tortuous, distended veins, seen and palpable through the skin. They function as secondary channels after partial or complete occlusion of a principal vein. The shape and nature of the collateral circulation is important as it indicates the location of the primary obstruction. Infrared photography clearly delineates the pattern and some spectacular results have been obtained with occlusion of axillary, subclavian and iliac veins, superior and inferior vena cava and in portal hypertension. Venous stasis caused by failure of the right ventricle to expand and contract in a normal manner will sometimes show in infrared photographs of the extremities, but frequently marked lymphoedema masks the 'pooled' venous blood.

### 14.4.2 Arterial disease

Peripheral vascular disease and arteriosclerosis are evidenced by ischaemia, ulceration or even gangrene of the extremities which require accurate colour photographs.

In the short term, poor supply of oxygenated blood results in cyanosis which needs accurate colour photography (it may be helpful to include some normal coloured skin, e.g. a nurse's hand, to act as a reference tone). In the long term, finger clubbing develops which requires lateral as well as anterior views of the fingers. Clubbing most often occurs as a result of pulmonary pathology rather than vascular. Arteriolar spasm as in Raynaud's disease is evidenced by cold white fingers – this is not demonstrated by infrared photography but requires thermography (the same applies to Pernio). Emboli cause localized ischaemia, followed rapidly by cyanotic discoloration and gangrene – the same effects are seen on a more widespread basis with Buerger's disease. The effects of aortic bifurcation emboli are clearly seen in photographs of the feet. Arterio-venous fistulae are evidenced by great distension of the venous system at several points in the circulation of a limb, due to a direct shunt between the artery and vein. Infrared is often successful in delineating the site of the fistula. The pulsing aneurysm is clearly shown by placing two matchsticks over the pulsating area and allowing the lever principle to enhance the movement which is then recorded on cine film or television with strong cross-lighting. Localized ischaemia is also seen in polyarteritis nodosa where multiple nodules appear on the walls of the small arteries.

### 14.4.3 Blood dyscrasias

The most commonly photographed disorders of the blood are anaemia, haemophilia and leukaemia. Chronic anaemia has a number of possible causes, including lack of iron. There is pallor of the skin and conjunctivae general weakness; cutaneous and mucosal haemorrhages; enlarged swollen tongue with papillary atrophy; and koilonychia (spoon shaped nails, demonstrated most effectively by a drop of water which is held in the spoon). Haemophilia is a disturbance of the mechanism of blood clotting and causes excessive and spontaneous bleeding. One may be asked to photograph haemorrhage and ecchymoses anywhere on the body. Leukaemia is a neoplastic disease of leucopoietic tissue with uncontrolled production of leucocytes. Spongy bleeding of the gums and other haemorrhagic manifestations, including purpura, are often photographed, as are swellings of the abdomen due to hepato – and splenomegaly. Polycythaemia rubra vera is where a hyperplasia of the bone marrow causes a marked increase in the production of erythrocytes. The patient has a bright red facial flush, capillary engorgement with small red lesions affecting the head, neck and upper trunk, often with splenomegaly.

### 14.4.4 Skin manifestations

Evidence of vascular and blood disorders is often seen in the skin such as angiomas, lymphangiomas, purpura, telangiectasia and naevi. All these conditions are dealt with in Section 6 of the guide.

### 14.4.5 Cardiac disease

Cardiac failure is said to exist when the output of the heart is insufficient for the needs of the tissues. It may be acute or chronic. In chronic congestive cardiac failure one typically photographs distended neck veins, engorgement of the liver and oedema (especially of the legs), then later gross ascites may develop. The congenital cardiac malformations such as mitral stenosis, patent ductus arteriosus, arterial septal defect and Fallot's tetralogy all result in peripheral cyanosis, especially of fingers, lips and nose, and ultimately marked finger clubbing. Aortic incompetence is evidenced by peripheral vasodilation with pink, warm, extremities. Coarctation of the aorta is accompanied by dilated, tortuous, pulsating vessels, especially in the neck.

### 14.4.6 Lymphatic disorders

Lymphadenoma, or Hodgkin's disease, is a progressive painless neoplastic enlargement of lymphoid tissue throughout the body. In addition to general signs of anaemia, the enlarged lymph nodes, typically of the cervical region, should be photographed. Lymphoedema is a chronic unilateral or bilateral swelling of the extremities caused by obstruction of the lymphatic vessels or disease of the lymph nodes. It is critical to show both sides of the body in any photograph to ascertain whether the condition is unilateral or bilateral. The student should also remember that swollen lymph nodes may be consequent on nearby invasion, e.g. swollen axillary nodes with carcinoma of the breast.

## References


Epstein, B.S. (1939). Infrared photographic demonstration of superficial venous pattern in congenital heart disease with cyanosis. *Am. Heart J.*, **18**, 282–289

Fear, R. *et al.* (1962). Convenient visualization of venous patterns by infrared photography. *Arch. Intern. Med.*, **110**, 898–899

Hinshaw, M.D. (1942). Lesions of the superior mediastinum which interfere with venous circulation. *J. Lab. Clin. Med.*, **27**, 908–916

Jones, E. (1935). The demonstration of collateral venous circulation by infrared photography. *Am. J. Med. Scie.*, **190**, 478–485

Massopust, L.C. (1936). Infrared photographic study of the changing pattern of superficial veins. *Surg. Gynaecol. Obstet.*, **63**, 86–89

Missal, M. *et al.* (1965). Inferior vena cava obstruction. *Ann. Intern. Med.*, **62**, 133–161

Payne, R.T. (1934). Infrared photography of the superficial venous system. *Lancet*, **226**. 235–236

Snow, D. and Ollerenshaw, R. (1953). Postmortem examination of the coronary arteries. *Med. Biol. Illustr.*, **3**, 4–7

Walker, W. (1980). *A Colour Atlas of Peripheral Vascular Disorders.* (London: Wolfe Medical Publications)

## Practical projects

(1) Photograph any example of 'collateral circulation' in panchromatic and infrared black-and-white; then produce 10″ × 8″ display prints, along with a diagram to indicate which major vessels have been blocked.

(2) Using the principles outlined in Section 17 produce 5″ × 7″ prints of cross sections of a major artery and vein. Produce overlays for each print to label the salient features of each vessel.

(3) Produce a series of 35 mm teaching transparencies which illustrate the salient features of any blood or vascular disorder. Supply brief notes to accompany your pictures in the form of a simple story board which could form the basis of a tape–slide programme.

(4) Try to visit the E.C.G. department in your hospital and familiarize yourself with the basic technique and the different types of recording machine used. Study the output of the latter with a view to photographic reproduction.

## Examination questions

Q.1 Describe the photographs you would take to illustrate the following conditions:
(*a*) Carotid aneurysm
(*b*) Aortic bifurcation embolism
(*c*) Raynaud's disease
(*d*) Chronic anaemia
(*e*) Arterio - venous fistula.

Q.2 What is 'collateral circulation'? Describe the value of infrared recording techniques in illustrating such conditions.

Q.3 Briefly describe the mechanism of blood clotting. What is haemophilia and what photographs might you expect to have to take to record this condition?

Q.4 Discuss the factors you would consider, and the steps you would take, to ensure accurate colour rendition in colour prints of cases of cyanosis, ischaemia and jaundice.

Q.5 Describe with the aid of diagrams the circulation of the blood through the heart. What effect would a ventricular septal defect have and what photographs would you take to illustrate the clinical manifestations of such a defect?

*Multiple choice questions (any of the statements may be true or false)*

Q.6. Fallot's tetralogy is characterized by:
(*a*) Peripheral cyanosis
(*b*) Pulmonary stenosis
(*c*) Right ventricular hypertrophy
(*d*) Vasodilation
(*e*) Ventricular septal defect

Q.7 Cyanosis would be seen in the following conditions:

(*a*) Mitral stenosis
(*b*) Polycythaemia rubra vera
(*c*) Aortic incompetence
(*d*) Ichthyosis
(*e*) Coarctation of the aorta.

# Section 15
# Photography in the pathologies

**D. Tredinnick**, FRPS, AIMBI
Head of Medical Illustration
St Bartholomew's Hospital and Medical College, London

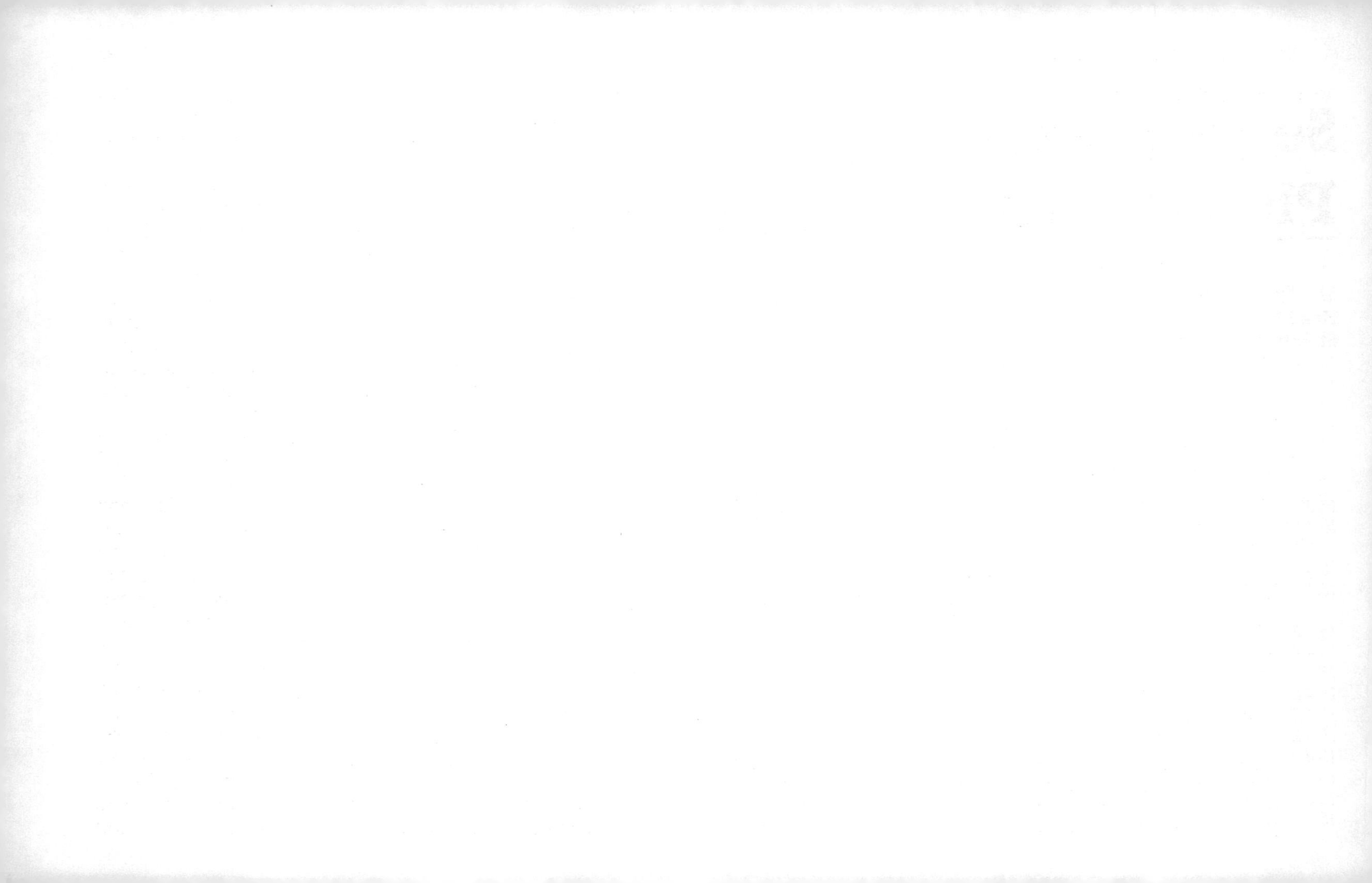

## 15.1 INTRODUCTION

This section groups gross pathological specimens together with laboratory preparations.

Gross specimens may involve both normal and pathological material, usually in the form of fresh or fixed anatomical specimens, including foreign bodies such as calculi. The laboratory preparations will have been prepared for diagnostic or research purposes and will vary from petri dishes, tubes and flasks to flat plates. The laboratories of microbiology, chemical pathology, haematology, immunology, virology and morbid anatomy will be the principal ones concerned and in large establishments and in universities these will have research units attached. Other sources of material for photography are:

(1) Operating theatre. Surgical specimens removed at operation may need to be photographed immediately and may link up with pathological states and abnormalities previously photographed.
(2) Post-mortem room. Apart from specimens obtained at post-mortem photographs of the cadaver may be required, to show organs and conditions *in situ*. (*see Section 1.5.4*). Forensic applications may need special documentation and these and other general investigations will be an indirect source of laboratory preparations needing photography.
(3) Animal house. Photographs of whole or part of an animal may be required.
(4) Pathology and anatomy museums. Photography is often required for teaching purposes, showing the exhibits as a whole (including the containers), or the specimen only, usually for publication, for use in a teaching programme or for video production.

## 15.2 SAFETY RULES AND TECHNIQUE

As a general rule it is wise to treat all fresh or partly fixed specimens as being capable of causing infection and all laboratory cultures as possibly pathogenic; i.e. producing disease. Therefore when handling such items it is essential that precautions are taken to protect patients, staff and the equipment from possible contamination or infection.

The laboratory service in the hospital will have its own safety rules in this respect, drawn up to conform (in the United Kingdom) to the Health and Safety at Work Act 1974, The Howie Report 1978 and the Code of Practice for the Prevention of Infection in Clinical Laboratories and Post-mortem Rooms 1978.

The safety rules will restrict the areas permitted to house certain classes of pathological material (categories A, B1, B2) even temporarily, making it necessary for any photography to be carried out in premises equipped for safe handling. Where local safety rules permit, photography of non-hazardous material may be carried out in the photographic studio; safe techniques of handling must nevertheless be adhered to.

Protective clothing must be worn and all specimens or preparations handled with disposable gloves, which should of course be removed before handling any apparatus. A useful method of working for the unassisted photographer is to keep one hand gloved for final arrangement of the subject, while the other ungloved hand can adjust the camera or lights. Any necessary instruments such as scissors, knives, probes and so forth must be kept solely for use with pathological material. *Never* use the same instruments, even if sterilized, in connection with patients. After use all instruments, cutting boards, backgrounds, rulers, plasticine, swabs, gloves or anything else which has come into contact, should be sterilized, cleaned with antiseptic solution or incinerated. The pathology services and safety officer (infection) should always be consulted regarding the handling techniques used, and in any case of uncertainty.

## 15.3 CARE IN HANDLING

All specimens and laboratory preparations need careful handling to avoid change or damage occurring through clumsiness, excessive heat or undue delay. When an organ or piece of tissue is removed from the body, a process known as autolysis, or breaking down of cell structure, takes place. This alteration in cell structure can so change the microscopical appearance that diagnosis can become uncertain or even impossible. Ideally the specimen should be placed in fixative immediately after it has been removed from the body. This, however, can alter the original appearance by removing the colour and sometimes distorting the shape. Therefore, on occasions when both colour and shape are to be recorded accurately the specimen has to be photographed in the fresh state.

It is of vital importance that autolysis is kept to a minimum, also that dehydration or haemolysis do not affect the gross specimen, so speed in photographing a fresh specimen is essential. Always have a readily accessible specimen set-up available and make sure the work is done with no waste of time and that the specimen is placed in a fixative as soon as photography is complete.

Some specimens, particularly membranes and tissues of the central nervous system are very fragile and will not stand much handling; great care must be taken when dealing with such material.

Laboratory preparations are often of a delicate nature or are not mounted on a firm support. For example, egg membranes or support gels may need to be transferred to glass or water prior to being photographed.

Organisms may be grown on substances compounded of organic and inorganic material and known as 'media'. When cultivated in this way they are said to grow '*in vitro*', i.e. outside the body. Some common media are agar, blood-agar and broth. They may be solid, semi-solid or fluid, transparent or opaque. They must be kept covered except during the photographic exposure and treated always with the greatest care.

## 15.4 PHOTOGRAPHIC TECHNIQUES FOR GROSS SPECIMENS

### 15.4.1 General

While it is possible to convert a copy stand to the photography of specimens and laboratory preparations, it is infinitely preferable for a separate set-up to be available, both for ease of working and also to comply with safety regulations.

### 15.4.2 Specimen table and camera mounting

The camera must be fixed to a vertical stand providing horizontal and vertical movement. The stand may be floor or wall-mounted but in any case all-round space must be allowed for placing lights in any direction relative to the specimen. The set-up is completed by a specimen table incorporating background illumination, including provision for a coloured background to be introduced.

### 15.4.3 Cameras and lenses

Any reliable 35 mm or stand camera with standard lenses can be used. For close up work, bellows or extension tubes with a lens in the 85–135 mm range are suitable. A macro lens of similar range is also useful.

### 15.4.4 Lighting

With the subject correctly orientated, its form, texture and structure can be shown by suitably arranged lighting. Usually this can be achieved with a simple two-lamp arrangement of modelling lamp at 45° and a suitably placed fill-in lamp, the two being modified to suit individual specimens. Tungsten sources should be used with care because of the possibility of damage to the specimen from heat generated by these lamps. Electronic flash tubes with integral modelling lights are preferable. These are particularly useful if the specimen has to be hand-held in order to demonstrate a special feature.

Care should be taken that the unavoidable highlights present in a fresh specimen should not obliterate any important features of interest. It is most important to keep obtrusive shadows to a minimum and to place any necessary ones in the correct viewing position, i.e. beneath the specimen as it lies in the correct anatomical position. Inattention to this point can cause a cavity to appear as a convexity and vice-versa. One way of achieving even illumination without specular highlights is to totally immerse the specimen in fluid but this is often difficult because the natural buoyancy of the specimen entails holding it submerged and usually air bubbles form as the liquid settles.

### 15.4.5 Background

The purpose of the background is to present a clean clinical appearance and to provide an effective contrast in order to better demonstrate important features of the specimen. Whatever material is used, it should be spotlessly clean and all blood or mucus seeping from a specimen should be removed from the background prior to taking the photograph. Never use absorbent material such as a dry theatre towel as background for a wet specimen.

White shadowless grounds can be obtained by supporting the specimen on glass above a transilluminated background, usually built-in to a specially constructed specimen table. The judicious use of black card surrounding the specimen, but not appearing in the final photograph, will cut down the amount of flare. The technique of background transillumination should be used with care, as the production of a photograph showing a specimen apparently suspended in mid-air because there is no background tone, *can* give rise to misinterpretation.

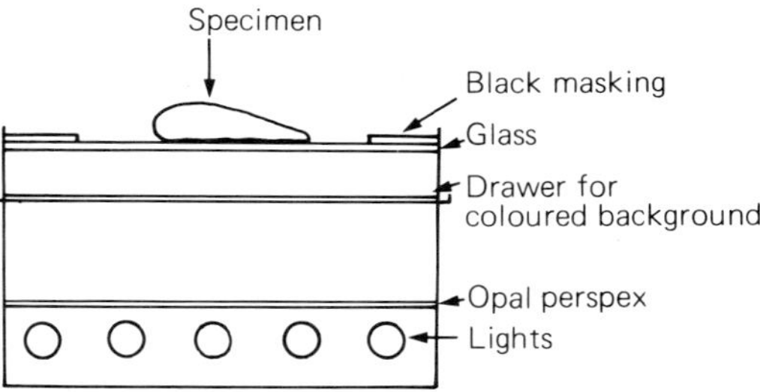


***Figure 15.1*** *A useful specimen support and background illuminator. Some method of controlling the output of the background lights, irrespecive of whether they are tungsten or electronic flash, is essential to avoid flare*

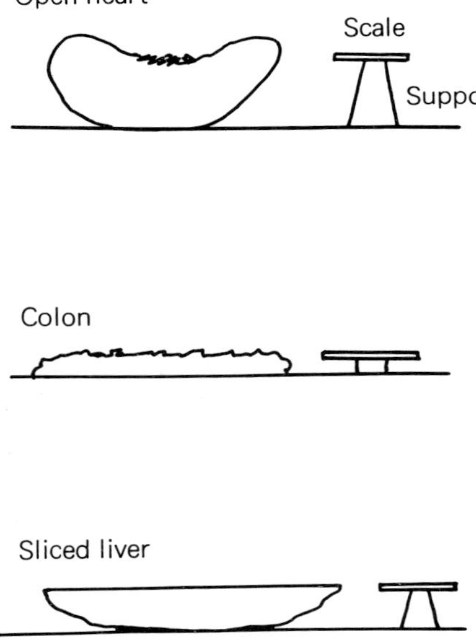


***Figure 15.2*** *Great care must be taken to ensure that the scale is placed in the plane of principal interest – not necessarily at the top of the specimen — and certainly not on the support glass*

### 15.4.6 Orientation and presentation

Gross specimens should be photographed in the accepted anatomical position, i.e. a stomach should be presented with, in the anterior/posterior view, the fundus at the top of the picture and the pylorus at the bottom left hand side.

On occasions it may be necessary to support the specimen in the required position. Plasticine and gauze are both useful for this purpose and can usually be hidden from view. Cotton wool should never be used as loose fibres tend to stick to the surface of the specimen and can be difficult to remove. The use of cork boards on which to pin out specimens, such as opened out intestine, is not recommended. Instead, cotton thread inserted with a surgical cutting needle can be placed at intervals along the side of the intestinal wall, and these can be retracted and fixed firmly outside the picture area. The threads can then be removed from the negative image before printing.

### 15.4.7 Scale

A clear, easily readable scale should be included in the picture area. If it is placed in the plane of critical focus this will demonstrate the size of the specimen. However, the effects of perspective and depth of subject mean that accurate measurements are not possible with this method. If accuracy is required for research purposes, the elimination of perspective is essential; one way of achieving this is by the use of a telecentric lens system (*see Section 20.2.1*).

### 15.4.8 Mounted specimens

Museum specimens are generally mounted in fluid-filled Perspex or glass containers. These should be positioned for photography in the upright position so that any air bubbles rise to the top of the container, and then left for half an hour so that any sediment sinks to the bottom. If the existing fluid is discoloured it should be replaced. Different techniques will be required depending on whether the container is to be included in the picture, or the specimen is to be shown alone.

Occasionally infrared or ultraviolet photographic techniques can be applied, with advantage, to the recording of gross specimens in order to show tissue changes not otherwise visible (*see Sections 18 and 19*).

### 15.4.9 Colour restoration

Occasionally it is possible to restore the

faded colours of a fixed specimen by soaking in alcohol but the photographer must always take advice from the pathologist before taking such action.

## 15.5 PHOTOGRAPHY OF CULTURE MEDIA

Cultures can be photographed with incident light or by transillumination. The relevant detail on any particular culture may require one type or the other, or a combination of the two. Thus it is most important for the photographer to be aware of the features to be recorded. These will include the colour, shape, size, distribution and composition of the colonies which have grown together with areas of inhibition or haemolysis. Cultures grown in tubes or bottles will need a different photographic set-up to those in dishes. Tubes may be displayed to advantage by suspending them by their necks. Lighting is difficult because if incident light is used, the reflections on the colonies, on the medium and on the glass support must be controlled so that characteristic detail of the culture is not lost. Some form of back lighting may be required to illuminate particles or turbidity seen in the media. When transillumination is used beneath a petri dish, flare can be eliminated by cutting a mask to accept the dish. Close up views of particular colonies may be required as well as a general view of the whole culture. Virus cultures may occasionally be recorded photographically and they require similar antiseptic precautions in handling. Mycological or fungal cultures are opaque and each individual type has a typical shape, size, contour and colour. Directional lighting is often required to show the elevations in the contour, though care must be taken not to throw a shadow of the edge of the petri dish on to the culture. Some cultures exhibit a characteristic colour; an example being the red underside of *Trichophyton rubrum*, but more often the texture and form are the important features.

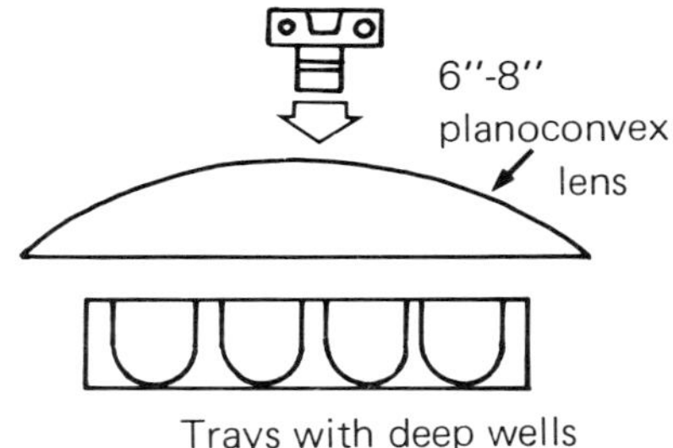


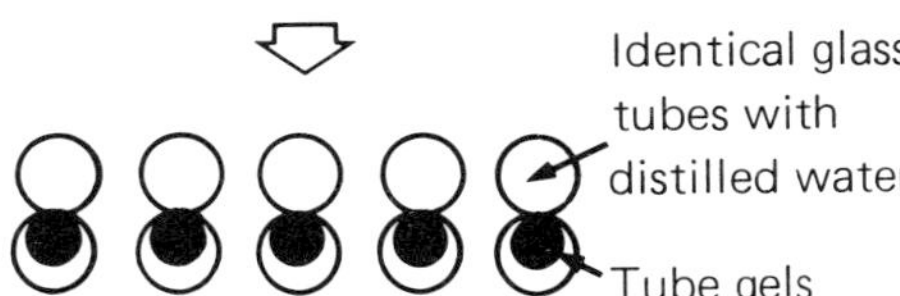


***Figure 15.3*** *(above) Plano-convex lenses or cylindrical lenses may be used to improve the geometry of the image when recording tray and tube gels*

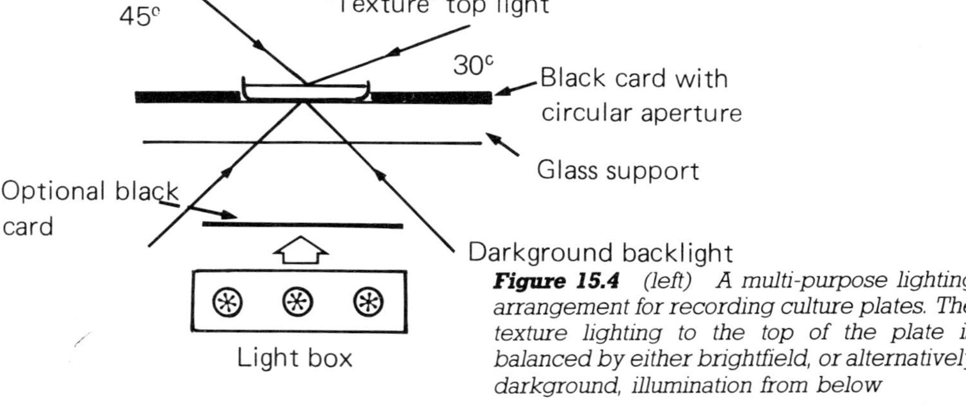


***Figure 15.4*** *(left) A multi-purpose lighting arrangement for recording culture plates. The texture lighting to the top of the plate is balanced by either brightfield, or alternatively darkground, illumination from below*

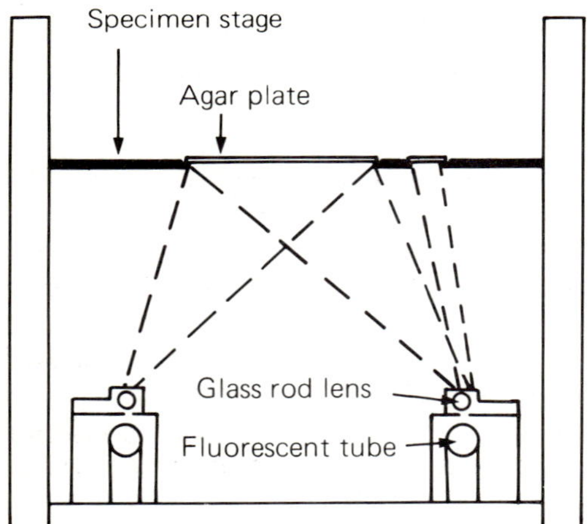


***Figure 15.5*** *Immunoelectrophoretic plates usually require darkground illumination. Fluorescent tubes masked by cylindrical rod lenses provide excellent lighting, especially when built into a housing as shown above*

## 15.6 IMMUNOELECTROPHORESIS PLATES

These plates can be presented in a number of forms and have their own special photographic problems. Usually a clear gelatine base on a glass slide or in a dish has several discs or channels cut into it which act as receptacles for test fluids (containing antigens for example) and precipitation bands are seen stretching between them. These bands consist of faint white deposits of varying strength and it is often difficult to see them within the clear gelatine; in many cases only the use of a darkground technique will reveal them. In order to further improve the contrast, a process film must be used. Scaling is important and slides and plates should be photographed to a standard scale on each occasion.

Immunologists often use the photographic negative as a research record but if a print is required care must be exercised to see that none of the precipitin bands are 'lost' in the printing stage.

## 15.7 CHROMATOGRAMS

The chemical pathologist and many other research workers use chromatography to separate out the individual components of a particular fluid, the end result being a series of deposits spaced on an absorbent paper or gel base. The latter are extremely fragile and should be mounted with considerable care on a glass plate for photography. The appearance is of a white or off-white base, which may be transparent or opaque, having deposits of varying density and colour. It can usually be photographed using flat copy lighting with occasional variations. Some deposits will not show up by normal photographic means but can be recorded by ultraviolet or fluorescence photography (*see Section 19*).

## References

Berry, J. *et al.* (1954). The photography of paper chromatograms. *Med. Biol. Illustr.*, **4**, 223–228

Brain, E. (1973). Photographing specimens immersed in fluid. *Ann. R. Coll. Surg. (Engl).*, **53**, 194-196

Burgess, C. (1975). Gross specimen photography – a survey of lighting and background techniques. *Med. Biol. Illustr.*, **25**, 159-166

Clayton, E.R. (1940). Infrared photography of gross specimens. *J. Tech. Meth.*, **19** 55–57

Drewello, E. (1954). Simultaneous photography of gross specimen and radiograph. *Dent. Radiogr. Photogr.*, **27**, 36-37

Ellis, J. (1977). Under-fluid gross specimen photography – recent observations. *J. Biol. Photogr. Assoc.*, **45**, 98-99

Ellis, J. (1978). Fibre-optic photography of polyacrylamide disc gels. *J. Biol. Photogr.*, **46**, 167-169

Fiske, P. (1974). Auxiliary cylindrical lenses for recording bands in narrow tubes. *Med. Biol. Illustr.*, **24**, 160-161

Geddes, N. (1980). Adjustable scale-supports for specimen photography. *J. Audiovis. Media Med.*, **3**, 142

Gillies, R. and Dodds, T. (1968). *Bacteriology Illustrated.* (2nd ed.). (Edinburgh: Churchill Livingstone)

Govan, A., McFarlane, P. and Callander, R. (1981). *Pathology Illustrated.* (Edinburgh: Churchill Livingstone)

Harrison, J. (1969). Some photographic techniques in bacteriology. *Image Dynamics*, **4**, 12–16

Harp, D. (1965). An adjustable scale stand for specimen photography. *J. Biol. Photogr. Assoc.*, **33**, 125-127

Jackson, R. (1968). Ultraviolet recording of thin layer chromatograms. *Vis. Sonic Med.*, **3**, 4–6

Kodak. (1982). *Using Photography to Preserve Evidence.* (Publication M2) (Rochester, NY: Eastman Kodak Ltd)

Lacey, B. and Hansell, P. (1954). Photography of bacterial colonies. *Med. Biol. Illustr.*, **3**, 206–211

Le Beau, L. (1973). Control of infectious hazards for the biophotographer. *J. Biol. Photogr. Assoc.*, **41**, 131-135

Le Beau, L. (1976). Effective lighting systems for photography of microbial colonies. (Part 1). *J. Biol. Photogr. Assoc.*, **44**, 4-14

Le Beau, L. (1980). Versatile and compact stage for photographing small laboratory subjects. (Part 2). *J. Biol. Photogr.*, **48**, 3-13

Le Beau, L. (1980). Photography of tubes and their contents based on image requirements and tube configuration. (Part 3). *J. Biol. Photogr.*, **48**, 93-107

Le Beau, L. (1980). Photography of polyacrylamide gels from disc electrophoresis. (Part 4). *J. Biol. Photogr.*, **48**, 141-144

Le Beau, L. (1981). Photography of compartmentalized plastic strips, trays, plates and slides used for microculture and serological reactions. (Part 5). *J. Biol. Photogr.*, **49**, 7-19

Lewin, K. and Morton, R. (1963). The preservation of human tissues in a fresh state. *Med. Biol. Illustr.*, **13**, 159–163

Marshall, R. (1957). Photographic background control. *Med. Biol. Illustr.*, **7**, 13-21

Martin, D. (1953). Care of specimens for illustration. *Med. Biol. Illustr.*, **3**, 216-223

Massopust, L. (1937). Infrared photography of gross anatomical specimens. *Arch. Path.*, **23**, 67–70

Mills, G. (1937). Infrared photography of gross specimens. *Radiogr. Clin. Photogr.*, **13**, 12–13

Murray, R. and Ollerenshaw, R. (1975). Large field darkground illumination. *Med. Biol. Illustr.*, **25**, 153-158

Paulson, R. (1971). Scales for scientific pictures. *Photogr. Applic.*, **6**, 16-32

Ruddick, R. (1982). The role of the medical photographer in forensic medicine. *Br. J. Photogr.*, **129**, 970-971

Simpson, K. (1974). *Forensic Medicine.* (7th ed.). (London: Edward Arnold)

Swindle, P. (1940). Infrared photography of specimens injected with red cinnabar. *J. Biol. Photogr. Assoc.*, **8**, 105–110

Symmers, W. (ed.). (1966). *Systemic Pathology.* (London: Longmans)

Vetter, J. (1960). An integrated method of preserving and photographing gross specimens. *J. Biol. Photogr. Assoc.*, **28**, 21-27

Vetter, J. (1969). Photographing gross specimens. *Lab Manag.*, **7**, 24-44

Vetter, J. (1983). The colour preservation and photography of gross specimens. *J. Audiovis. Media Med.*, **6**, 7-12

Weiss, C. (1968). Fungus photography : culture plates with ultraviolet fluorescence. *J. Biol. Photogr. Assoc.*, **36**, 145-153

Williams, A.R. (1977). Control of scale in specimen photography – a look at telecentric systems. *Med. Biol. Illustr.*, **27**, 55-62

Williams, L. (1969). Routine photography of clinical electrophoresis gels. *Med. Biol. Illustr.*, **19**, 105-108

Zweidinger, R. *et al.* (1973). Photography of bloodstains visualized by luminescence. *J. Forens. Sci.*, **18**, 296-302

## Practical projects

(1) Learn the various methods of sterilization with special reference to heat, chemical and radiation effects.

(2) Familiarize yourself with study of gross organ anatomy.
Make sure you understand the terms referring to views and aspects such as proximal and distal and that you can distinguish between a right and left kidney.

(3) Make rough sketches and annotate the following:
(*a*) Heart and great vessels.
(*b*) Respiratory tract.
(*c*) Digestive tract.
(*d*) Genito-urinary tract.
(*e*) Inferior aspect of the brain.
(*f*) Medial view of one hemisphere.
(*g*) Longitudinal section of a femur
(*h*) Coronal section of a kidney.
(*i*) Microscopic section of skin.
(*j*) A P view of uterus and ovaries.
(*k*) The vertebral column.

(4) Photograph as many specimens as you can – vary the backgrounds and lighting as necessary. Keep the results in a properly indexed album along with notes on your technique, condition of the specimen, diagnosis, etc.

(5) Photograph in colour a culture plate to show sensitivities to antibiotics of a specific organism.

(6) Photograph a blood agar culture of, for example, *H. influenzae*, to show particularly the areas of haemolysis.

(7) Photograph any broth culture to bring out the turbidity (*E. coli* is a good example). Experiment with different lighting arrangements to obtain a good result. Produce in a medium of your choice.

(8) Photograph any culture which is enhanced by the use of invisible radiation (e.g. a UV culture of *B. diphtheriae* on telluric acid medium by infrared, or a culture of *Ps. pyocyanae* or *H. pertussis* by ultraviolet). Produce a matched 'control' print and submit along with notes on your technique and results.

### Examination questions

Q.1 You decide to produce a 15 minute tape – slide programme on some aspect of the photography of pathological specimens as part of your own staff training. Select objectives and describe the sequence of illustrations you would use to achieve your aim.

Q.2 Describe the problems of handling and the photography of a fresh specimen of tuberculous kidney which has already been cut.

Q.3 Discuss under the following headings the major problems in the photography of viral cultures (egg membranes):
(*a*) Handling
(*b*) Lighting,
(*c*) Backgrounds.

Q.4 What is a chromatogram? How may invisible radiations be employed in the photography of chromatograms?

Q.5 Discuss with the aid of diagrams the principles of darkground illumination as applied to the photography of precipitin bands (Ouchterlony plates). Describe one other technique which is suited to recording such plates.

Q.6 With photography in mind, name two pathological conditions which affect the following organs, (*a*) brain, (*b*) heart, (*c*) lung, (*d*) colon and (*e*) kidney. Briefly describe the appearance of three of the conditions which you have named and the technique which you would use to record them.

Q.7 You are asked to provide a regular service for photography of bacteriological cultures in petri dishes. You will receive a minimum of two per day for recording as colour transparencies.
(*a*) Describe the apparatus and materials needed, giving your reasons.
(*b*) Discuss both the photographic and specimen handling techniques you would use.

Q.8 Distinguish between the following:
(*a*) *Vivo* and *vitro*,
(*b*) Necrosis and gangrene,
(*c*) Bacteria and viruses,
(*d*) Infection and infectious,
(*e*) Benign and malignant tumours.

*Multiple choice questions (any of the statements may be true or false).*

Q.9 The following are disorders of the kidney:
(*a*) Wilms tumour.
(*b*) Cholecystitis.
(*c*) Renal calculus.
(*d*) Hypernephroma.
(*e*) Adrenal necrosis.

Q.10 You are asked to make a black-and-white photograph of a whole brain specimen with haemorrhagic areas on the cortex surrounded by yellow staining.
(*a*) A scale should be placed in contact with the background.
(*b*) If the specimen is laid directly on an X-ray illuminator, the exposure for the background is immaterial provided that it will produce black on the negative.
(*c*) Correct perspective on a final 10″ × 8″ print would be obtained by using a 6″ lens and a 4″ × 5″ negative.
(*d*) You would see the optic chiasma from an inferior view.
(*e*) The stained area will be well contrasted from the cortex by using a yellow filter and panchromatic film.

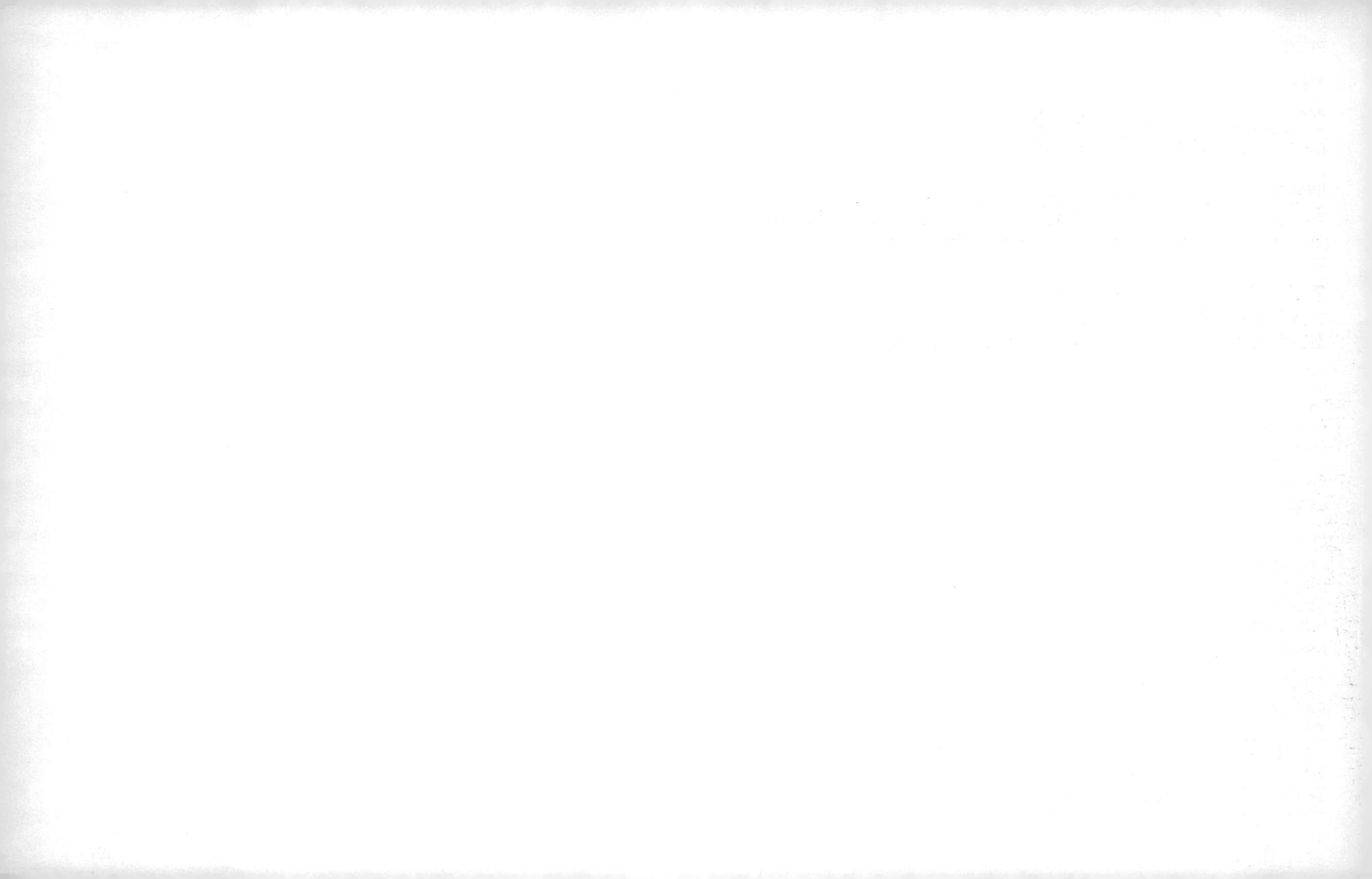

# Section 16
# Photomacrography

**R.R. Phillips**, FBIPP, FRPS
Head of Medical Illustration
Middlesex Hospital and Medical School, London

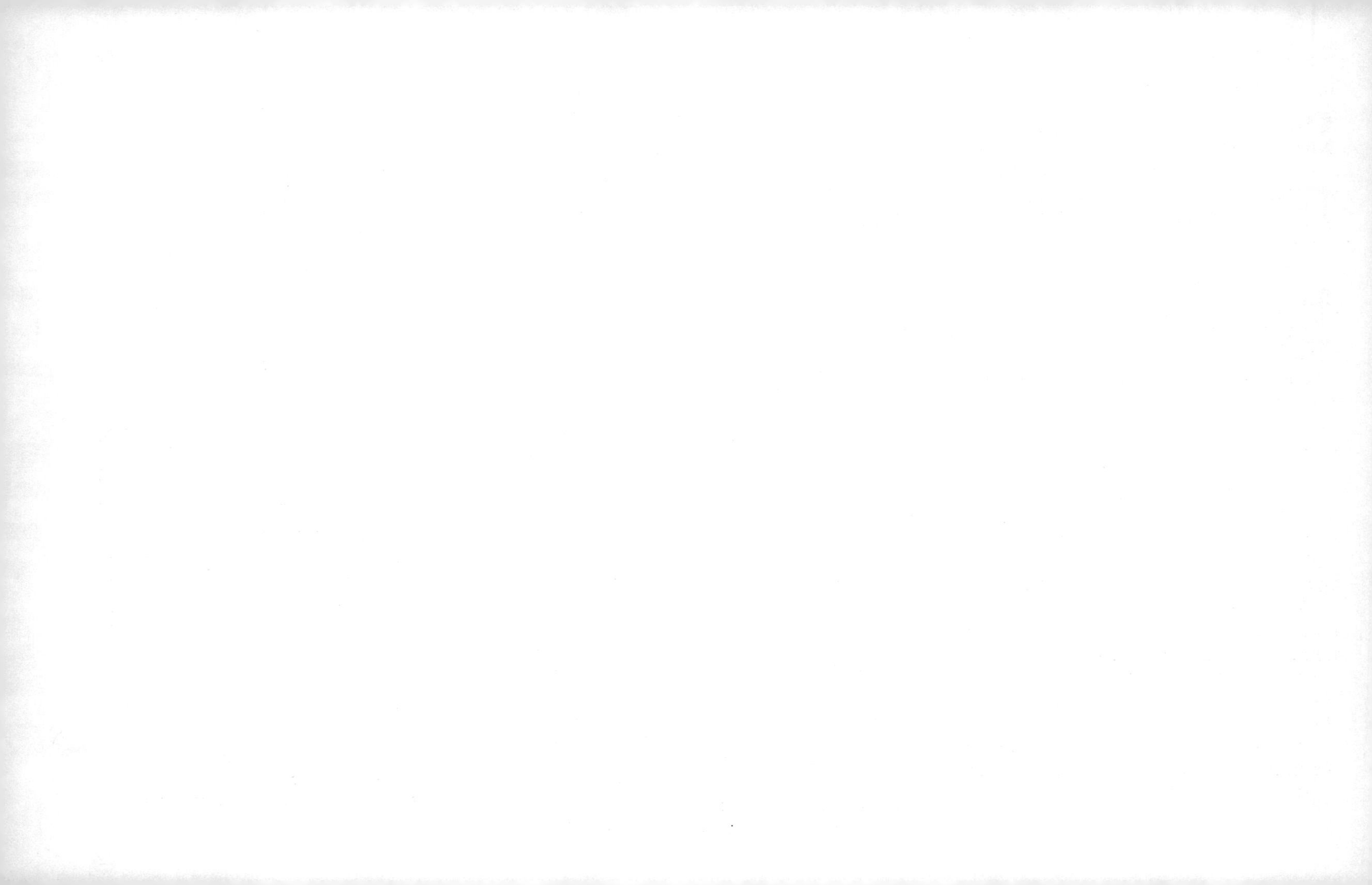

## 16.1 INTRODUCTION

Photomacrography is photography where the image size is greater than the object size; it fills the gap between close-up photography and photomicrography. The degree of magnification may be between one and twenty five times.

Another definition is based on the optical system used. Historically the simple microscope consisted of an objective lens only, as opposed to the compound microscope with objective lens and eyepiece. Photography with the simple microscope became known as photomacrography and with the compound microscope, photomicrography.

Much medical photography especially in the fields of dermatology, dentistry, ophthalmology and pathology falls into this category – only general principles will be covered here. The student should refer to other sections as appropriate.

Note that whilst 'macrophotography' and 'photomacrography' mean the same thing 'microphotography' and 'photomicrography' are very different procedures – the former being the production of very small photographic images of large objects, especially for example, in the production of microelectronic circuits.

Photography in this range of magnification has always presented technical problems, but the perfection of the single-lens-reflex camera, computer designed macro lenses and computerized electronic flashguns has made the task very much simpler.

## 16.2 OPTICAL CONSIDERATIONS

### 16.2.1 Lenses

Ordinarily photography produces an image smaller than the original objects photographed and camera lenses are designed to produce their optimum results under these conditions, i.e. with the object conjugate considerably longer than the image conjugate. Photomacrography requires an opposite set of conditions.

Specially made lenses such as the Leitz *Summar* or Zeiss *Luminars* are preferable for good quality photomacrography, but carefully selected normal camera lenses may be mounted and used in reverse to give excellent results. Variable bellows extensions facilitate continuously variable changes of magnification. Whether high quality short-mount special lenses or normal camera lenses are used, comprehensive practical tests must be carried out on each, in order to

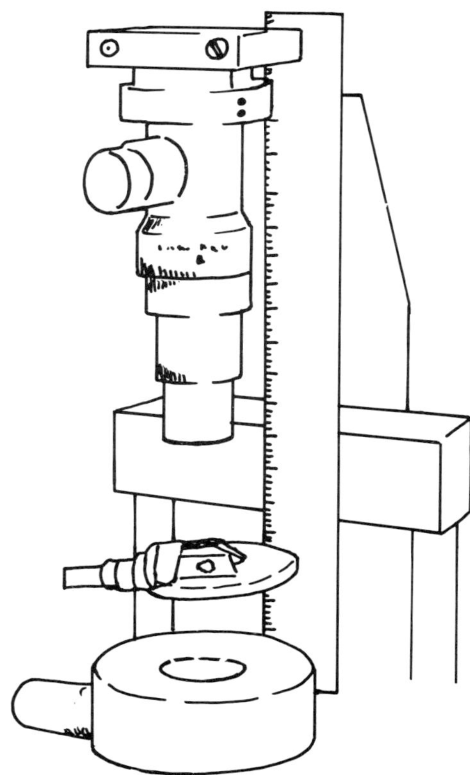

***Figure 16.1*** *The Zeiss Tessovar zoom-lens system for photomacrography complete with rotating stage and transillumination condenser*

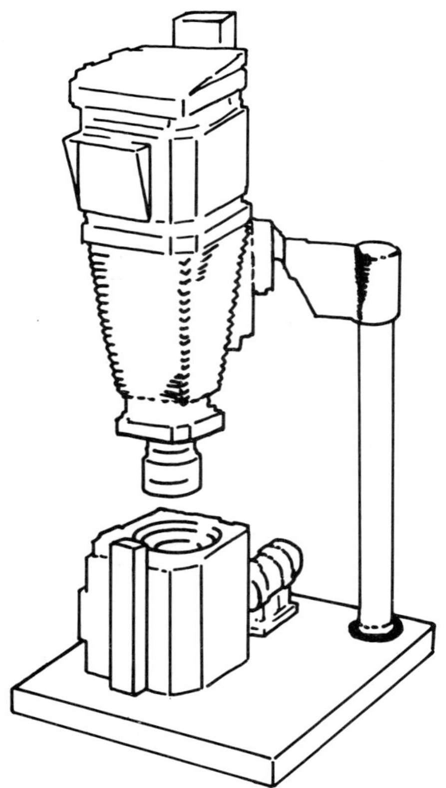

***Figure 16.2*** *The large format vertical macrocamera such as a Nikon Multiphot or Leitz Aristophot*

determine the aperture which produces optimum results (stopping down too far drastically reduces resolution). The so-called 'macro' or 'micro' lenses supplied by many 35 mm camera manufacturers will produce an image of 1:1 without further extension. Higher magnifications are achieved by using bellows attachments, but even these lenses should then be reversed for better correction of aberrations and increased performance.

Photomacrographic zoom systems such as the Zeiss *Tessovar* offer an easily used, compact and variable method of producing magnification from ×0.8 to ×14 (on 35 mm film). Such equipment produces acceptable results with the minimum amount of setting up. Various manufacturers supply vertical large format macrocameras as complete systems, e.g. Nikon *Multiphot* and Leitz *Aristophot*, based on optical bench principles. These have the advantage of being very rigid at long bellows extension, and have a wide range of accessories purpose built for macro work such as specimen stages with rack and pinion focussing and built in condensers for Köhler illumination. Both these types of camera have been reviewed in the literature and the student should be familiar with them.

### 16.2.2 Formulae

Probably the most important factor in choosing lenses for photomacrography is the scale of reproduction required. The scale or magnification ($M$) is defined as the ratio of the linear size of the object ($O$) to the linear size of the image ($I$).

$$M=\frac{I}{O}$$

As the lens to film distance ($V$) and the lens to object distance ($U$) are in a fixed relationship,

$$M=\frac{V}{U}$$

Various components may then be derived from these equations:

$$I=\frac{O\times V}{U},\ O=\frac{U\times V}{V},\ V=\frac{I\times V}{O},\ U=\frac{O\times V}{I}$$

The relationship between the extension required ($V$), the focal length of lens ($F$), and magnification ($M$) is given by:

$V = \mathrm{F}\quad (I+M)$

This is the single most useful formula in macrophotography, as it enables one to calculate magnification from focal length and extension or *vice versa*.

The object distance $U$ can also be calculated from the formula:

$$U = \frac{F\quad (I+M)}{M}$$

This is usually of great importance in photomacrography because the object distance, or 'free working distance' is the space between the subject and camera lens. As magnification increases this distance decreases. The object distance determines the space available for lighting or lens accessories and will also be important in ophthalmic and dental work where it is inadvisable to approach the subject too closely.

As magnification increases the object distance approaches closely the focal length of the lens, whereas the image distance gets very large. It is for this reason that focussing in photomacrography is very difficult. Undoubtedly the best technique is to preset the image distance for a given magnification and move the whole camera/lens assembly back and forth to focus.

### 16.2.3 Depth of field

In photomacrography depth of field is always limited, so obtaining maximum depth becomes especially important. Depth of field is dependent only upon the magnification and the *f* number used. Stopping down the lens increases depth of field but may also decrease resolution due to diffraction. In macro work if greater depth of field is required it may be better to obtain it by lowering the magnification and using a longer focal length lens – then subsequently enlarging the negative more to obtain the longest focal length consistent with the magnification required and the extension available.

### 16.2.4 Exposure

The *f*-stops engraved on a lens are calibrated for the lens focussed on infinity. At very close ranges some exposure compensation is necessary; the simplest formula for this is:

$$E = (1 + M)^2,$$

where $E$ is the exposure factor and $M$ the magnification, e.g. for a magnification of ×5 the exposure factor would be ×36.

Supplementary close-up lenses do not require an increase in exposure because the magnifications achieved are low ( a 3 dioptre lens fitted to a standard 50 mm lens only gives 1:6) and because they effectively lower the focal length thus increasing exposure at any set aperture. Such lenses are rarely used in medical photomacrography (the exception being the Nikon *Medical Nikkor* lens).

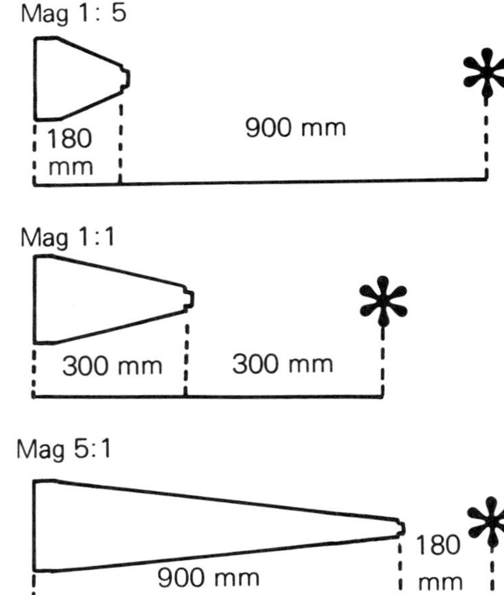


***Figure 16.3*** *The relationship between image distance and object distance at different magnifications. As magnification increases so the object distance gets very small and the image distance gets very large. Hence the need to move the whole camera back and forth to obtain accurate focussing*

## 16.3 LIGHTING

Because the object is small and the distance between object and objective short, special lighting arrangements are necessary for both opaque and transparent objects. In the latter respect, it should be noted that histological sections may sometimes be photographed using the condenser enlarger whose optical system fulfils both the illumination requirements and the correct conjugate proportion for photomacrography.

### 16.3.1 Incident light (opaque objects)

The broad principles of photographic lighting still apply, but must be achieved in a miniaturized form using one or more of the following light sources:

(1) Miniature focussing light or small electronic flash sources, used with or without a reflector or small 'flood' lamp as a fill-in.
(2) Small annular light unit (electronic flash or fluorescent tube) mounted around the objective.
(3) Ring of small individually switched lamps, in suitable reflector, also around the objective.
(4) Fibre-optics – flexible, small, cold source.

The use of standard studio lighting is contra-indicated since the large scale of the lamp in relation to the size of the subject will fail to produce crisp shadows or small sharp highlights.

### 16.3.2 Transmitted light (transparent subject)

Best results are obtained by using a system incorporating a small light source and a suitable diameter condenser. The image of the light source is focussed by the condenser onto the iris diaphragm of the lens. This produces a bright even field of illumination. Image quality is determined by rigidity, focus and control of the diaphragm. Excess diffraction must always be avoided. Dark-ground illumination may be used with most photomacrographic techniques and follows standard principles.

## 16.4 SPECIAL TECHNIQUES

***(1) Immersion***. One technique for increasing depth of field is to immerse the subject to be photographed in a fluid of higher refractive index than air. Increasing the refractive index increases the depth of field. Any liquid may be used but water ($n$=1.33), glycerol ($n$=1.47.) and cedar oil ($n$=1.51) are the most

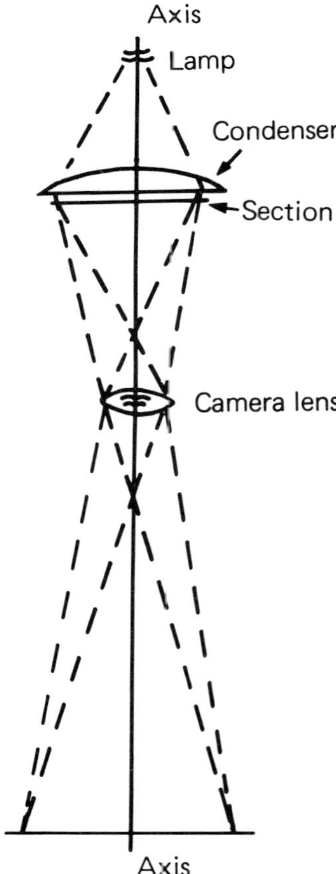


***Figure 16.4*** *The optical arrangement for recording large macro-sections of histological preparations. Note that this optical arrangement is found in a condenser enlarger and these can be used with great success*

useful. One has to be particularly careful about air bubbles in the fluid especially as it warms up. Another advantage of fluid immersion is that surface reflections are entirely eliminated but the very 'flat' lighting can be a disappointment. Immersion can give a small specimen such as a biopsy a more natural appearance, but this buoyancy can be a problem with larger specimens causing them to have to be fixed to the base of the container.

***(2) Light scanning.*** Another way to increase the apparent depth of sharp focus is to illuminate the subject with a narrow slit of light which is restricted to those parts of the subject which will be in sharp focus. A series of exposures are then made by moving the subject backwards or forwards during the exposure. A sufficiently large number of exposures need to be recorded to avoid any unevenness in the beam lighting. The technique is not suitable for hollow concave objects or ones which will move between exposures.

## 16.5 APPLICATIONS IN MEDICAL PHOTOGRAPHY

(1) Clinical photography to show, for example, fine textural changes in the skin, conditions affecting the hair shaft or details of blood vessels in the eye or nail fold.

(2) Fine small detail in pathological specimens.

(3) Bacterial and mycological cultures, for surface appearance, growth structure and colony pattern.

(4) To show fine instruments (micro surgery) and also micro electronic equipment detail.

(5) Histological sections of whole or part of specimen, frequently to supplement higher power photomicrography.

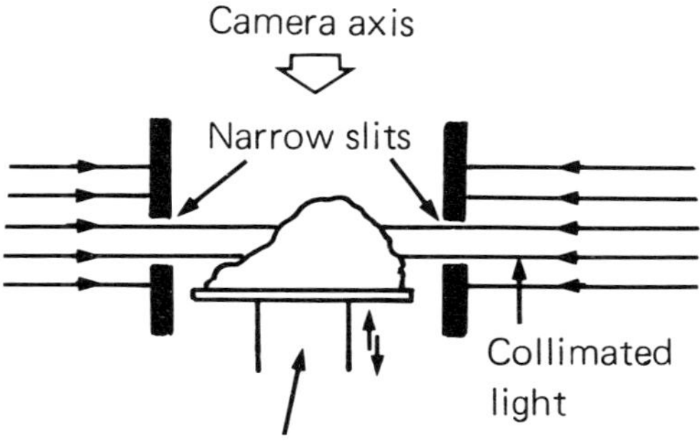


***Figure 16.5*** *The light-scanning method of obtaining infinite depth-of-field photomacrography*

## References

Bracegirdle, B. (1971). The Zeiss Tessovar and photography in the macro range. *Med. Biol. Illustr.*, **21**, 215-222

Brackenbury, W. and Steward, J. (1963). Macroscopic appearances of mucosal biopsies from the small intestine. *Med. Biol. Illustr.*, **13**, 220-227

Cory, L. (1962). Rapid focussing of single lens reflex cameras at very close range. *J. Biol. Photogr. Assoc.*, **30**, 81-83

Crooks, H. (1954). Photography of epidermal ridges and superficial blood capillaries of the fingers. *Med. Biol. Illustr.*, **3**, 198–205

De Veer, W. (1979). Photomacrography of microsections with a modified Illumitran copy set-up. *J. Biol. Photogr.*, **47**, 127-129

Hill, B. (1974). Low power photomicrography and photomacrography using the Nikon Multiphot system. *Med. Biol. Illustr.*, **24**, 153-159

Kodak. (1977). *Close-up Photography and Photomacrography.* (Publication N12) (Rochester, NY: Eastman Kodak Ltd)

Williams, A.R. (1977). Immersion techniques for increasing depth of field. *Brit. J. Photogr.*, **124**, 5

## Practical projects

(1) Produce photomacrographs at ×5 and ×15 (primary magnification) of a transparent subject which requires brightfield illumination. Submit exhibition quality 12″ × 10″ black-and-white prints and colour transparencies of the same field.

(2) Photograph a small, flat, moist subject such as the cut surface of an orange to show the structure and texture. Experiment with various lighting arrangements. Produce a colour projection tranparency and then convert it to a black-and-white print via internegative.

(3) Photograph a small highly reflective object such as a micro-surgery instrument,
(*a*) the whole instrument
(*b*) at high magnification to show some detail, e.g. a cutting edge.
Produce two matched colour prints along with diagrams of your lighting technique and a description of your method.

(4) Photograph any active animal, e.g. moth, fish, mouse, spider, fly at ×2–×5 magnification on a colour transparency. (The subject must be living, unanaesthetized, untranquilized and unrefrigerated).

(5) Produce a photomacrograph at ×10–×20 of any subject which requires reflected and transmitted light simultaneously. Produce in a medium of your choice but include records of reflected light only and transmitted light only.

## Examination questions

Q.1 With the aid of diagrams compare a simple microscope with a compound microscope. Briefly describe the arrangement for critical illumination with a simple microscope.

Q.2 Describe at least two techniques for increasing depth of field in photomacrography. Be sure to give any advantages/disadvantages.

Q.3 Explain the relationships between aperture, focal length, depth of field and resolution in photomacrography. Suggest criteria for selecting the focal length of lens to be used.

Q.4 Draw a ray diagram for photomacrography of a transparent subject at 1:1 magnification with critical illumination.

Q.5 What factors determine 'free working distance' in photomacrography and why is this distance of importance in medical work? Calculate the free working distance for a 50 mm lens at a magnification of ×4.25.

Q.6 Discuss the factors affecting image quality in photomacrography.

Q.7 Why is normal studio lighting unsuitable for opaque macroscopic subjects? Describe fully the equipment which you would choose for the task.

Q.8 Describe fully the photomacrography of either:
(*a*) The epidermal ridges,
(*b*) The capillaries of the cuticle, or
(*c*) The gingival margin.

*Multiple choice questions (any of the statements may be true or false)*

Q.9 In photomacrography:
(*a*) The object distance approaches the focal length as the magnification increases.
(*b*) The magnification is equal to the image distance divided by the object distance.
(*c*) The extension required is equal to the focal length multiplied by the magnification.
(*d*) The use of supplementary (close-up) lenses shortens the effective focal length.
(*e*) Exposure needs to be increased by a factor equivalent to the magnification squared.

Q.10 You are asked to photograph at a magnification of ×10 a histological section of monkey brain which has been silver stained.
(*a*) No precautions against infection are necessary.
(*b*) Best results will occur from using a dark-field lighting technique.
(*c*) If using an asymmetrical lens not designed for photomacrography it should be reversed on the camera.
(*d*) The image distance can be calculated by dividing the desired magnification by the object distance.
(*e*) It is important to insulate both camera and specimen from vibration.

# Section 17
# Photomicrography

**R.R. Phillips**, FBIPP, FRPS
Head of Medical Illustration
Middlesex Hospital and Medical School, London

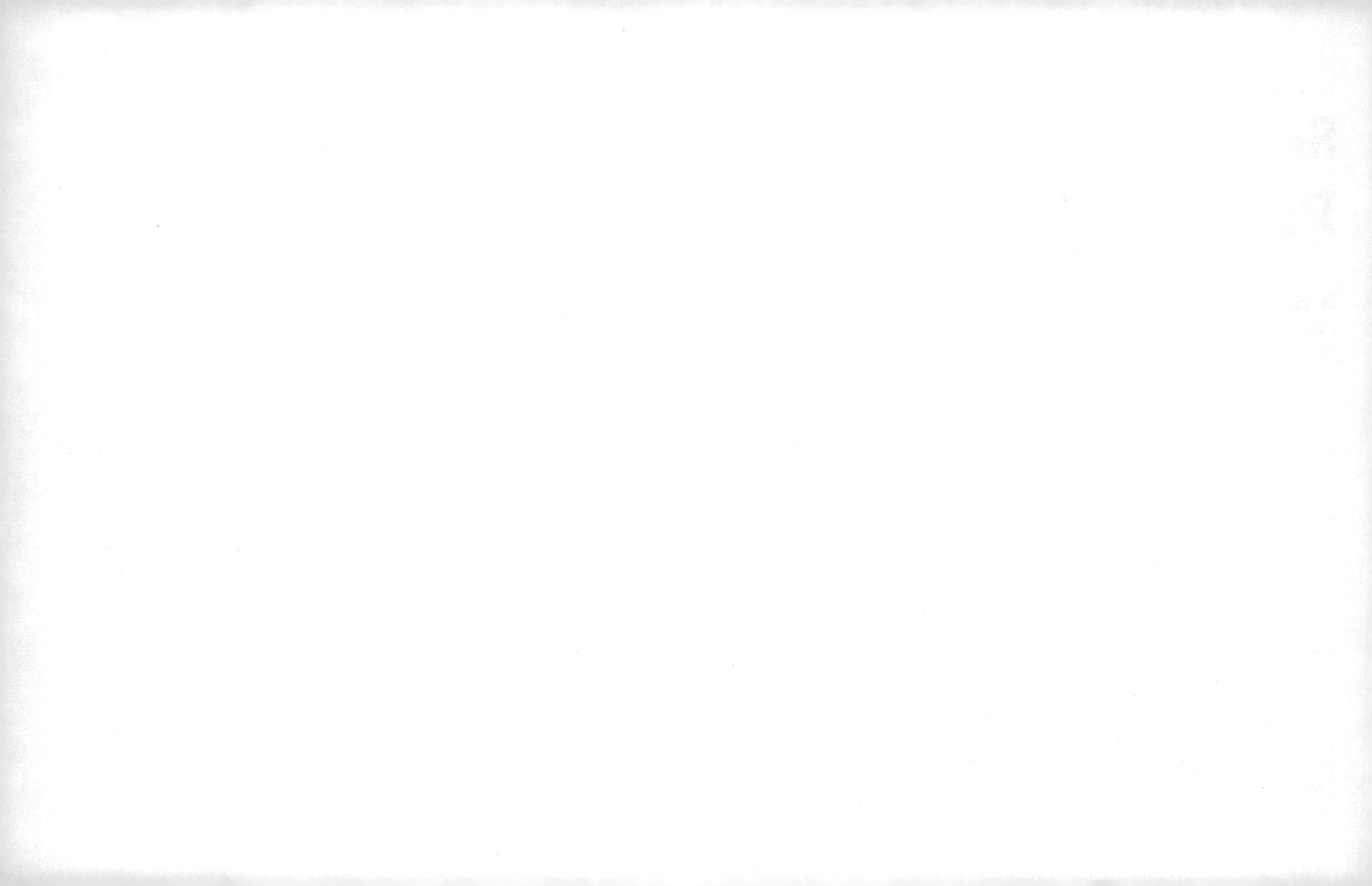

## 17.1 DEFINITION

Photomicrography is the photography of small preparations by means of a compound microscope and a camera system. Magnification may range from ×30 to ×1000.

Photomicrography should not be confused with microphotography which involves making extremely small photographic images of large objects as in the production of micro-electronic circuits.

## 17.2 INTRODUCTION

With the advent of advanced automatic photomicrographic apparatus, this technique is usually carried out within departments of pathology, or where numerous and varied techniques are required a specialist photomicrographic unit is established. Medical photographers are therefore seldom called upon to produce photomicrographs routinely, but their advice may be constantly sought to help improve quality and to trace faults. A working knowledge of microscopes and current photomicroscopes is therefore essential. Main areas of trouble include colour temperature of system and films to use; correction filters and the mired shift; reciprocity failure in fluorescence work; use of substage and field diaphragms and identifying the plane of intruding dirt: the interpretation of exposure meter readings (spot or integrated) and exposure controls manipulation.

The interested student will also gain much by personal contact with laboratory staff who will be able to give background information on slide preparation, staining and nomenclature.

Since the subject is too large to be covered adequately in a single section of this book, and fortunately this is the one area of medical photography where many excellent comprehensive texts do exist, the student is advised to consult these specialist publications with particular reference to the basic areas of study mentioned below.

## 17.3 ESSENTIAL AREAS OF STUDY

***(1) The compound microscope*** – general principles, diffraction theory and resolution, magnification, depth of field, depth of focus. A working knowledge of all the main mechanical and optical components, their names and their functions. The optical path through a compound microscope – two stage magnification. Mechanical and optical tube lengths.

***(2) Objectives*** – main types and their

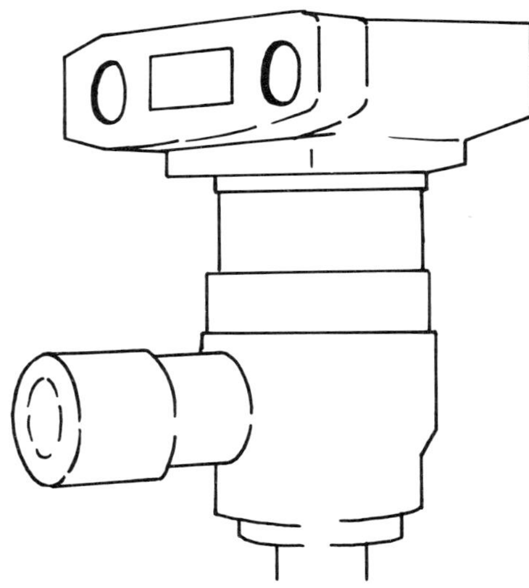

***Figure 17.1*** *The simplest arrangement for obtaining photomicrographs is an attachment which fits onto the microscope eyepiece and carries a parfocal camera and viewing piece*

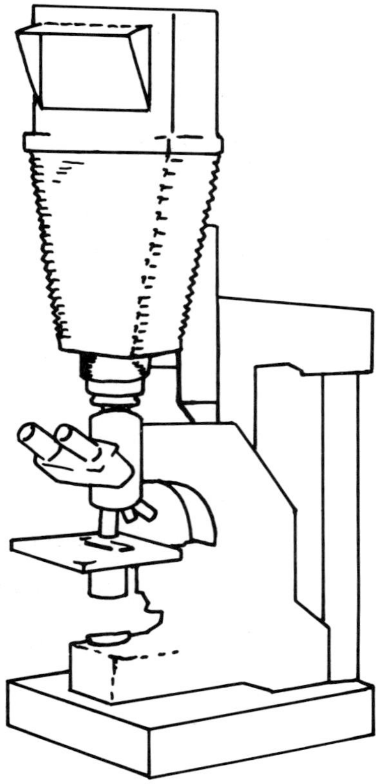

***Figure 17.2*** *Large format cameras are especially made on rigid vertical stands for attachment to laboratory microscopes*

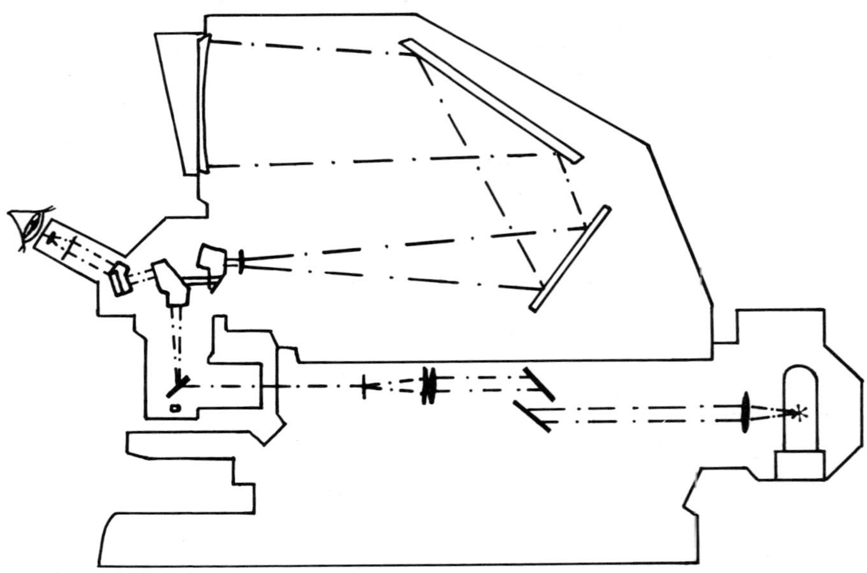

***Figure 17.3*** *The complex and expensive photomicroscope is purpose-built for photomicrography and has many refinements such as choice of several illuminants. They usually have built-in 35 mm and large format cameras with automatic exposure assessment*

merits, focal lengths, numerical apertures and magnifications. Resolution and 'useful' magnification. Field curvature and aberration correction, correction for coverslip thickness, working distance. Oil and water immersion objectives.

***(3) Oculars*** – main types and their suitability for photographic use, range of magnifications. Bertrand lenses.

***(4) Substage condensers*** – common types in use, focal lengths and numerical apertures, relationship with objectives, specialist condensers.

**(5) *Light sources*** – those in current use, including tungsten–halogen, coiled tungsten filament, xenon arc, electronic flash, Considerations of colour temperature and colour photography.

**(6) *Methods of illumination*** – Nelsonian or critical illumination, Köhler illumination. The complete optical aligning of lighting and microscope components achieved by careful application of Köhler illumination is the basis of all high quality photomicrography. The student must be completely familiar with this technique.

**(7) *The camera*** – problems of stability, vibration, shutter position, camera distance from exit point of ocular, types in use – including large format systems and 35 mm systems.

**(8) *Determination of magnification*** –calculation formulae, scaled grids and stage micrometers.

**(9) *Types of film*** – choice of emulsion, monochromatic and colour, with particular reference to the control of contrast and range of acceptance.

**(10) *Exposure determination*** – screen metering, spot and integrated measuring, automatic exposure controls and their potential problems.

**(11) *Filtration*** – Use of correction and didymium filters for colour photography. Applications of normal photographic filtration principles to increase or decrease image contrast with the various stains in monochrome reproduction.

**(12) *Routine applications*** – to produce photographs of stained histological sections, blood and bone marrow films, bacteria and fungi.

**(13) *Special techniques*** – the student must be familiar with the principles and practice of:

(a) Dark ground (dark field)
(b) Polarization,
(c) Phase contrast,
(d) Fluorescence,
(e) Interference,
(f) Epi-illumination,
(g) Optical staining, e.g. Rheinberg,
(h) Cine and time-lapse,
(i) Infrared and ultraviolet, and
(j) Stereomicroscopy.

**(14) *Electron microscopy*** – principles and practice and photographic problems involved, including scanning electron microscopy.

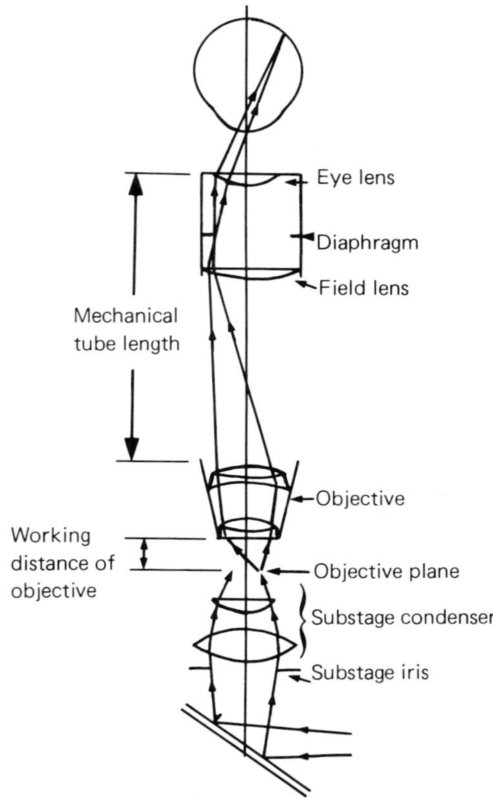


***Figure 17.4*** *The optical pathway of the compound microscope*

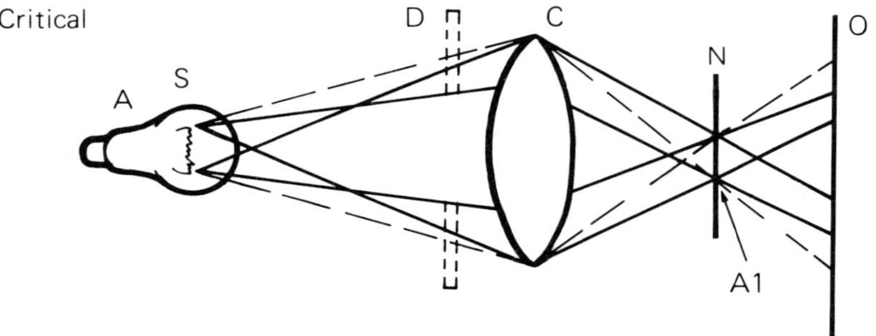


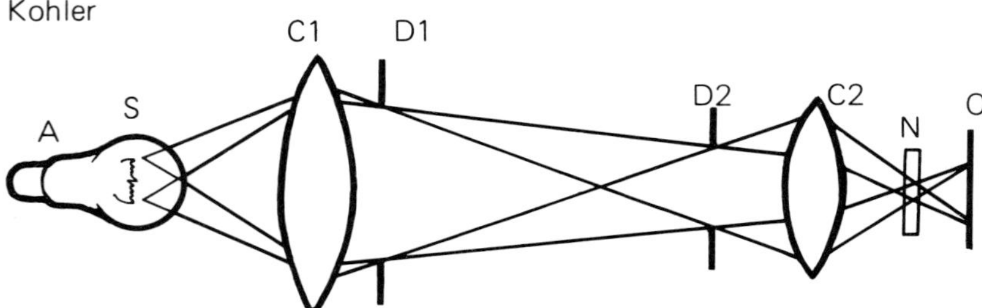


***Figure 17.5*** *The two standard forms of illumination used in photomicroscopy. In critical illumination (above) an image of the sources is focussed in the subject plane (N) whereas in Köhler illumination an image of the source (S) is focussed in the plane of the substage diaphragm D2. The field diaphragm D1 controls the diameter of the cone of illumination. Köhler illumination gives evenly illuminated specimens, maximum resolution, minimum light scatter and the most efficient use of the light source*

## 17.4 KÖHLER ILLUMINATION

It is imperative that the student is able to set up this type of illumination on any photomicroscope almost without having to think about it. Practice is the only way to achieve this level of competence. Use the test questions below to assess performance:

(1) Where does the first real image of the filament occur?
(2) If the image of the filament at the field stop is not in sharp focus how do you adjust this?
(3) How do you centre the lamp?
(4) What is the function of the field stop?
(5) Where does the first image of the lamp diaphragm appear?
(6) How can you demonstrate that the field diaphragm is in the plane of the specimen?
(7) After centring and focussing the image of the lamp filament onto the field diaphragm what do you do next?
(8) When viewing the objective back plane what images should you be able to see here?
(9) Where are the three locations that a real image forms of the field diaphragm?

(10) How far should the field diaphragm be closed?
(11) Where do you see a sharp image of the substage (or aperture) diaphragm?
(12) What is the effect of closing the substage diaphragm too far?
(13) How is the image of the field diaphragm centred?
(14) Where and how do you focus a sharp image of the field diaphragm?
(15) Where is the Ramsden disk or exit pupil? and what images are located here?
(16) What observations can be made by looking at the rear focal plane of the objective?
(17) What is the function of the Bertrand lens?
(18) What are the two most common methods of determining the correct setting for the substage diaphragm?
(19) What observations can be made by removing the eyepiece?
(20) What is the function of the substage condenser?

The student should be able to answer all of the above questions without hesitation.

## 17.5 PREPARATION OF THE MICROSCOPE SLIDE

Most histological materials examined on the photomicroscope are prepared by sectioning them into very thin slices, staining them and mounting them in a mounting medium between a glass slide and a cover glass. Before sectioning the specimen usually has to be fixed and hardened – ethyl alcohol with 1% acetic acid is very popular for this but it does cause cell shrinkage. It is of great advantage to have an understanding of the common stains and of the colour produced by staining and counter-staining of specific tissues and the mounting of sections. The thickness of the section, density of staining and thickness of the cover slip are important factors in the image quality.

In general a good section is very thin (1 or 2 $\mu$m), well stained (or heavily stained for low power work), mounted in a clear mounting medium of high refractive on a thin slide, with a high quality thin glass çoverslide.

A bad section is thick (5 $\mu$m), understained for lower powers or overstained for high powers, uneven thickness or staining, thick microslides or coverglasses (or worse still plastic), mounted in a medium with a colour cast.

The actual processes of cutting and staining sections are not the concern of the photographer, but it is wise to have some understanding of the procedure. Undoubtedly the most commonly encountered stains are haematoxylin and eosin which appear as magenta and pink, respectively, but many others will be found in medical practice such as:aniline blue, basic fuchsin, congo red, crystal violet, eosin yellow, methyl green, neutral red, safranin orange, and toluidine blue. The advanced student should know the transmission characteristics for these dyes and the appropriate filters to render each satisfactorily in monochrome. The basic student should remember the colours of 'H and E' (haematoxylin and eosin) and that a Wratten number 58 (green) filter enhances the rendition and separation of these two dyes in monochrome, and that a didymium filter does the same in colour photography.

## References


Hoffman, R. (1979). Photomicrography using the modulation contrast system. *J. Biol. Photogr.*, **47**, 111-116

Klosevych, S. (1966). Photomicrography – the importance of cover glass thickness. *J. Biol. Photogr. Assoc.*, **34**, 1 and 101

Klosevych, S. (1974). Microscopy and photomicrography – Part 1. (Image formation and optics, aberrations and magnification.). *J. Biol. Photogr. Assoc.*, **42**, 123-131

Klosevych, S. (1974). Microscopy and photomicrography – Part 2. (Objectives, aberrations, resolving power, condensers.). *J. Biol. Photogr. Assoc.*, **42**, 147-160

Klosevych, S. (1975). Microscopy and photomicrography – Part 3. (Abbe and Köhler illumination.). *J. Biol. Photogr. Assoc.*, **43**, 30-38

Klosevych, S. (1975). Microscopy and photomicrography – Part 4. (Phase contrast, interference and filters.). *J. Biol. Photogr. Assoc.*, **43**, 51-69

Klosevych, S. (1975). Microscopy and photomicrography – Part 5. (Dark field, polarized light, epi-illumination and fluorescence techniques.). *J. Biol. Photogr. Assoc.*, **43**, 119-139

Klosevych, S. (1975). Microscopy and photomicrography – Part 6. (Conclusion and bibliography.). *J. Biol. Photogr. Assoc.*, **43**, 187-189

Kodak. (1973). *Electron Microscopy and Photography.* (Rochester NY: Eastman Kodak Ltd)

Kodak. (1975). *Photomicrography Colour Film 2483.* (Publication P302) (Rochester, NY: Eastman Kodak Ltd.)

Kodak. (1980). *Photography through the Microscope.* (Publication P2) (Rochester, NY: Eastman Kodak Ltd.)

Lawson, D. (1972). *Photomicrography.* (London: Academic Press)

Loveland, R. (1970). *Photomicrography; a Comprehensive Treatise.* (2 volumes) (New York: John Wiley)

Smith, A. and Bruton, J. (1978). *A Colour Atlas of Histological Staining Techniques.* (London: Wolfe Medical Publications)

Vetter, J. (1963). The production and use of Rheinberg colour differential filters. *J. Biol. Photogr. Assoc.*, **31**, 15-18

Vetter, J. (1974). A systematic approach to colour photomicrography – Part 1. (The microscope, optics and alignment.). *Med. Biol. Illustr.*, **24**, 74-85

Vetter, J. (1974). A systematic approach to colour photomicrography – Part 2. (Cameras and photographic techniques.). *Med. Biol. Illustr.*, **24**, 140-152

Weakley, B. (1972). *A Beginner's Handbook in Biological Electron Microscopy.* (Edinburgh: Churchill Livingstone)

Weiss, C. (1976). Optical staining of colourless specimens with infrared colour film. *J. Biol. Photogr. Assoc.*, **44**, 86-87

Williams, A.R. (1978). Incident illumination photomicrography. Part 1. *J. Audiovis. Media Med.*, **1**, 15-18

Williams, A.R. (1978). Incident illumination photomicrography. Part 2. *J. Audiovis. Media Med.*, **1**, 85-87

## *Practical projects*

(1) Really study the texts cited in the bibliography. All students should be at least familiar with *Photography Through the Microscope* by Kodak and advanced students should consult the excellent publications by Lawson, Loveland, Klosevych and Vetter.

(2) Practice setting up Köhler illumination on all types of microscope and at all magnifications from very low power to very high power oil immersion.

(3) Photograph a normally stained section at medium power (*a*) with the substage diaphragm wide open, (*b*) closed to the optimum point, and (*c*) closed well beyond the optimum point. Produce a series of black-and-white prints and commment on your results.

(4) Take photomicrographs of at least five different stain combinations in monochrome at medium power. Demonstrate the use of filters to enhance the rendition of the various stains. Submit a series of 'control' and 'filter' prints accompanied by notes on your technique.

(5) Produce two photomicrographs of the same section by Köhler illumination, (*a*) low power (primary magnification × 20), (*b*) high power (primary magnification × 50). Demonstrate your knowledge of the filtration, film and processing techniques associated with photomicrography that produce a matching pair of reproduction quality black-and-white prints. Indicate magnification by the addition of a bar scale upon each print.

(6) Photograph an unstained section (or very thinly stained), (*a*) with conventional bright-field transmission, (*b*) with dark ground illumination, (*c*) with Rheinberg technique, (*d*) with phase contrast, and (*e*) with interference technique (or as many of those techniques as you have access to). Submit a series of colour transparencies with notes on your technique.

(7) Photograph at medium power a well stained H and E section, (*a*) as a 10" × 8" black and white print, (*b*) as a 35 mm colour transparency, and (*c*) as a 10" × 8" colour print. Pay particular attention to filtration and colour rendition.

## *Examination questions*

Q.1 Write brief notes on the following:
(*a*) Apochromatic objective,
(*b*) Nicol prism,
(*c*) England finder,
(*d*) Numerical aperture,
(*e*) Mechanical tube length,
(*f*) Didymium filter.

Q.2 Discuss the following specialized photomicrographic techniques:
(*a*) Phase contrast,
(*b*) Interference contrast,
(*c*) Optical staining, e.g. Rheinberg.

Q.3 Compare and contrast the following:
(*a*) Apochromatic and planapochromatic objectives,
(*b*) Mechanical and optical tube length,
(*c*) Numerical aperture and focal length,
(*d*) Huygenian and negative eyepieces,
(*e*) Aplanatic and achromatic condensers.

Q.4 With the aid of simple diagrams describe the setting up of Köhler illumination.

Q.5 Using the information engraved on most objectives how can you determine the type or purpose of the objective? magnifying power? NA? aberrations corrected? Cite specific examples.

Q.6 Provide diagrams and notes to describe, (*a*) the image-forming pathway and (*b*) the illuminating pathway of a compound microscope. What is (i) Köhler illumination, (ii) critical illumination?

Q.7 Describe fully the use of ultraviolet radiation in photomicrography.

Q.8 Using a simple diagram describe how the transmission electron microscope works. What peculiarities are there in the way that photographic emulsions respond to the electron beam?

*Multiple choice questions (any of the statements may be true or false)*

Q.9 In Köhler illumination:
(*a*) The image of the filament is formed at the substage diaphragm,
(*b*) The image of the field diaphragm appears in the plane of the specimen,
(*c*) The effects of moving the substage diaphragm can be monitored by looking at the objective's rear focal plane,
(*d*) The substage diaphragm is focussed with the substage condenser,
(*e*) The specimen must be sharply focussed before a sharp image of the field diaphragm is set.

Q.10 In photomicrography:
(*a*) Fluorite objectives are used for ultraviolet work,
(*b*) Achromatic condensers are corrected for spherical aberration,
(*c*) Nicol prisms are used for phase contrast techniques,
(*d*) Didymium filters enhance the rendition of certain tissue stains in colour photography,
(*e*) Spherical aberration can be corrected by changing mechanical tube length.

# Section 18
# Infrared photography

**R.J. Lunnon**, MPhil, FBIPP, FRPS, AIMBI, SBStJ
Director of Medical Illustration
Institute of Child Health and Hospitals for Sick Children

## 18.1 INTRODUCTION

One important function of medical photography is to extend the range of spectral visualization of the human eye: infrared photography is therefore acting as an investigative tool, discovering new facts about clinical cases. The range of infrared radiation applicable to photography extends from the termination of the red part of the spectrum at about 700 nm to a wavelength of about 900 nm, this limit being set by the sensitivity of the photographic emulsion. Other infrared sensitive surfaces such as cathode ray tubes may be used to visualize the infrared image. Infrared photography does not record heat – this is the province of thermography. Black-and-white infrared photography can be defined as the technique of focussing an infrared image with a conventional camera lens onto an emulsion sensitive to infrared radiation. These emulsions are sensitive to violet, blue and red light as well as to infrared; therefore a filter has to be used over the camera lens (or sometimes the light source), to block the unwanted visible light rays. The subject producing the image reflects or transmits varying amounts of the infrared radiation falling on it; or it may emit luminescence in the infrared region when lit with visible light.

## 18.2 APPLICATIONS

In some fields of clinical investigation extensive work has been reported on the use of medical infrared photography; other areas of application are still untouched and await the attention of the research orientated medical photographer. Space permits only a brief review of applications – the keen student is urged to consult the more comprehensive texts.

Infrared radiation has two useful properties when used for medical photography; firstly, its ability to penetrate the superficial layers of the epidermis and to reveal structures beneath them and secondly, the reflection and absorption characteristics differ from those of the visible spectrum. These two properties form the basis of all the reported applications.

***Venous studies***. Venous blood absorbs infrared heavily, whereas oxygenated blood reflects infrared well; thus vascular disorders such as varicose veins or venous obstruction are clearly delineated. Only the superficial veins can be recorded due to the limited depth of penetration. The sinuous curved stems of varicose veins are clearly seen and the changing pattern of superficial vessels in the breasts and abdomen due to pregnancy have been mapped. When one of the main venous trunks of the body is obstructed a 'collateral' circulation develops to circumvent the problem. These engorged and distended cutaneous veins stand out more vividly in an infrared photograph, and obstruction of the femoral, subclavian and portal veins, the vena cava and mediastinal tumours are classic examples of applications for infrared photography. Others have reported the usefulness of the technique for studying venous patterns in congenital heart disease and pericardial effusion, in thrombotic conditions and in venous stasis, and for hypertension. A great deal of work has been done on the vascular patterns of the female breast during pregnancy or in neoplastic disease. The vascular changes in diabetic patients have been mapped by infrared as have postprandial engorgements of veins. The clarity of the venous record obtained depends upon various factors such as the thickness of subcutaneous fat, the thickness of the vessel walls and the depth of the vessel from the skin surface.

***Ophthalmology***. In cases where an opaque cornea is obscuring the pupil, its size, shape and position can be revealed by infrared photography. Dark brown pigmented irides often record lighter in tone than blue ones, the deeply pigmented trabeculae often registering the lightest. Infrared colour film has been used to penetrate a vitreous humour clouded with blood to provide a record of the fundus. Similarly, cataracts have been penetrated to record retinal changes in retinitis pigmentosa, and melanotic lesions become strongly emphasized in the false colour record. Scleral melanosis can be distinguished from associated vascularities and vascular lesions of the choroid have been recorded through the retina. Infrared radiation has been used to record the diameter of the pupil in numerous studies of physical and physiological effects in both human and animal subjects (since the eye does not see infrared the pupil does not respond to this radiation).

***Gross specimens***. There is increased detail and differentiation between silicotic and pneumoconiotic lesions from the surrounding lung tissue. Injection techniques using mercuric sulphide (red cinnabar) into arteries and suspended carbon (Indian ink) into veins can be used to record these vessels as white (reflecting infrared) or black (absorbing infrared) respectively. The translucent amniotic membrane is penetrated to reveal details of the foetus. It is possible to distinguish between otherwise visually similar substances, for example, silver sulphide deposits and melanin granules in localized argyria. Various tissues exhibit very strong infrared luminescence such as human teeth, bilirubin, artery lining and adrenal cortex.

***Dentistry***. Enamel photographs darker than dentine, although there is some evidence to show that this situation is reversed with pre-carious chalky degeneration. In the healthy living tooth the condition of the incisal edge can be clearly seen. Uneven areas of thin enamel appear light in tone. The vascular network of the oral mucosa does not show well in the infrared record and the dorsum of the tongue and hard palate are too heavily stratified for sufficient penetration.

***Dermatology***. Infrared records are able to show the healing process under deep seated lesions such as lupus vulgaris and eczema, hair stubble in shaved areas and tattoo patterns obliterated to visual examination. Xanthomata record very clearly with infrared photography. Full details of dermatological applications will be found in *Section 6.6*.

***Oncology***. Infrared photography has been much used in the study of tumours, especially for delineating the increased blood supply to breast tumours, and for differentiating between benign and malignant pigmented lesions of the skin.

***Liver pathology***. Much work has been done on the relationship between cirrhosis of the liver and collateral circulation and infrared photography is useful in the early detection of this.

***Transilluminography***. There are conflicting reports on the value of infrared photography for transillumination techniques. Some workers reported that there was little to be gained especially with transilluminating the breast, whilst others reported much enhanced recording particularly with infant skulls.

## 18.3 BLACK-AND-WHITE INFRARED TECHNIQUE

Because infrared photography is a visible interpretation of an invisible state a control photograph must always be taken in visible light to provide the clinician or researcher with an exact comparison of the rendering of the subject.

### *Lighting*

Though tungsten lamps, such as photoflood and quartz iodine lamps, are rich in output of infrared radiation excessive heat is a serious drawback in their use. Electronic flash tubes, however, emit infrared in sufficient quantity to take clinical photographs at small apertures – this source is therefore the usual choice for this type of photography.

Infrared photographs reveal density differences due to variations in the absorption characteristics of tissues, and any shadows cast by the lighting will cause confusion. Therefore, the subject must be evenly illuminated, using several sources of radiation. Some workers go so far as to recommend the use of a white room or tent to obtain diffuse enough lighting. Illumination drops off very quickly with increasing angle in infrared work so dark edges to the subject appear all too easily unless special care is taken to light these areas. Bear in mind also that different backgrounds reflect infrared more or less successfully – a well lit pure white background might reproduce dark grey on infrared. Many photographers prefer to work with an unlit black background.

### *Filters and emulsions*

A visually opaque infrared transmission filter (Wratten 87 or 88A) must be used over the camera lens in a 'light tight' mount. This requires the use of either a focussing frame or a technique whereby the image is focussed visually then the filter quickly flipped over the front of the lens and an exposure made before the subject has a chance to move. To overcome this difficulty it is possible to use a deep red filter such as a Wratten 25 or 70 which will still absorb the violet and blue light but pass enough red light to see the subject. In practice however, focussing through these very dark red filters is very difficult, and it is more reliable to focus in visible light and quickly filter the lens.

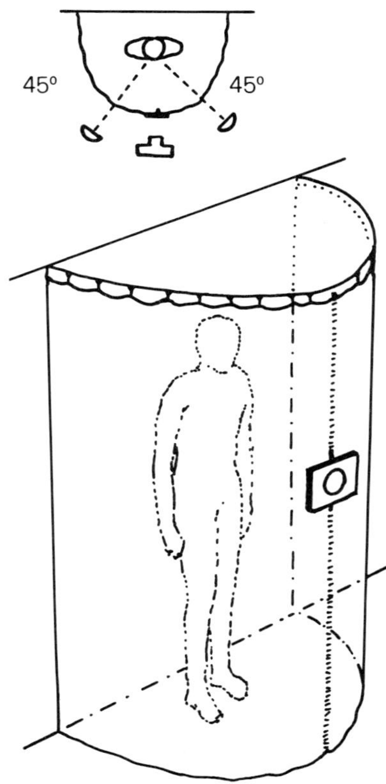


***Figure 18.1*** *(after Gibson) A white muslin tent can be hung from a ceiling mounted track so that when illuminated from the sides it gives very even lighting across the subject*

Black-and-white infrared sensitive emulsions are available in sheet film and 35 mm sizes, e.g. Kodak High Speed Infrared film. These films are very sensitive and will enable small apertures to be selected. As a general rule an infrared negative of a clinical subject should look fairly dense but serious overexposure must be avoided. Infrared materials are contrasty which generally helps in depicting veins etc. but as explained above great care needs to be taken with lighting ratios – soft flat lighting is required. The shelf life of infrared emulsions is severely limited, even when refrigerated, so great care must be taken to ensure that only fresh stock is used.

### *Equipment*

Unfortunately infrared radiation is able to penetrate leather and thin layers of many plastics and also through some cloth focal-plane shutters. Metal dark slides, film cassettes and shutters are therefore essential. All equipment to be used for infrared work should be tested first.

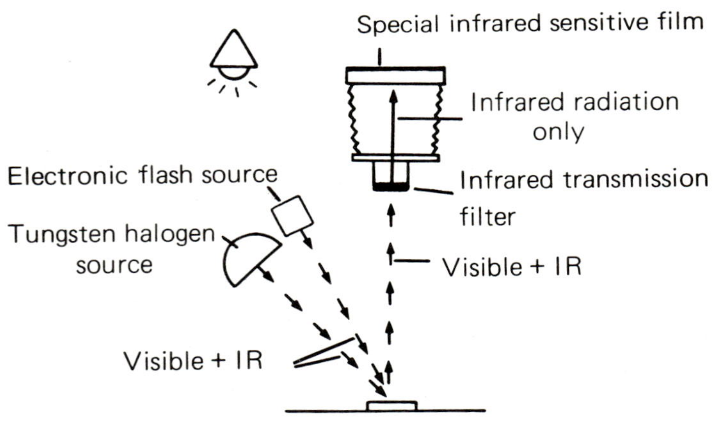


***Figure 18.2*** *The basic arrangement for photographic recording of the infrared image*

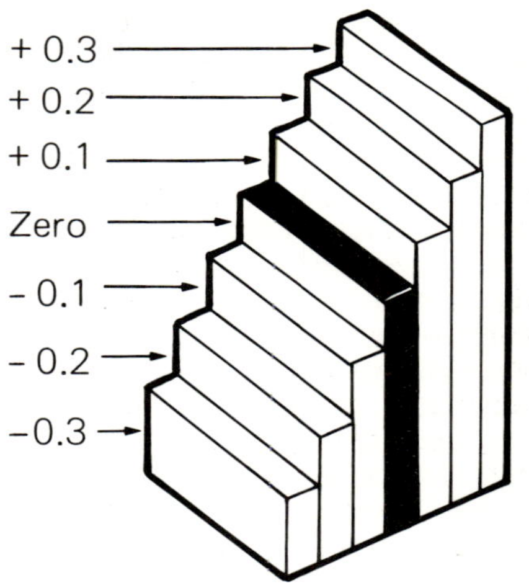


***Figure 18.3*** *A simple test for establishing focus shift. If the camera is focussed with visible light onto the zero 'step' it is a simple matter to note which step is recorded sharply by the infrared record*

### ***Focus shift and optical quality***

Standard photographic lenses are suitable for infrared photography but the infrared image is displaced beyond the visible focus. At low magnifications and using small apertures this displacement or shift is accommodated within the depth of focus of most lenses. Correction for shift becomes necessary when the depth of focus does not include the infrared focus, and this occurs when magnification of the image decreases depth of focus, significantly. When correction for shift becomes necessary, empirical methods, such as increasing the image conjugate by 1/250th of the focal length may be used, but it is better to conduct a focus test at various magnifications thus arriving at an exact determination of shift for the individual lens in use.

Many lenses which have been corrected for wavelengths in the visible spectrum give an image of poorer quality when used in the infrared range. This occurs even when the optimum infrared focus has been obtained and it is further diffused by scatter of radiation in the tissues.

### ***Printing technique***

Printing infrared negatives is very difficult because there are no accepted standards of what the subject should look like – no-one has ever seen it! Basically the technique is to print for the detail and ignore the flesh tones. The print should be just dark enough to show the faintest details or structures, and just contrasty enough to show them clearly. The quality of the finished print can be enhanced immeasurably by using an unsharp mask in contact with the negative during printing. This performs several roles – auto-dodging shadow areas, enhancing fine detail, by allowing a more contrasty grade of paper to be used. The unsharp positive area mask should be such that the lightest area presents a density of about 0.5. Contrast should be such that the ratio of darkest to lightest area is approximately 25% of the same ratio on the negative.

## 18.4 COLOUR INFRARED TECHNIQUE

Infrared colour photography is accomplished by using Kodak Infrared Ektachrome film. This is a so-called false colour film in that the three emulsion layers are sensitive to green, red and infrared instead of the conventional blue, green and red. Infrared Ektachrome is also sensitive to blue so a deep yellow (Wratten 12) filter must be used over the camera lens. On processing a yellow positive image records in the green sensitive layer, and positive images of magenta and cyan appear in the red and infrared sensitive layers, respectively. Many biological subjects appear with characteristic colours such as melanin which records red–brown, arterial blood which reproduces green, cholesterol and collagen which reproduce blue and so on. Many publications testify to the usefulness of this film, but at the time of going to press its future is in serious doubt – the film is for the E4 process only and there are no plans to market an E6 version. Colour infrared film has been used for all of the applications reported for black-and-white, and many-workers feel it reveals additional information.

## 18.5 NON-PHOTOGRAPHIC RECORDING OF INFRARED IMAGES

Thermography applied to medical subjects reveals the slight changes in temperature which may be associated with pathological disturbances. Examples are the surveying of the female breast to locate tumours which produce a temperature above that of the surrounding tissue, or the recording of the cold ischaemic fingers of the patient exhibiting Raynaud's phenomenon.

Infrared television may be used for observation purposes, e.g. animal behaviour patterns in the dark, or simply to visualize a clinical condition to predict whether full photographic recording with infrared would be profitable. Camera tubes with sensitivity extended into the infrared region must be used.

Infrared radiation may also be recorded by an image converter tube and if required, the resultant image can be recorded photographically from the fluoroscopic screen.

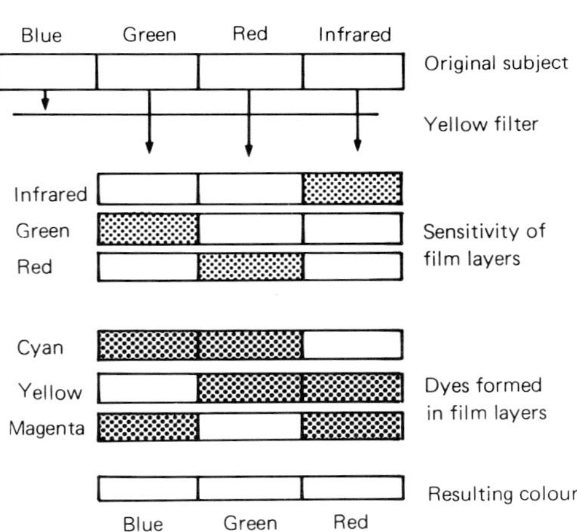


***Figure 18.4*** *Colour infrared film is a 'false colour' system recording green, red and infrared*

## 18.6 INFRARED LUMINESCENCE

Blue and ultraviolet fluorescence techniques are well known and documented in medical photography, but infrared luminescence because it occurs in the invisible part of the spectrum is rather less well known. Infrared emission is excited by using blue-green light. Blue-green filters are placed over the light source and a visually opaque infrared transmitting filter over the camera lens. A Corning 9780 cyan filter coupled with a Corning 3966 heat absorbing filter are placed over the lights. Alternatively, a 13% solution of copper sulphate in a glass cell may be used. Exposures are very long and the results totally unpredictable. The technique and results of tests on a variety of specimens have been fully reported in the literature.

### References


Bean, W. (1958). *Vascular Spiders and Related Lesions of the Skin.* (Springfield: Charles C. Thomas)

Blackburn, I. *et al.* (1975). Infrared time-lapse photography: a technique for analysing night movement in affective patients. *J. Psych. Res.*, **12**, 69-73

Casida, L. (1968). Infrared colour photography: selective demonstration of bacteria. *Science*, **159**, 199-200

Choromokos, E., Kogure, K. and Noble, J. (1969). Infrared absorption angiography. *J. Biol. Photogr. Assoc.*, **37**, 100-104

Clayton, E. (1940). Infrared photography of gross specimens. *J. Tech. Meth.*, **19**, 55–57

Cubberly, M. (1976). Infrared photography as a diagnostic tool in ophthalmology. *J. Biol. Photogr. Assoc.*, **44**, 80-85

De Ment, J. and Cuthbertson, R. (1951). Comparitive infrared photography in dental science. *Dent. Radiogr. Photor.*, **24**, 28–34

Dent, R. (1941). The photographic aspect of light reflection from human skin. *J. Lab. Clin. Med.*, **26**, 1852-1857

Epstein, B. (1939). Infrared photographic demonstration of the superficial venous pattern in congenital heart disease with cyanosis. *Am. Heart J.*, **18**, 282-283

Ford, R. (1974). Infrared photography of transilluminated infant skulls. *J. Biol. Photogr. Assoc.*, **42**, 94-102

Friedman, J. *et al.* (1958). Infrared photography of the oral mucosa. *N.Y. J. Dent.*, **28**, 7-9

Gibson, H.L. (1961). Post-prandial intensification of venous pattern. *Med. Radiogr. Photogr.*, **37**, 16-17

Gibson, H.L. (1962). The photography of infrared luminescence. *Med. Biol. Illustr.*, **12**, 155-166

Gibson, H.L. (1963). The photography of infrared luminescence. (Part 2). *Med. Biol. Illustr.*, **13**, 18-26

Gibson, H.L. (1963). The photography of infrared luminescence. (Part 3). *Med. Biol. Illustr.*, **13**, 89-90

Gibson, H.L. (1964). Diffuse lighting for clinical infrared photography. *Med. Radiogr. Photogr.* **40**, 38-41

Gibson, H.L. (1978). *Photography by Infrared: its Principles and Practice.* (New York: John Wiley)

Gibson, H.L. *et al* (1965). New vistas in infrared photography. *J. Biol. Photogr. Assoc.*, **33**, 1-5

Gilder, R. and Rutherford, A. (1970). Diffuse lighting for infrared photography in medicine. *Med. Biol. Illustr.*, **20**, 227-230

Gorman, W. and Hirscheimer, A. (1939). A study of the superficial venous pattern in pregnant and non-pregnant women by infrared photography. *Surg. Gynaecol. Obstet.*, **68**, 54-56

Handelsman, M. *et al.* (1962). Skin vascular changes in diabetes mellitus. *Arch. Intern. Med.*, **110**, 70-72

Haxthausen, H. (1933). Infrared photography of subcutaneous veins: demonstration of concealed varices in ulcer and eczema of the leg. *Br. J. Dermatol.*, **45**, 506-509

Hinshaw, H. and Rutledge, D. (1942). Lesions in the superior mediastinum which interfere with venous circulation. *J. Lab. Clin. Med.*, **27**, 908-909

Jankelson, I. *et al.* (1954). Symposium on cirrhosis of the liver: correlation between needle biopsy of the liver and infrared photography of the abdomen in cirrhosis. *Am. J. Gastroenterol.*, **21**, 9-12

Kodak. (1972). *Kodak Infrared Films.* (Publication N17) (Rochester, NY: Eastman Kodak Ltd)

Kodak. (1974). *High Speed Infrared Film 2481.* (Publication M9) (Rochester, NY: Eastman Kodak Ltd)

Kodak. (1977). *Applied Infrared Photography* (Publication M28) (Rochester, NY: Eastman Kodak Ltd)

Lowenstein, O. (1956). Pupillography. *Am. Med. Assoc. Arch. Ophthalmol.*, **55**, 565-567

Marshall, R. (1978). A densitometric study of an uneven development effect in infrared film. *J. Audiovis. Media Med.*, **1**, 117-120

Marshall, R. (1979). Infrared recording of neural tube defects. *J. Audiovis. Media Med.*, **2**, 92-94

Marshall, R. (1982). A television method for measuring infrared and ultraviolet reflections of pigmented lesions. *Med. Biol. Illustr.*, **5**, 51–55

Marshall, R. (1982). Infrared photographic photometry with an instant film. *J. Audiovis. Media Med.*, **5**, 69-71

Massopust, L. (1936). Infrared photographic study of the changing pattern of the superficial veins in a case of human pregnancy. *Surg. Gynaecol. Obstet.*, **63**, 86

Massopust, L. (1950). Infrared photographic studies of the superficial thoracic veins in the female. *Surg. Gynaecol. Obstet.*, **91**, 717-719

Mills, G. (1937). Infrared photography of gross specimens. *Radiogr. Clin. Photogr.*, **13**, 12–13

McCarty, G. (1976). Intra-oral infrared colour photography of radiotherapy patients. *J. Prosth. Dent.*, **35**, 327-330

Mimura, S. *et al* (1981). A new gastrocamera technique using infrared film. *Endoscopy*, **13**, 40-43

Morton, R. and Miller, S. (1981). Infrared transillumination using photography and television (videodioscopy). *J. Audiovis. Media Med.*, **4**, 86-90

Ogg, A. (1958). Examination of the eye with infrared radiation. *Br. J. Ophthalinol.*, **42**, 306-309

Ronchese, F. (1937). Infrared photography in the diagnosis of vascular tumours. *Am. J. Surg.*, **37**, 475-477

Rosenbloom, M. (1953). Infrared photography of the breast: report on a survey of vascular patterns of normal breasts with possible application to cancer detection. *J. Obstet. Gynaecol.*, **2**, 603-607

Stevenson, J. (1981). Penetration of eschar by infrared photography. *J. Audiovis. Media Med.*, **4**, 141-143

## Practical projects

(1) Photograph (*a*) the inner aspect of an arm, (*b*) a chest, (*c*) a leg and (*d*) a brown eye, with infrared black-and-white film and also with a panchromatic 'control' film. Mount the photographs as a series of comparison prints and make full notes of your technique and any difficulties encountered in each case.

(2) Photograph a female chest (preferably with a neoplasm) with infrared and panchromatic films. Make an unsharp area mask and produce an exhibition quality pair of prints. Submit your negative and mask with the prints.

(3) Using either black-and-white or colour infrared film photograph any patient whose diagnosis indicates to you that this technique might be of value. Write short notes on your results, equipment and methods.

(4) Photograph the venous structure of a colleague's arm – note the effects on detail of overexposure and of developing the film to different gammas.

(5) If your hospital has a thermography unit ask to see the equipment and its use on a variety of patients.

## Examination questions

Q.1 Describe fully the technique of infrared photographic recording of venous collateral circulation. What factors are particularly relevant in achieving good image quality?

Q.2 What is 'false colour infrared photography'? Describe its application to medical photography.

Q.3 Under the headings lighting, emulsions, filters, developing and printing discuss the technique of infrared photography.

Q.4 Discuss the value of infrared photography to the following specialities:
(*a*) Dentistry,
(*b*) Dermatology,
(*c*) Ophthalmology,
(*d*) Oncology.

Q.5 Distinguish between thermography and infrared photography. Describe the importance and application of each to medical practice and research.

Q.6 Infrared photography may be used to study the movements of animal or human subjects in the dark. Describe this technique fully.

Q.7 Give two medical conditions which require the use of infrared recording. For one of the conditions named explain your working technique.

*Multiple choice questions (any of the statements may be true or false)*

Q.8 Parts of the electromagnetic spectrum outside the visible range can be of value in medical photography but:
(*a*) Short wavelength ultraviolet radiation is harmful to the eyes.
(*b*) Colour infrared film is sensitive to red, green and infrared only.
(*c*) Ultraviolet fluorescence photography is never used to record venous blood patterns.
(*d*) Television tubes cannot be made to 'see' infrared radiation.
(*e*) The infrared region extends beyond the visible region of the spectrum for approximately 200 nm.

Q.9 In infrared photography of patients:
(*a*) High speed infrared films have two areas of sensitivity – one in the UV/blue region and one in the infrared.
(*b*) Infrared Ektachrome has three emulsions, sensitive to blue, red and infrared, respectively.
(*c*) A Wratten 87 filter is always used for black-and-white infrared.
(*d*) A Wratten 25 filter must be used with infrared colour film.
(*e*) The camera lens needs to be adjusted by 1/200th of its focal length so that the image forms nearer the lens.

# Section 19
# Ultraviolet photography

**R.J. Lunnon**, MPhil, FBIPP, FRPS, AIMBI, SBStJ
Director of Medical Illustration
Institute of Child Health and Hospitals for Sick Children, London

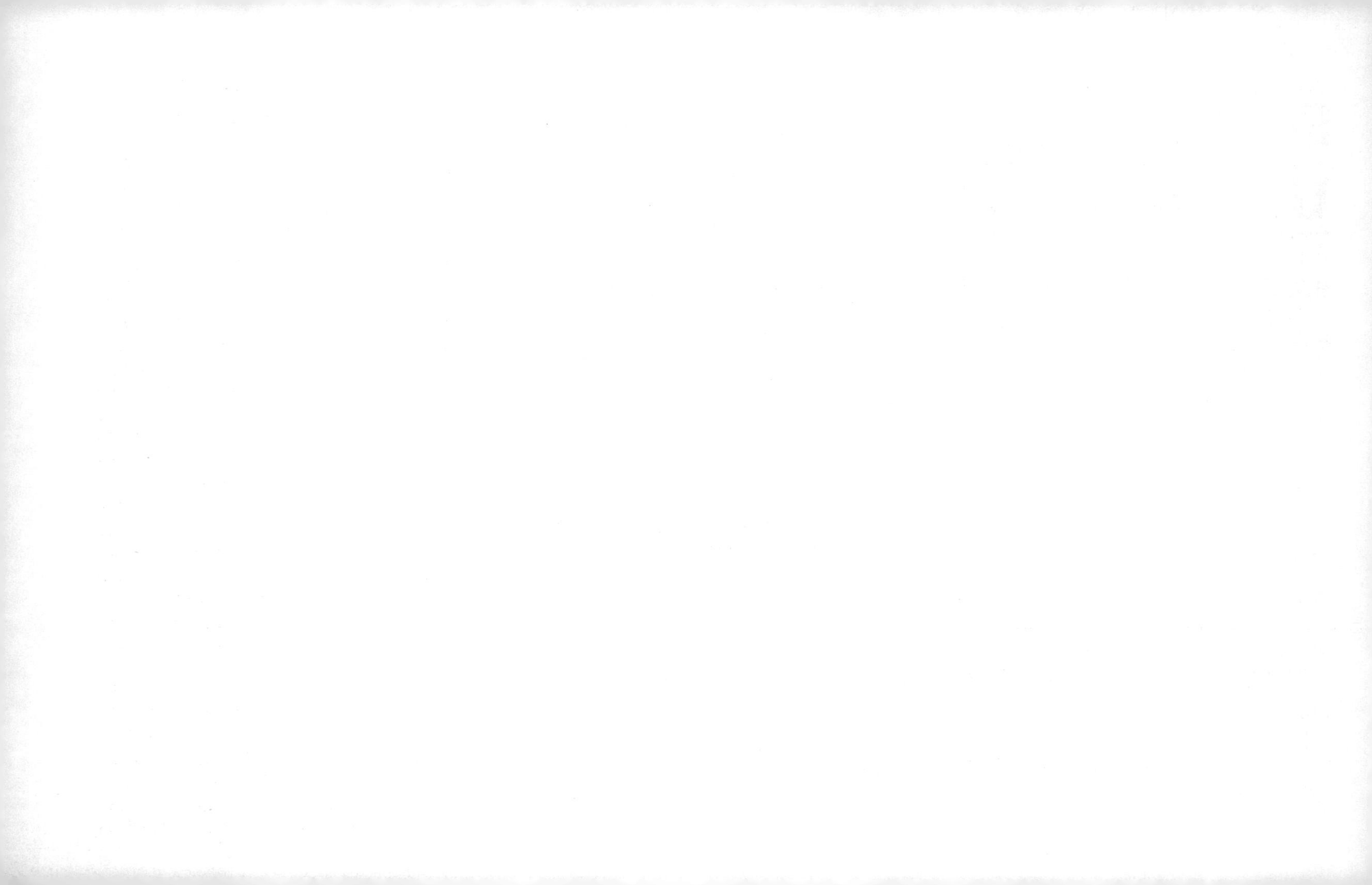

## 19.1 INTRODUCTION AND DEFINITIONS

The ultraviolet spectrum extends from approximately 10 nm to 400 nm, overlapping X-rays at the shorter wavelengths and running into the violet end of the visible spectrum. The ultraviolet spectrum is further sub-divided into 'near UV', or 'black light' ranging from 320 to 380 nm' 'middle UV' ranging from 200 to 320 nm and 'vacuum UV' between 10 and 200nm. Photography is restricted to the 320–400 nm region when using conventional glass lenses. Fluorite or quartz lenses extend the range to 150 nm, however below 250 nm a special low gelatin emulsion must be used since conventional emulsions absorb the shorter wavelengths.

Like infrared, the use of ultraviolet radiation is particularly important in that it enables the clinician to obtain 'new' information about his patient. UV photography has applications in diagnosis, documentation and research. It should be noted that because reflected ultraviolet photography is a visible interpretation of an invisible state, a control photograph taken in visible light must always be taken to provide an exact comparative rendering of the subject. Dermatologists particularly use the 'Wood's light' routinely for examining patients, so are most familiar with the ultraviolet technique and request it most often. The good clinical photographer will be alert to, and prepared for, the opportunities to use ultraviolet techniques in any area of medicine.

There are two quite distinct forms of 'ultraviolet photography', (a) reflected or direct ultraviolet photography and (b) ultraviolet fluorescence photography. In reflected ultraviolet photography the exposure is made using only ultraviolet radiation. In ultraviolet fluorescence photography, the exposure is made by the visible radiation which is produced when the subject is irradiated with ultraviolet, mainly in the 350–400 nm band.

## 19.2 APPLICATIONS OF REFLECTED ULTRAVIOLET PHOTOGRAPHY

Many substances reflect/absorb ultraviolet radiation in a completely different way to that for visible light. Some materials which are jet black to visible light reflect ultraviolet so effectively they record as white using reflected UV technique. Most biological subjects react rather less dramatically but the principle is applied widely. Tone and colour differences so slight that they are barely discernible often become very clear in UV.

(a) Slight changes in pigment of skin show more clearly than by conventional methods. Unpigmented skin reflects UV strongly, whereas melanin absorbs it very heavily. The extent of hypo- and hyperpigmentary conditions is clearly delineated. Applications include vitiligo, pigmented naevi, halo naevi, malignant and benign melanomas, melasma/chloasma, albinism, scleroderma, keratin plugs, moles and freckles. Although there are some comprehensive studies reported, much research needs to be done on how different conditions record with this method.

(b) There is greatly enhanced detail and resolution in the surface of the body tissues. The ultraviolet radiation does not penetrate the skin surface and become scattered in the same way as visible light. Reflected UV maps the surface blood vessels of the sclera, conjunctiva and some visceral surfaces of internal organs with exceptional clarity. Disturbances in the skin surface texture as in ichthyosis or poikiloderma are shown very clearly.

(c) In chromatography and certain forensic investigations reflected UV technique may be used to photograph ultraviolet-absorbing chemicals.

(d) In photomicrography, transmitted ultraviolet radiation is used to produce increased resolving power and to differentiate biological tissue through selective absorption.

(e) Photographs of old museum specimens lacking in contrast can be much improved by utilizing the reflected UV technique.

The student must appreciate that the effects of UV reflection technique are unpredictable and cannot be 'seen' with the naked eye. The pigmentary disturbance which will only become evident to the patient in mid-summer can be 'mapped' in mid-winter. Some workers have used television systems to be able to see in 'real time' whether reflected UV technique would be of value in recording certain patients.

## 19.3 APPLICATIONS OF FLUORESCENCE TECHNIQUE

Some substances absorb energy from radiation striking them by raising their orbiting electrons to higher energy levels. These electrons then slip back into their normal orbits and release energy again as light, the wavelength of the 'exciting' radiation being different from that of the 'emitted' light. This phenomenon is known as 'fluorescence'. Fluorescence may be a natural property of biological material e.g. fungal infections or it may be induced by the application/injection of a fluorescent dye.

Do not confuse fluorescence photography with reflected ultraviolet photography – the techniques are completely different. Also the student should be aware that although ultraviolet will stimulate emission from 'fluorescein' dye, its maximum excitation occurs at 460 nm in the visible blue region – it is not strictly speaking therefore a *UV* fluorescence technique. Indeed with certain applications, e.g. fluorescence angiography of the retina, fluorescein staining of corneal abrasions or contact lens fitting, it would be undesirable to use ultraviolet since the subject would develop a marked conjunctivitis. For convenience, however, fluorescein photography is usually discussed as an ultraviolet fluorescence technique.

Applications include:

(a) Photography of diagnostic fluorescence of *Tinea capitis* (microsporum canis infection) and *Erythrasma* (microsporum minutissimum), and some other fungal disorders (*see Section 6.6*).

(b) Some chemicals in chromatograms fluoresce, so demonstrating their presence and situation.

(c) Injection of fluorescent dyes can be used to delineate, for example, ischaemic tissue, blood vessels of the retina, or to outline parts of the body served by certain vascular pathways. Fluorescein drops may also be used to assess the accuracy of corneal scarring (*see Section 8.4.7/8*).

(d) Many normal and pathological tissues may fluoresce and thus reveal their characteristics and contour, e.g. the 'live coal' fluorescence of epidermoid carcinoma, or the bright red fluorescence of urine from a patient with porphyria. Much work has been done, for example, in evaluating the female gynaecological status by studying the fluorescence of the vulva.

(e) Fluorescent marker dyes can be used to delineate treatment areas for radiotherapy for example, or to study bone disease, or to distinguish between a drug preparation and a placebo.

(f) Fluorescence microscopy, particularly in the study of neoplastic disease, is now commonplace.

(g) In bacteriology some cultures of

organisms fluoresce, e.g. *H. pertussis.*

## 19.4 SOURCES OF ULTRAVIOLET RADIATION

*Incandescent sources*

The sun has a peak emission at 480 nm but emits approximately 10% of its radiation as ultraviolet. Atmospheric absorption prevents it being a useful UV source.

Tungsten lamps are very inefficient as UV sources but have been used by some workers in the past.

High intensity carbon-arcs have their peak emission at 390 nm and are a good source of UV.

*Gas discharge lamps*

Mercury vapour discharge lamps of low, pressure emit about 90% of their output as a single line at 254 nm, whereas medium and high pressure lamps emit a continuous spectrum in the near UV with lines at 365 nm and blue and green wavelengths. green wavelengths.

*Fluorescent tubes*

Domestic fluorescent tubes are poor sources of UV but specially coated tubes are available with peak emissions around 360 nm – the background visible light is usually filtered off with a Wood's glass envelope.

*Electronic flash*

The xenon flash tube is an excellent source of UV with emission in the range 350–450 nm. Portability and short duration/high output, make it the obvious choice in medicine. Normal guide numbers do not apply. Many modern flash tubes are 'gold coated' to filter out the 'unwanted' ultraviolet radiation – although at least one major manufacturer sells uncoated tubes especially for ultraviolet work.

## 19.5 SAFETY FACTORS

There is potential danger to both patient and operator – wavelengths of ultraviolet in certain bands, particularly 280–310 nm cause severe burning and acute conjunctivitis. When continuous sources emit shorter wavelengths than 350 nm, precautions to protect patient and photographer are essential. Conjunctivitis and skin erythema only appear 4 or 5 hours after exposure to UV, so that there are no warning signs to alert the operator that he is exceeding a safe dosage. With an electronic flash source, the time of exposure is so short that no danger arises under normal conditions.

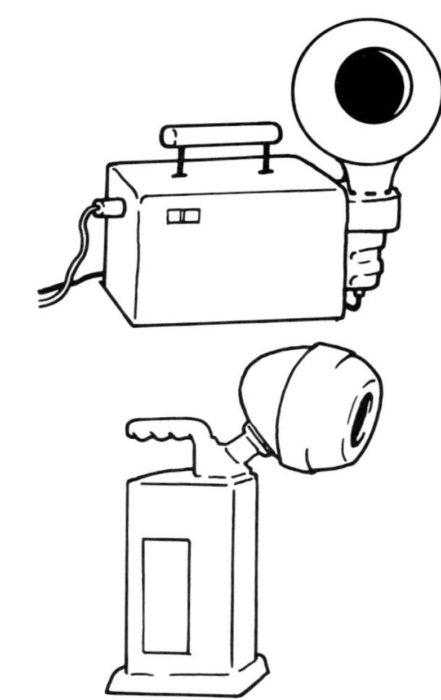

**Figure 19.1** *Two typically used continuous ultraviolet sources*

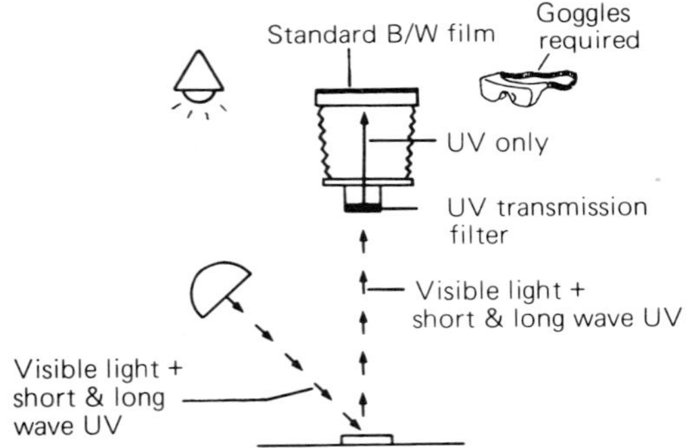


***Figure 19.2*** *Reflected ultraviolet method with continuous ultraviolet source*

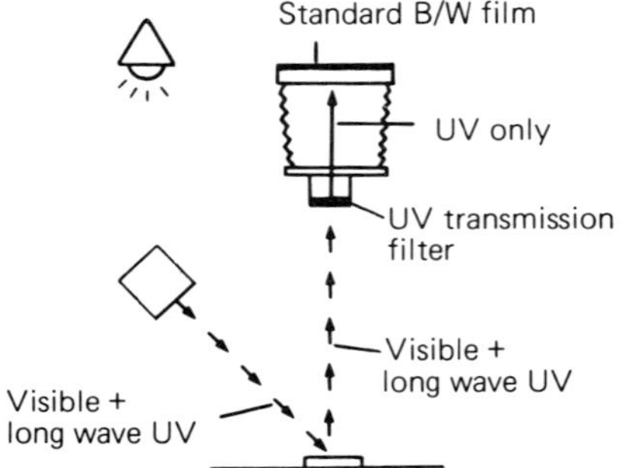


***Figure 19.3*** *Reflected ultraviolet method with electronic flash*

## 19.6 REFLECTED ULTRAVIOLET METHOD

This demands that only UV radiation reaches the film. The simplest method is to fit an optically flat ultraviolet transmission filter over the lens in a light-tight mount (*see Filter section*). Visible radiation given by the ultraviolet source can thus be ignored because it is absorbed by the filter. Note that when focussing is carried out through the taking lens, this must be done before the filter is attached. When using a hand-held single-lens reflex camera some form of flap filter mechanism must be devised for rapid positioning.

Another method is to use an ultraviolet transmission filter fitted over the light source. This may be of rolled glass but in this case the photography will have to be undertaken in a darkened room to avoid any visible radiation affecting the film.

Close-up photography (larger than half size) in ultraviolet will need an adjustment of the image conjugate to account for 'focus shift'. The focus shift is the difference between the visible focus and the ultraviolet focus which in some lenses is sufficient to need realignment of the focal plane. Note that with some modern compound lenses the image conjugate may need to be *increased*. As for infrared work practical tests must be carried out for any individual lens at set magnifications for optimal results.

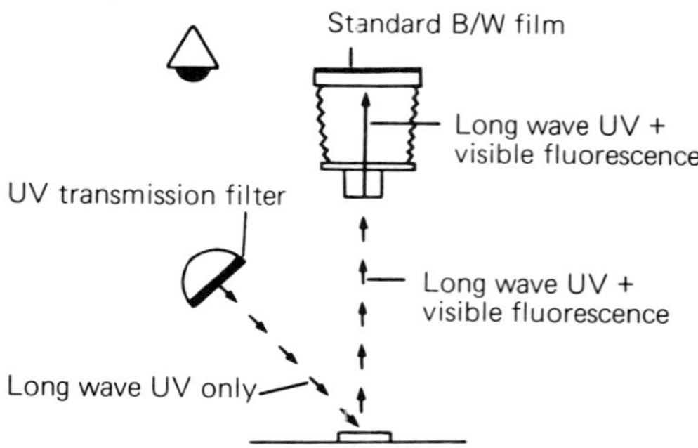


***Figure 19.4*** *Reflected ultraviolet method with a filter over the light source. This method requires darkroom conditions*

## 19.7 FLUORESCENCE METHOD

In the fluorescence technique, ultraviolet radiation stimulates the subject to emit visible radiation (fluorescence) and it is this image that is recorded.

The first step is to ensure that only ultraviolet radiation reaches the subject and the ultraviolet transmission filter (*see Filter section below*) is fitted over the source. At this stage it should be noted that the subject is (a) reflecting UV radiation, (b) reflecting any ambient or focussing lights and (c) emitting its own fluorescence.

The next step therefore is to fit an ultraviolet-absorbing filter over the lens and this will eliminate (a), the reflected UV radiation. It only remains for the focussing light to be turned off immediately prior to exposure, eliminating (b), all other visible light having been excluded. The film emulsion can now only be affected by the fluorescence (c). In practice, some of the surround may show even though it does not fluoresce, but should the filtration be perfect, there may be difficulty in orientating some subjects. This of course can be overcome by providing a low level of overall illumination, but it must be carefully balanced so as to avoid swamping the fluorescent areas.

The efficiency of any filter combination for fluorescence work can be tested by photographing a specularly reflecting metal object. Ideally the specular reflection from the source should be entirely absorbed by the barrier filter on the camera.

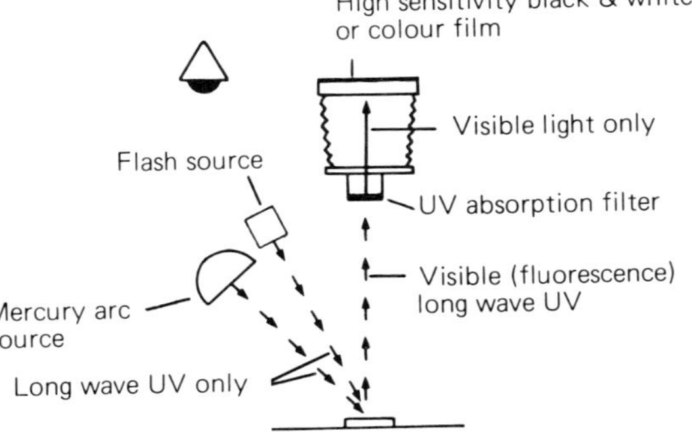


***Figure 19.5*** *The fluorescence method of ultraviolet photography*

## 19.8 FILTERS

Filters for reflected ultraviolet photography must transmit only wavelengths of radiation in the 350–400 nm band and as a consequence are visually opaque. Such filters are manufactured in rolled glass form or as optical flats, e.g. Wratten 18A/18B or Chance OX1/OX7. The rolled glass filter can only be used over the source whilst the optically flat filter is utilized in a light-tight mount on the lens.

The ultraviolet transmission filter mentioned above is also used over the source for fluorescence photography. In addition an ultraviolet absorption filter must be fitted over the lens, e.g. Wratten 2A/2B/2E. Ultraviolet absorption filters are also obtainable as gelatin sheet but care must be taken to ensure that the absorbing quality has not faded (this fading does not occur with glass UV-absorbing filters). Sometimes a pale cyan filter is needed in fluorescence work to offset the slight red/infrared leak of the UV-transmitting filter.

As mentioned earlier, fluorescein dye responds primarily to blue stimulation and the Wratten 47A has been especially formulated to provide efficient excitation. This is used in conjunction with a Wratten 2B and varying degrees of yellow filtration depending on how much blue background illumination is acceptable.

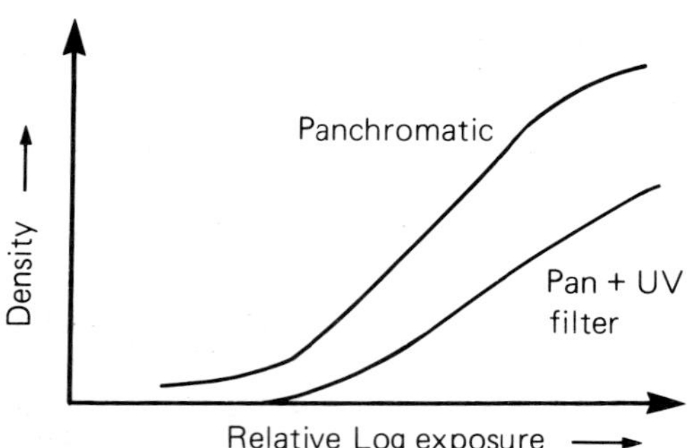


***Figure 19.6*** *The gamma/lambda effect shows that contrast falls as the wavelength of light used is reduced. The effect is of considerable importance in ultraviolet photography*

## 19.9 EMULSIONS

All photographic emulsions are sensitive to ultraviolet but note that their sensitivity does not relate to their sensitivity to visible light. For example, a blue-sensitivity copy film may have a greater relative speed to UV radiation than a fast hypersensitized panchromatic emulsion. The choice of emulsion is also influenced by the need to compensate for some loss of contrast which may occur due to reciprocity law failure and to the gamma/lambda effect. Loss of contrast can usually be compensated by choosing an emulsion of high contrast and by considerably increasing development. (The gamma/lambda effect is that contrast falls as the wavelength of light used gets shorter).

Emulsions for fluorescence work must be highly sensitive as light intensities are very low – they should be sensitive to the colour of fluorescence being produced.

## 19.10 EXPOSURE ESTIMATION

Exposure is difficult to calculate; intensities are always low and subject reflectance characteristics unpredictable. Exposure tests are always necessary. As a rough guide, using a 100 joule electronic flash at 18″ with 50 ASA film will give apertures of approximately f/5.6 for reflected UV and f/1.8 for fluorescence. It is always necessary to bracket exposures. In fluorescence work a spot photometer may have sufficient sensitivity and measure a conveniently small area to be practical. In the case of very long exposures, allowance must be made for reciprocity failure which in the case of colour films will affect colour balance. With some fluorescence there is also the problem of exhaustion extinction – the longer the subject is irradiated the weaker the fluorescence becomes.

Test subjects may be used to establish exposure in fluorescence work. A card on which Vaseline, fluorescent nail varnish and stencil correcting fluid have been smeared will provide a good test subject and levels of fluorescence can be judged alongside the test object and exposures estimated.

## References


Bailey, N. (1961). Blacklight photography of the eye. *Contacto.* **5**, 91-96

Benson, R. and Vogel, M. (1955). The principles of identification and measurement of vulvar fluorescence. *J. Clin. Endocrinol.*, **15**, 784-800

Callender, R. (1975). Fluorescence macrophotography. *Br. J. Photogr.*, **122**, 964

Cameron, J., Ruddick, R. and Grant, J. (1960). Ultraviolet photography in forensic medicine. *Forens. Photogr.*, **2**, 23-28

Costello, M. and Luttenberger, L. (1944). Fluorescence with the Wood filter as an aid in dermatologic diagnosis. *N.Y. J. Med.*, **42**, 1778-1784

Drury, D. and Bullough, P. (1970). Improved photographic reproduction of bone and cartilage specimens using ultraviolet illumination. *Med. Biol. Illustr.*, **20**, 57-58

Feindel, W. *et al* (1967). Intracarotid fluorescein angiography: a new method for examination of the epicerebral circulation in man. *Can. Med. Assoc. J.*, **96**, 1-7

Grossman, J. *et al.* (1981). A simple technique for fluorescein photography. *Plast. Reconstr. Surg.*, **67**, 257-258

Hansell, P. (1961). Ultraviolet radiations. In *Medical Photography in Practice* Linssen. E.F. (ed.). (London: Fountain Press) P. 175–192

Klosevych, S. (1971). Fluorescence photomacrography. *J. Biol. Photogr. Assoc.*, **39**, 163-164

Le Cover, M. (1972). Documenting radiation portals by use of ultraviolet illumination. *J. Biol. Photogr. Assoc.*, **40**, 9-12

Lindenstam, B. (1959). The use of ultraviolet light in dental photography. *Med. Biol. Illustr.*, **9**, 26-31

Lunnon, R. (1959). Direct ultraviolet photography of the skin. *Med. Biol. Illustr.*, **9**, 150-154

Lunnon, R. (1968). Clinical ultraviolet photography. *J. Biol. Photogr. Assoc.*, **36**, 72-78

Lunnon, R. (1976). Reflected ultraviolet photography of human tissues. *Med. Biol. Illustr.*, **26**, 139-144

Lunnon, R. (1979). Direct or reflected ultraviolet photography. *Photogr. J.*, **119**, 380-386

McIntyre, D. (1967). The stimulation of fluorescein in external ophthalmic photography. *J. Biol. Photogr. Assoc.*, **35**, 155-157

Moore, G. *et al.* (1950). Biophysical studies of methods utilizing fluorescein and its derivatives to diagnose brain tumours. *Radiology*, **55**, 344-362

Mustakallio, K. and Korhonen, P. (1966). Monochromatic ultraviolet photography in dermatology. *J. Invest. Dermatol.*, **47**, 351-353

Ronchese, F. (1953). The fluorescence of ulcerated epidermoid carcinoma under the Wood's light. *Med. Radiogr. Photogr.*, **29**, 6-8

Ruddick, R. (1974). A technique for recording bite marks for forensic studies. *Med. Biol. Illustr.*, **24**, 128-129

Ruddick, R. (1977). Ultraviolet fluorescence technique for improved tone separation of low contrast specimens. *Med. Biol. Illustr.*, **27**, 47-48

Ruddick, R. (1979). Ultraviolet fluorescence photography. *Photogr. J.*, **119**, 381-385

Rutherford, A. (1973). Ultraviolet fluorescence photography in ophthalmology. *Med. Biol. Illustr.*, **23**, 204-205

Schaefer, D. and Baldwin, E. (1970). The photography of fluorescein dye fluorescence in surgery. *J. Biol. Photogr. Assoc.*, **38**, 70-74

Tredinnick, W.D. (1961). Further advances in fluorescence colour photography. *Med. Biol. Illustr.*, **11**, 16-21

## Practical projects

(1) Use the ultraviolet fluorescence technique (using colour film) to photograph (*a*) some Vaseline smeared onto the back of the hand (*b*) normal teeth in occlusion, anteriorly. Write a description of your technique and comment on your results.

(2) Photograph a pathological specimen of your own choice, e.g. slice of lung, kidney section etc., using black-and-white reflected and fluorescence techniques. Record the normal visual appearance using panchromatic film. Produce a matched set of three prints and write comments on the differences.

(3) Photograph normal skin (*a*) with visible light and (*b*) with reflected ultraviolet technique. Note the difference in surface detail recorded.

(4) Produce an 8″ x 10″ exhibition quality print of any hyper-or-hypo pigmentary condition. Submit a 'control' print and your negatives along with a full description of your technique.

(5) Photograph either a fluorescent bacterial culture or a fluorescent chromatogram with both reflected and fluorescence techniques. Note the similarities and differences in the results.

## Examination questions

Q.1 Discuss the importance of the following in ultraviolet photography.
(*a*) Gamma/lambda effect
(*b*) Focus shift
(*c*) Reciprocity failure

Q.2 Describe fully a practical technique for recording the reflected ultraviolet appearance of vitiligo.

Q.3 Describe the usefulness and application of fluorescence photography in (*a*) ophthalmology and (*b*) dermatology

Q.4
(*a*) List the radiation sources available for ultraviolet photography.
(b) What are the biological hazards associated with UV?
(*c*) Why should a control photograph always accompany a reflected UV record?

Q.5 Discuss the value of ultraviolet photography in clinical medicine.

Q.6 It is sometimes said that 'the characteristics of paper chromatograms are best revealed by ultraviolet'. Comment on this statement. Describe how you might photograph such characteristics.

Q.7 Draw a diagram to explain how the electromagnetic spectrum is filtered for (*a*) reflected ultraviolet photography, (*b*) fluorescence photography and (*c*) infrared photography. Give several examples of applications for each technique in medicine.

Q.8 Give two medical conditions which require the use of reflected ultraviolet technique. For one of the conditions named explain your working technique.

*Multiple choice questions (any of the statements may be true or false).*

Q.9 With the technique of reflected ultraviolet photography:
(*a*) Surface texture recording is much enhanced,
(*b*) Scleral blood vessels are clearly delineated,
(*c*) Wavelengths from 10 to 200 nm are used,
(*d*) The gamma/lambda effect helps to increase contrast,
(*e*) It is possible to work in normal room lighting.

Q.10 Fluorescence photography may be of value in recording the following:
(*a*) Epidermoid carcinoma
(*b*) Porphyria
(*c*) Corneal scarring
(*d*) Pityriasis versicolor
(*e*) Ischaemia.

# Section 20
# Endoscopic and cavity photography

**Dr P.N. Cardew**, MRCS, LRCP, FRPS, FBPA, AIMBI
Director of Audio-visual Communications
St Mary's Hospital and Medical School, London

## 20.1 INTRODUCTION

Although photography or television through endoscopes is in general carried out by a surgeon, the medical photographer is often involved as an adviser on photographic aspects and must have a knowledge of the theory and practical aspects of the subject.

## 20.2 DEFINITION

Endoscopic and cavity photography merge into each other but a working definition can be taken as endoscopic photography being concerned with tubes whose length is greater that the width, while cavity photography is concerned with apertures or tubes whose diameters are greater than their depth.

## 20.3 ENDOSCOPIC PHOTOGRAPHY

### 20.3.1 Applications and instruments

The recording of appearances within the body as seen through the natural orifices or through surgical openings. The following are the more commonly employed instruments:

(1) The *otoscope* for viewing the eardrum.

(2) The *rhinoscope* may be an anterior instrument for seeing into the nasal cavity through the nostril or a retrograde version which sees the nasopharynx when inserted via the mouth behind the soft palate.

(3) The *laryngoscope* and *bronchoscope* are used for the respiratory tract.

(4) The *oesophagoscope* and *gastroscope* are used for the upper digestive tract, the latter needing to be flexible to accommodate to the thoracic curvature.

(5) The *cystoscope* is passed through the urethra to inspect the urinary bladder.

(6) The *proctoscope*, the *sigmoidoscope* and the *colonoscope* are all passed through the anus to examine respectively the rectum, the lower and the upper colon.

(7) The *arthroscope* for viewing internal joint structures, especially the knee.

(8) The *laparoscope* is passed into the peritoneal cavity via an incision in the abdominal wall. Visualization is aided by inflation of the peritoneal cavity. Extensive use is made of the laparoscope to examine and operate on the Fallopian tubes, ovaries and associated structures. It is also used an an amnioscope to penetrate the wall of the pregnant uterus. *See also Section 12.1.4.*

(9) Continual progress is being made to develop instruments to pass into the smaller and more inaccessible body cavities, such as the ureter, pelvis of the kidney, bile ducts and cerebral ventricles.

### 20.3.2 Optical principles and illumination

Endoscopes can be broadly divided into three groups: (a) the open-tube type, (b) those which incorporate a telescopic system of lenses and (c) fibrescopes.

Involved in all endoscopic photography are the problems of (1) illuminating the subject, (2) providing a view for the operator and (3) taking a photograph. All these functions must be carried on simultaneously and it should be realized that increased efficiency in any of these requirements is obtained only at the expense of the other two. Whatever system is used, there is a theoretical maximum to the amount of light that can be collected by an endoscopic optical system, since the diameter of the scope limits the diameter of the lens, irrespective of whether it is situated distally as in a telescopic or fibre optic system, or proximally as in an open tube endoscope. The light-

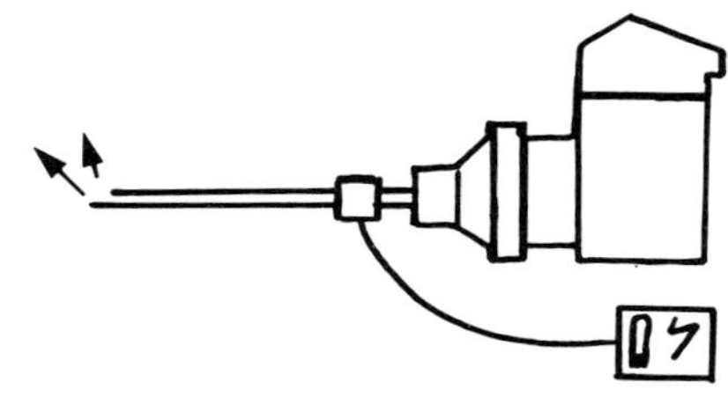

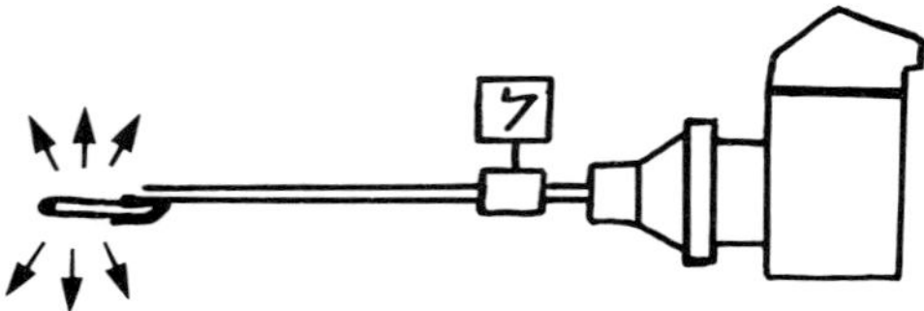

***Figure 20.1*** *Extra-corporeal flash (above) gives a poorer quality of illumination than intra-corporeal flash (below), which tends to give crisper detail*

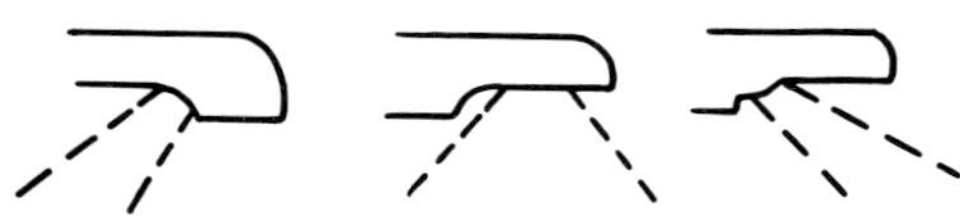

***Figure 20.2*** *The three most commonly used types of endoscopic illumination: retrograde, lateral or right-angle and fore-oblique*

conducting path is similarly limited. If the optical system has been designed to take the maximal advantage of the possible diameter of the scope, then the brightness of the image-forming rays at the film plane can only be further increased by either increasing the efficiency of the light source or by using a shorter focal length objective lens with a resulting smaller image. Since modern illumination systems operate at or near their maximum practical efficiency, it follows that the possible image size through a particular instrument is a function of film speed and of the exposure time. With the small endoscopes, the image size may be severely restricted. To fill a 35 mm frame requires 12 times more light than an 8 mm frame. A compromise may sometimes be reached by using a smaller image on a larger format. The practical benefits of using 16 mm stock may be retained by accepting an image size which only fills half the frame. In the case of television a smaller but brighter image may have to be accepted.

### 20.3.3 Open tube endoscopes

With the development of modern efficient optical systems, the open tube endoscope is obsolete. The principles are similar to those of cavity photography (c.f.) and the main problems were mechanical due to the difficulty of using heavy equipment attached to open tube endoscopes which needed delicate handling when in use on patients. In expert hands using endoscopes shorter than 8″ and of ½ ″ diameter, superb results could be obtained, but their use was limited to the larynx and rectum and so they have been abandoned for telescopic or fibre optic systems.

### 20.3.4 Telescopic endoscopes

In this system the objective lens is situated at the distal end of the scope. The lens is of short focal length, resulting in an angle of view of up to 90°. This may be combined with a right angle or oblique prism which permits the scanning of a wide field. The image produced by the objective lens is then repeatedly transferred along the endoscope through a series of lenses and emerges from the eyepiece as a parallel beam. Any camera objective lens with its focus at infinity, set in the axis of this beam, will then produce a sharp image. The depth of field of the telescope objective lens is sufficiently great to avoid the necessity for any focussing mechanism. Modern developments in optics have made possible good recording through telescopes of only 3 mm in diameter.

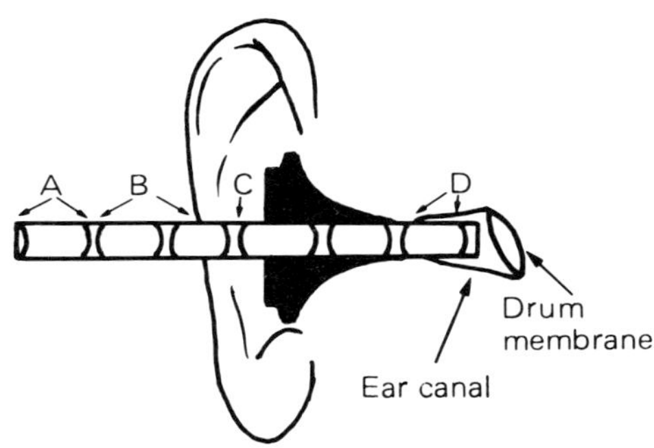


A - eyepiece, B - rod - lens relay system,
C - air gap, D - objectives.

***Figure 20.3*** *The relationship between the speculum and the viewing optics for otoscopy*

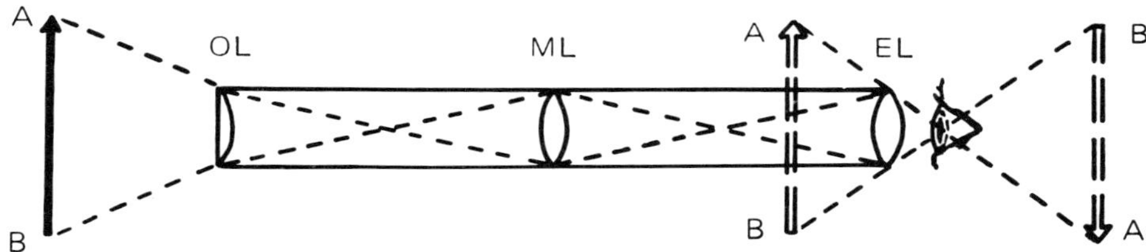


***Figure 20.4*** *The principle of the direct telescopic endoscope. The image is inverted by the lens OL, is again inverted by the repeater lens ML, and seen upright by the eye through EL. The photographic image, however, is inverted.*

The light source is external to and separate from the scope, the filament image being focussed by a condenser lens onto a fibre light-guide which runs adjacent to, or is split to encircle the telescope and light guide; this is not often possible in practice as the endoscope may need to accommodate biopsy forceps, irrigating systems and other ancillary refinements for surgery.

### 20.3.5 The fibre optic endoscope

The image-forming fibre-optic system is similar to the light guide system, but differs from it in that the geometry of the fibres at the distal and proximal ends of the cable are identical. An image produced on the distal end by an objective lens will therefore result in an identical image at the proximal end of the scope however much the fibres may have been bent (short of breaking) in their passage from end to end. The advantage of flexibility allows pictures to be taken of otherwise inaccessible organs, such as the upper colon and the pelvis of the kidney, the fundus of the stomach and distal bronchi.

The image produced by a fibrescope is inferior to that of the telescope since it

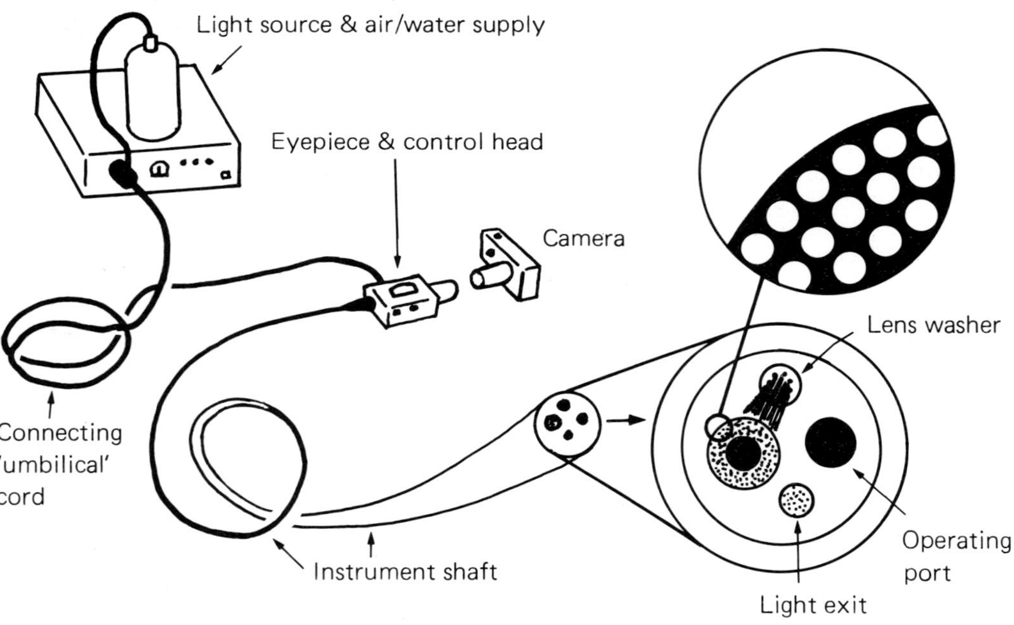


***Figure 20.5*** *Fibre-optic endoscopy. A separate control box houses the cold-light source and electronic flash along with air and water supply. The control head houses all the 'steering' controls for the scope, the air and water valves and the camera/eyepiece assembly. The distal end of the scope (shown in two stages of enlargement) contains the coherent bundle of fibres used for imaging, the incoherent bundle used for lighting, a lens washer and operating port. This last facility is used to insert loops, needles and other surgical instruments. The camera itself is normally a very simple film holder – typically 35 mm half-frame or 16 mm*

suffers from a granularity, being composed of discrete elements each corresponding to a single fibre surrounded by a sheath of glass of lower refractive index. This sheath around each fibre is essential to an image forming system in order to preserve total internal reflection and thus prevent leakage of light from one fibre to another. The separation between picture elements has a theoretical minimum of about 15 μm. The objective lens at the distal end of the endoscope forms an image on the input plate of the fibre bundle which behaves like a block maker's half tone screen so that the resolution of the emergent rays at the exit face of the bundle is limited by the number of fibres in the endoscope. The quality is fair for a ½″ cable diameter, such as in a colonoscope, but falls off greatly when the diameter is reduced to ureteric dimensions.

### 20.3.6 Photographic attachments to endoscopes

Much endoscopy involves delicate surgical manoeuvres and the attachment of a camera to the eyepiece or at the proximal end of an open tube scope may create practical difficulties in manipulation by the surgeon. Weight should be minimal and if a heavy camera has to be used, then a counterweight suspension system must be employed. For reasons of safety, any method of attachment must be capable of quick release. The camera, whether still or cine, must incorporate a reflex viewing system so that the subject can be kept under continuous observation.

Camera weight presents less of a problem when used with a fibrescope since the proximal end of the flexible instrument insulates the patient from any camera movements.

### 20.3.7 Exposure and image quality

The medical photographer will, in practice, be involved mainly in an advisory capacity since the actual photography is normally carried out by the surgeon. A frequent question asked concerns exposure determination. Most endoscopic systems are working at the limit of their light transmitting power and are designed to use the fastest available colour emulsions. With a continuous light source, as opposed to flash, a balance must be struck between the longest exposure that is feasible for the particular circumstance and the increasing loss in quality due to using faster emulsions, possibly combined with forced processing. With a view that involves considerable depth such as in the peritoneal cavity, it may only be possible to obtain a correctly exposed image at one particular plane, closer objects being over-exposed and the more distant being under-exposed. Under these conditions, the right compromise can only be reached by experience. With cinematography the exposure is determined by the taking speed and again a compromise must be achieved between emulsion speed and the acceptable amount of speeding up of subject movement.

The photographer may be asked to test the definition of a telescopic system. Make sure that the aperture of the objective lens on the camera is not greater than the emergent beam from the telescope. However, there is no advantage in stopping down further than this diameter. Do not forget that optics of cystoscopes are designed to work in a water-filled bladder and these conditions must be reproduced for a test object.

### 20.3.8 Television

The overwhelming advantages of direct viewing on a monitor screen are leading to film recording being replaced by the television camera and videotape. The endoscopic image is very effective on a television screen. This is probably due to the relatively low definition of a 625 line monitor screen. The surgeon is in fact accustomed to seeing image definition of this quality.

## 20.4 CAVITY PHOTOGRAPHY

### 20.4.1 Applications

These include (a) intra-oral, (b) the anterior nasal view and photography of the ear drum being examples of small cavities and (c) some surgical operative views.

### 20.4.2 Intra-oral

The shape of the mouth well illustrates the classic problems of cavity photography. Although not particularly deep, the aperture formed by the lips is slightly less than the diameter of the interior of the mouth thus making it difficult to obtain a single view of the whole mouth.

As with endoscopy, there is the requirement to illuminate, view and photograph down the same axis, all simultaneously. The illuminating system must provide a continuous source for focussing as well as flash (in the case of stills) for making the exposure. A reflex camera meets the other two requirements. The choice of focal length of lens is important.

Short focal length lenses give the

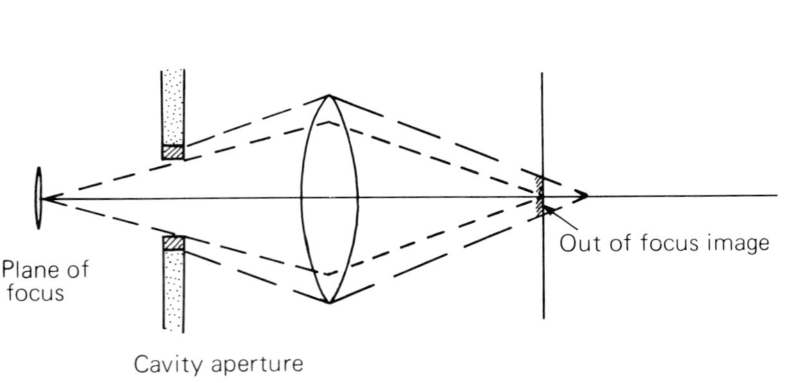


***Figure 20.6*** *A large diameter lens to illuminate/photograph any cavity can cause out-of-focus reflections which degrade the true image*

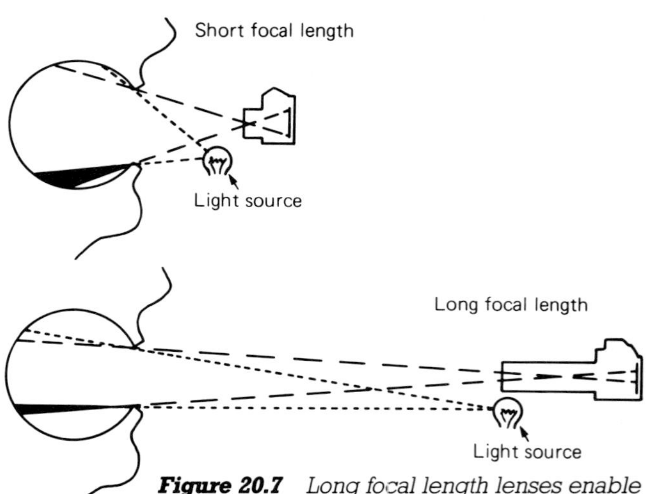


***Figure 20.7*** *Long focal length lenses enable the illumination to more closely cover the area being photographed but have the disadvantage that less of the cavity is recorded*

widest field of view but make it difficult to achieve axial illumination due to physical limitations of space. The long focal length lens is convenient for providing illumination but the field of view is more restricted. Any system is a compromise between these two extremes.

Lighting may be either a single small source adjacent to the lens or alternatively a ringflash. The small source gives the best result as the size and extent of the highlights on the moist mucous surface is minimal and the slight degree of offset from the axis helps to reveal small detail. However, shadowing from the lips is inevitable. This will not occur when using a ringflash which is more fool-proof as an illuminant but it tends to give a 'flat' image.

### 20.4.3 The nose and eardrum

These are examples of small cavities whose size presents an added problem. Not only is the conventional camera cumbersome when used with these subjects but the lens size mitigates against obtaining good results. When photographing any cavity or down an endoscope, the lens diameter should never exceed the proximal aperture of the cavity. The outer diameter of the lens not only serves no useful purpose but contributes out-of-focus reflections which degrade the true image.

Successful pictures can only be

obtained with apparatus whose lens and lighting system is of the appropriate scale. In practice commercial equipment such as the Kowa fundus camera must be used.

## References


Alberti, P. (1975). Still photography of the larynx – an overview. *Can. J. Otolaryngol.*, **4**, 759-765

Berci, G. (1976). *Endoscopy*. (New York: Appleton-Century Crofts)

Chen, B. *et al* (1979). Otoscopy and photography : a new method. *Ann. Otol. Rhinol. Laryngol.*, **88**, 771-773

Chole, R. (1980). Photography of the tympanic membrane – a new method. *Arch. Otolaryngol.*, **106**, 230-231

Chole, R. (1982). *A Colour Atlas of Ear Disease*. (London: Wolfe Medical Publications)

Cockel, R. (1973). Gastric photography. *Med. Biol. Illustr.*, **23**, 26-30

Hahn, C. and Kitzing, P. (1978). Indirect endoscopic photography of the larynx. *J. Audiovis. Media Med.*, **1**, 121-130

Hawke, M. (1982). Telescopic otoscopy and photography of the tympanic membrane. *J. Otolaryngol.*, **11**, 35-39

Hearnsberger, P. (1976). The Kowa RC-2 fundus camera for biomedical photography. *J. Biol. Photogr. Assoc.*, **44**, 44-46

Holinger, P., Brubaker, J.D. and Brubaker, J. (1975). Open-tube, proximal illumination mirror, and direct laryngeal photography. *Can. J. Otolaryngol.*, **4**, 781-785

Jeffreys, N. (1966). Kowa retinal camera used for cavity photography. *Med. Biol. Illustr.*, **16**, 200

Jensen, D. (1981). Laparoscopy advances in biopsy and recording techniques. *Gastroint. Endosc.*, **27**, 150-155

Karlan, M. (1979). Photographic documentation techniques. *Ear, Nose, Throat J.*, **58**, 21-25

Katzenberg, B. (1979). Photographing otolaryngological microsurgery. *J. Biol. Photogr.*, **47**, 55-58

Katzenberg, B. (1981). Endoscopic photography in otolaryngology. *J. Biol. Photogr.*, **49**, 101-107

Kilbourne, S. (1982). Photography through the operating microscope. *J. Biol. Photogr.*, **50**, 9-13

Morton, R. (1982). Photography the fibrescope. *J. Audiovis. Media Med.*, **5**, 137-140

Morton, R. and Bain, D. (1983). Photography as an aid to the study of otitis media. *J. Audiovis. Media Med.*, **6**, 4-6

Morton, R. and Munro, A. (1975). Photoproctoscopy with the Kowa fundus camera. *Med. Biol. Illustr.*, **25**, 102-103

### *Practical projects*

(1) If you have not already done so you should complete project 1, listed under section 12 'Photography in Genito-urinary medicine and Gynaecology'.

(2) Visit your endoscopy unit and ask if you might be shown the endoscopes and how they work.

(3) If circumstances allow, borrow an arthroscope (or bronchoscope) and familiarize yourself with its operation. Take a series of photographs of the inside of a cavity (the inside of a partially clenched fist or the inside of the mouth). Make notes on your results and any special problems you encounter.

(4) Duplicate the images obtained from (*a*) a straight rod endoscope, (*b*) a fibrescope so as to obtain full-frame 35 mm colour transparencies. Make notes on the quality of the resulting images.

(5) Advanced students should consult a comprehensive text on endoscopy such as *Practical gastrointestinal endoscopy* by Cotton and Williams (Blackwell, 1980)

### *Examination questions*

Q.1 With the aid of diagrams describe the photography of the eardrum.

Q.2 Describe the use of the following instruments:

(*a*) Otoscope,
(*b*) Bronchoscope
(*c*) Gastroscope,
(*d*) Cystoscope,
(*e*) Colonoscope,
(*f*) Arthroscope.

For one of these give a full description of the optical arrangement used for photography.

Q.3 Compare and contrast the telescopic endoscope with the fibreoptic endoscope. Give examples and diagrams where necessary.

Q.4 Discuss the factors affecting image quality in photo-colonoscopy.

Q.5 Discuss fully the relative merits of a single small light source and ringflash for photography of the oral cavity.

Q.6 Describe two different techniques for photography of rectal lesions, giving their relative advantages/disadvantages.

Q.7 Why is the image from an endoscope so small? What factor precludes optical enlargement of the image? Describe one method of photographically enlarging the endoscopic image.

*Multiple choice questions (any of the statements may be true or false).*

Q.8 The following are fixed tube telescopic endoscopes:

(*a*) Cystoscope,
(*b*) Laryngoscope,
(*c*) Laparoscope,
(*d*) Proctoscope,
(*e*) Amnioscope.

Q.9 In endoscopic photography:

(*a*) An open tube endoscope is used to photograph the larynx.
(*b*) An arthroscope is especially designed to photograph inside the major arteries.
(*c*) A flexible fibrescope works on the principle of total internal reflection.
(*d*) The camera is attached to the distal end of a colonoscope.
(*e*) Early methods of intra-gastric photography required the patient to swallow the complete camera.

# Section 21
# Cine and television for the photographer

**Dr P.N. Cardew**, MRCS, LRCP, FRPS, FBPA, AIMBI
Director of Audio-visual Communications
St Mary's Hospital and Medical School, London

## 21.1 INTRODUCTION

The medical photographer is primarily concerned with still photography, film and television being adjuncts to his other work. It is only possible in a single chapter to draw attention to the differences between the still and moving pictures and highlight their special applications in medicine. Any photographer intending to undertake the more elaborate aspects of film or television should study the specialized texts on these subjects as well as those on sound recording.

## 21.2 APPLICATIONS

(1) Records of any subject involving movement or change in appearance, e.g. a patient's gait, the microscopic appearance of tissue cultures, the recording of animal experiments and endoscopic appearances. Such records may be used for teaching or research. In the latter case they may also be subjected to frame-by-frame analysis.
(2) Demonstration of techniques, e.g. surgical operations, laboratory procedures, clinical techniques.
(3) More complex teaching films, such as the exposition of a subject or a film designed to teach an attitude towards a subject.
(4) Film loops for short sequences and the study of repetitive action.
(5) Live television demonstrations to large audiences of small scale procedures or from hazardous sites such as autopsy rooms.
(6) Television recording of students' performance for training, assessing and providing feedback.

## 21.3 FILM OR TELEVISION?

The kinetic arts include both cinematography and television. As technical advances in the latter have developed, the characteristics distinguishing film from television have become blurred, and indeed many medical users will refer to a 'film' when meaning a video tape. One reason is the ease with which television can display images from all sources on a monitor or television set. These may come live from a camera or be tape recordings of television images, of film, of tape/slide programmes or of computer-generated images, either radiological or graphic. Television thus can be seen to have a dual function, being both a recording medium and a transmitting medium.

Often a decision has to be made as to whether to use film or television for some specific purpose. It may be that the question is resolved by the availability of existing equipment but where a choice can be made the advantages and drawbacks of each system should be understood. The following are the salient features of each.

### 21.3.1 Film – the pros and cons

Educational film systems may be of 8 mm or 16 mm gauge and both share the following attributes. The equipment is simple and reliable. Unlike television, the photographic image is permanent and is not at the mercy of changing standards of video tape formats. Operating costs are heavy. Film magazines are fixed in size so that the maximum length of 'take' is limited to 10 minutes and may be much shorter. This means that careful planning and scripting is essential. Since the results of filming are not seen until after processing, technical excellence must be ensured and departures from a tight script are fraught with danger. In general only one camera can be used, inserts having to be filmed sequentially and subsequently edited in. Synchronous live sound is possible but only with elaborate equipment and requires post-production editing.

Film is well suited to handling time compression or expansion. Time lapse photography and high speed recording are easy with suitable equipment and of course animation depends largely on the use of the stop frame camera.

*16 mm film*

16 mm film has become the standard work horse of the documentary film world, with the result that production apparatus of every degree of sophistication is readily available. When a production is undertaken which involves sound and where optical effects such as superimposition or dissolves are necessary and from which many copies may be required then 16 mm must be used. Original shooting costs will be high as will be the hire of post-production facilities, but when considered in relation to the potential numbers of viewers they may well be justified.

Although for 'in house' use 16 mm film may well be on the decline it still has one great advantage – 16 mm projectors exist in hospitals and educational institutions throughout the world. They can project a picture of adequate size for the largest audience, the format is universally standardized and even the domestically recorded magnetic commentary stands a high chance of being shown successfully.

*8 mm*

Where picture definition is concerned, the 8 mm gauge falls between 16 mm film and television. For pictures on a screen of up to 3 ft there is little difference between an original 8 mm film and a 16 mm print. However, few 8 mm projectors can give enough light for a picture in excess of 4 ft so the audience size is limited. Camera size and equipment costs are only slightly less than with 16 mm, but running costs are but a quarter. Editing is fiddly at this size and post production equipment scanty.

Copies are not very satisfactory and the addition of sound is usually limited to a magnetic track. 8 mm projectors with sound facilities are far from universal so that the showing of such a film outside one's home institution may not be possible. For all these reasons the use of 8 mm film is best confined to silent records where little editing needs to be done and viewing is to take place locally.

### 21.3.2 Television – the pros and cons

The very wide range of applications of television and the relative ease of its use are the most important factors to be exploited in the medical and educational fields. At one extreme it can compete with the sophistication of a full scale 16 mm film production while at the other extreme it may provide a magnifying glass to enlarge a 2″ kymograph trace onto a 26″ monitor. In the first instance the apparatus will be very costly and involve a production team with an electronic maintenance engineer to run it, while in the second case monochrome cameras and monitors are cheap and can be operated by any laboratory technician. The technically unskilled can rapidly learn to use a television camera because the monitor provides instant feedback of adjustments to camera and lighting. This valuable feature is not just of benefit to the amateur or indeed to an expert camera team but can be of great value to the presenter. A demonstrator or surgeon having a monitor within his field of view can ensure, as the recording is being made, that the audience will clearly see the procedure. In addition any videotape recording can be instantly played back for further checking.

This importance of instant viewing cannot be over estimated since it widens the scope of making visual records to situations that would not be practical when using film.

Video tape costs are not only negligible when compared with film costs but tape can be reused many times. There is virtually no limit on the length of a continuously recorded sequence so that it becomes economic to record many hours of tape in order to capture an occurrence lasting only a few seconds.

Sound and picture are both recorded on the same tape so that problems of synchronization do not arise.

In the more elaborate 'production' situation, where two or more cameras are used, most of the editing takes place at the time of making the record. Post-production work may be kept to a minimum with the finished result being available in a matter of days.

Editing has to be carried out by copying selected sequences. This has the disadvantage of quality loss, the amount being dependent on the sophistication of the equipment used and on the excellence of its maintenance. Unlike film, the editing process does not mutilate the original master so that it is quite feasible to produce several versions for differing purposes.

Although the running costs of television would seem to be low, the capital cost is very high. The quality of picture image is fairly closely linked to equipment costs. Furthermore, the rapidity of development in electronics means that standards rapidly change and may make equipment obsolescent in 3 or 4 years. The situation is most serious in the case of videotape recorders since when new standards are introduced recordings made to the old standard can only be used so long as the manufacturers will continue to service and make available parts for the old machines. Thus archival material is continuously at risk unless it is transferred to film.

In comparison with equipment for film making, television apparatus is unreliable and needs constant maintenance. A film camera that has not been used for months or even years will function perfectly well when needed at a moment's notice but a television camera is unlikely to do so. Many electronic components change their 'values' in response to alterations in temperature during a period of non-use and as the complex circuits involved are sensitive to these small differences, adjustments have to be made to the circuits before optimal results can be obtained. Furthermore, these adjustments should not be attempted until the equipment has had a suitable chance to warm up and dry out. The moral is that all such equipment works best when in constant use.

For all these reasons it must be realized that television is most cost-effective when used heavily. The occasional user will find himself suffering with unreliable and obsolescent equipment.

## 21.4 STILL OR MOVING PICTURES – THE ESSENTIAL DIFFERENCES

### 21.4.1 Lighting

(a) When lighting a film subject, the arrangement has to be satisfactory for all the likely actions that will take place. This often means that a simpler lighting scheme has to be adopted than would be the case in 'still' shot. A key light to one side of the camera, filler flood on the other and a back light opposite the key light will meet many requirements.

(b) Since the subject moves, the lighting may have to cover a much larger area than with a still picture. In the case of a gait recording the area may be very large, even illumination both in width and depth being needed. To avoid excessive amounts of lighting, the cinematographer must work with fast film and maximum apertures.

(c) Surgical operations pose two problems – specular reflections and the illumination of cavities. The solution to both is to use but a single light source. The scialytic lamp should be extinguished and replaced with a single spot light as near as possible to the camera axis. This will

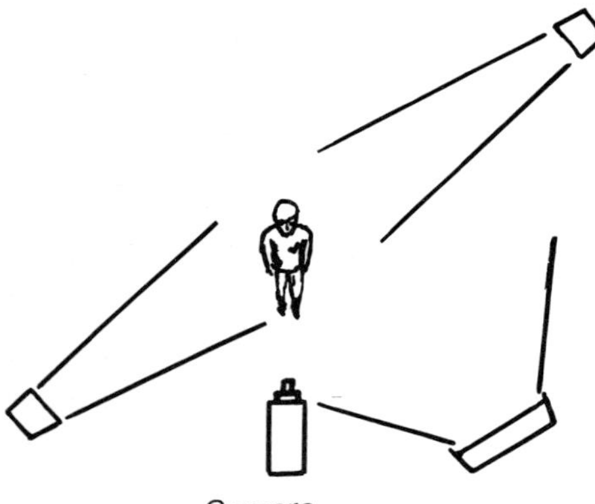


***Figure 21.1*** *A simple lighting arrangement for a 'talking-head' shot*

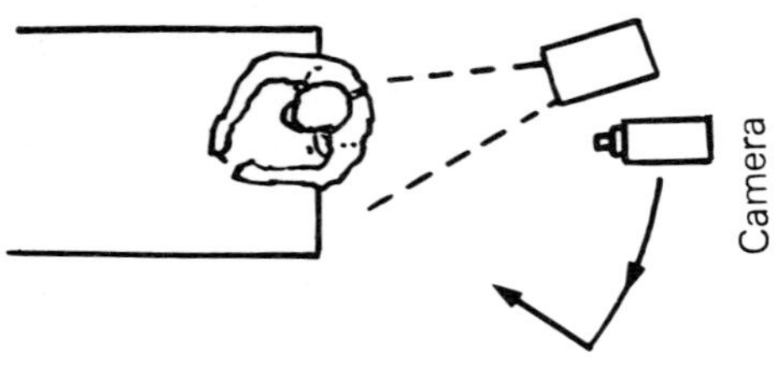


***Figure 21.2*** *A single light source aimed across the surgeon's shoulder will suffice for much surgical cinematography*

reduce specular reflections to a minimum.

The light source will also provide illumination for the surgeon so that if a cavity is involved, light source, surgeon and camera should all lie as far as possible in the same axis. An arrangement such as this encourages the surgeon to keep his hands from encroaching on the camera viewpoint since the light path is obscured first.

Light sources used in the operating theatre should always be equipped with heat-filters. When filming the unconscious patient an intense light source which is not adequately heat-filtered may cause direct burns. The anaesthetized patient is deprived of his natural withdrawal reflex while the surgeon may not appreciate the degree of heat since he wears rubber gloves and his hands may only occasionally be in the direct beam, particularly if working mainly with instruments.

### 21.4.2 Lenses

A 'normal' lens for 16 mm film is of 25 mm focal length and about half this for 8 mm film. This is about twice the equivalent length of a standard lens on a still camera: the reason being that the viewer in the centre of the audience of an average lecture theatre would see roughly the same perspective. The use of a shorter focal length gives the effect of unpleasant distortion particularly should the camera be angled up or down. However the relatively narrow angle of view may make filming a full length figure impossible in a studio designed for still photography so that a 10 mm lens may have to be used. Modern cine cameras frequently use a zoom lens with focal length ranging from 10 to 100 mm (5–50 for 8 mm) as a standard. They should be fitted by the manufacturer and not be removed by the user, since the back focal distance is critical if they are to remain parfocal at all settings. Often they fail to focus sufficiently closely for medical work and this must be overcome by the use of supplementary lenses and not by extension tubes which would negate the use of the zoom facility.

### 21.4.3 Camera supports

A pan and tilt head is essential for filming. Some form of damping must be provided for smooth operation and this is aided by a long handle for easy control. When filming surgical operations a greater degree of downward tilt is required than many heads provide. A wedge may be needed to achieve this and a counterweight is useful to balance the overhanging camera.

Remember that for filming, as opposed to still pictures, the photographer may need to operate the camera continuously for long periods and must be comfortably supported at a suitable height to see through the viewfinder. With a television camera this is less important, provided that a monitor screen can be arranged for convenient viewing by a floor level operator, and that the camera controls can be adjusted for access from a low level.

## 21.5 SCRIPTING AND EDITING

*Although the following section refers to cinematography it is equally applicable to recorded television.*

The most important way in which cinematography differs from still photography is in the necessity of planning pictures and organizing the results of shooting to form a coherent whole. Scripting and editing are the means by which this is done. The scriptwriter plans the intended sequences while the editor assembles and arranges the resulting material. If a script were carried out exactly as planned the editor's task would be a simple mechanical exercise. However much medical filming can only be roughly scripted so that editing assumes great importance – it is as vital to a cinematographer as composition is to a still photographer.

The viewer of a film is at the mercy of the producer in a way that does not occur when looking at a set of still pictures. In the latter case the viewer can flip through them or browse at his own inclination. The film audience however is in the hands of the editor who controls how much of each action is shown and the general rate of presentation. The film maker must judge his audience correctly if he is not to bore them by showing too much for too long or confuse them by cutting too tight.

'Real time' is not the same as 'film time' and the editor's job is to convert one into the other without the viewer being aware of it. Here are some examples. A pathologist wants to demonstrate the 'rapid' sedimentation of a suspension in a test tube. He says it only lasts 1 minute. A single close up of this would be useful as a research record from which measurements could be made, but a continuous shot 1 minute long shown to a audience would give the impression of extreme slowness. Either some form of cut away shot might be introduced to hide the fact that only the beginning and end of the sequence were used, or the shot should be planned as a half frame sequence to be married to the other half frame which would record a 'normal' sedimentation as a comparison. Both would need to be speeded up about four times for the movement to be detectable on the screen. Another common example is the surgical operation lasting an hour which can be shown in 10 minutes on film. If the camera operator has included a sufficient number of close-ups and long shots the editor can hide the missing 50 minutes without the audience being aware of the loss.

Alteration in time scale may have to be planned to reveal rapid movements more clearly. Slow-motion is particularly valuable when magnification is involved (speed also being magnified) such as occurs when filming an eye in close-up to show the movements of nystagmus. An example of time-lapse or speeded-up movement is given above and the technique is much used in conjunction with the microscope to show bacterial growth and tissue cultures.

Timing is of importance when cutting from long shots to close-ups. This is particularly so with rhythmic movements such as a patient's gait. The exact point in the cycle must be chosen if an apparent jump backwards or forwards is to be avoided.

These are some obvious examples where the time factor is of the greatest importance. However there is no shot, however simple, in which the editor can avoid considering timing. Every shot has a relationship to the adjoining shot and a beginning and end which must be precisely determined. To use a shot as it came off the camera is as crude as if a photographer presented the customer with an unmasked or untrimmed print.

## 21.6 FACTS, FIGURES AND STANDARDS

### 21.6.1 Film running time

The 35 mm gauge is confined to the film industry. For 'in house' productions, 16 mm sound film is taken as standard. It is always projected at 24 frames per second, although when shot for television 25 fps taking speed may be used.

| | | | | |
|---|---|---|---|---|
| 1 Reel = | 400 ft | = | 10 minutes approx. |
| | 100 ft | = | 2½ minutes |
| | 36 ft | = | 1 minute |
| | 1 ft | = | 1⅔ seconds |
| | 1 ft | = | 40 frames |
| | 1 ft | = | 7 syllables of commentary |

### 21.6.2 Sound advance

On combined prints the sound track is ahead of the picture (projector sync).

| | |
|---|---|
| 16 mm optical | 26 frames |
| 16 mm magnetic | 28 frames |
| 8 mm magnetic | 56 frames |
| Super 8 magnetic | 18 frames |
| Super 8 optical | 22 frames |

### 21.6.3 Television standards

Standards, particularly in relation to tape recorders, change so rapidly with the development of new formats that the student must regard this information as only partially complete. The number of standards and formats should forewarn users and producers of the difficulties in ensuring that any tape recording made in any one institution can be successfully shown in another, let alone in another country. Although commercial organizations can transfer recordings from one standard to another, this is costly for a single showing.

### 21.6.4 Video tape formats

The 2″ Quad and 1″ C format are unlikely to be used 'in house'.

The ¾″ Umatic cassette system is widely used in hospitals and medical schools. It corresponds to 16 mm film and is the workhorse for making original recordings.

The BVU system uses the same cassettes but is not compatible with Umatic. It has been designed to give higher quality for broadcast work. Do not confuse these similar formats.

½″ VHS and Betamax domestic systems are being increasingly used and neither is compatible with the other. These formats resemble 8 mm film – quality is good enough for making recordings from which copies will not be needed and for making final show copies from Umatic originals.

There are other ½″ and even ¼″ formats but their limited distribution makes them unsatisfactory for institutional use. This situation will, however, change and the student must obtain up-to-date information.

Obsolescent but still used is the ½″ EIAJ reel system and its associated cartridge recorder.

### 21.6.5 Colour systems

In addition to tape recorder standards, the greatest obstacle to compatibility across national boundaries is the variety of systems to encode colour signals. There are three main systems and some countries have adopted modifications of these.

(1) NTSC. Used in the USA and associated countries; is designed for a 60 Hz field rate and 525 lines.
(2) PAL. The UK system and parts of Europe; uses a 50 Hz field rate and 625 lines.
(3) SECAM. The French system (also used in many parts of Europe) is similar in rate and line standards to PAL but otherwise the coding system is not compatible.

Triple standard VTRs and monitors can be obtained but the results cannot be relied upon to give satisfactory colour particularly if the tape supplied is not of high quality. A monochrome result may have to be accepted.

## References


Baddeley, W. (1973). *The Technique of Documentary Film Production.* (London: Focal Press)

Berger, M. (ed.). (1970). *Videotape Techniques in Psychiatric Training and Treatment.* (USA: Brunner-Mazel)

Brodbeck, E. (1974). *Handbook of Basic Motion Picture Techniques.* (Englewood Cliffs, N.J: Prentice-Hall)

Burder, J. (1979). *The Technique of Editing 16 mm Film.* (London: Focal Press)

Burton, A. (1971). *Cinematographic Techniques in Biology and Medicine.* (London: Academic Press)

Fielding, R. (1977). *The Technique of Special Effects Cinematography.* (London: Focal Press)

Foss, H. (ed.). (1980). *Video Production Techniques.* (2 volumes) (London: Kluwer Publishing)

Guest-Lee, S. (1979). Fundamentals of television in medicine – part 1. *J. Audiovis. Media Med.*, **2**, 64-66

Guest-Lee, S. (1979). Fundamentals of television in medicine – part 2. *J. Audiovis. Media Med.*, **2**, 118-121

Guest-Lee, S. (1979). Fundamentals of television in medicine – part 3. *J. Audiovis. Media Med.*, **2**, 152-155

Guest-Lee, S. (1980). Fundamentals of television in medicine – part 4. *J. Audiovis. Media Med.*, **3**, 23-26

Halas, J. and Manvell, R. (1976). *The Technique of Film Animation.* (London: Focal Press)

Herskovitz, A. and McDermott, I. (1979). Video transfer for the photographer. *J. Biol. Photogr.*, **47**, 137-142

Johns, M. (1974). Some aspects of medical cinematography. (Part 1 – Master cutting and commentary recording.). *Med. Biol. Illustr.*, **24**, 63-70

Johns, M. (1975). Some aspects of medical cinematography. (Part 2 – Basic principles of picture editing.). *Med. Biol. Illustr.*, **25**, 211-219

Jones, P. (1972). *The Technique of the Television Camera.* (London: Focal Press)

Kodak. (1975). *Television Film Editing and Splicing Techniques.* (Publication H-40.8.). (Rochester, NY: Eastman Kodak Ltd)

Kodak. (1976). *Care and Handling of Television Film.* (Publication H-40.9.) (Rochester, NY: Eastman Kodak Ltd.)

Kodak. (1976). *Basic Production Techniques for Motion Pictures.* (Publication P-18.) (Rochester, NY: Eastman Kodak Ltd.)

Kodak. (1977). *Motion Picture Prints from Colour Originals.* (Publication H-25.) (Rochester, NY: Eastman Kodak Ltd.)

Kodak. (1977). *Splicing for the Professional.* (Publication H-50:1) (Rochester, NY: Eastman Kodak Ltd.)

Kodak. (1977). *Magnetic Sound Recording for Motion Pictures.* (Publication S-75L). (Rochester, NY: Eastman Kodak Ltd.)

Kodak. (1978). *The Business of Film making.* (Publication H-55L.) (Rochester, NY: Eastman Kodak Ltd.)

Kodak. (1978). *Using Films for Television.* (Publication H-40.11.) (Rochester, NY: Eastman Kodak Ltd.)

Kodak. (1979). *The World of Animation.* (Publication S-35.L.) (Rochester, NY: Eastman Kodak Ltd.)

Kodak. (1979). *Techniques of Telecine Video Operation.* (Publication H-40.13.) (Rochester, NY: Eastman Kodak Ltd.)

Kodak. (1979). *Making Television Pictures from Films and Slides.* (Publication H-40-12.) (Rochester, NY: Eastman Kodak Ltd.)

Kodak. (1980). *Surgical Motion Picture Photography.* (Publication M3-719.) (Rochester, NY: Eastman Kodak Ltd.)

Kodak. (1980). *Film Sound Recording and Reproduction.* (Publication H-40.15.) (Rochester, NY: Eastman Kodak Ltd.)

Kodak. (1982). *Professional Motion Picture Films.* (Publication H-1L.) (Rochester, NY: Eastman Kodak Ltd.)

Kodak. (1982). *Cinematographer's Field Guide.* (Publication H-2L.) (Rochester, NY: Eastman Kodak Ltd.)

Kodak. (1982). *The Book of Film Care.* (Publication H-23L.) (Rochester, NY: Eastman Kodak Ltd.)

Manville, R. and Huntley, J. (1975). *The Technique of Film Music.* (London: Focal Press)

Mascelli, J. (1973). *The Five C's of Cinematography.* (USA: Cine Grafic)

Michaelis, A. (1955). *Research Films in Biology and Medicine.* (London: Academic Press)

Millerson, G. (1972). *The Technique of Lighting for Television and Motion Pictures.* (London: Focal Press)

Millerson, G. (1974). *The Technique of Television Production.* (London: Focal Press)

Myers, R. (1981). A systematic approach to medical motion picture production. (Part 1). *J. Biol. Photogr.*, **50**, 15-29

Myers, R. (1982). A systematic approach to medical motion picture production. (Part 2). *J. Biol. Photogr.*, **50**, 15-29

Myers, R. (1982). A systematic approach to medical motion picture production (Part 3). *J. Biol. Photogr.*, **50**, 47-58

Myers, R. (1982). A systematic approach to medical motion picture production. (Part 4). *J. Biol. Photogr.*, **50**, 83-94

Nisbett, A. (1976). *The Technique of the Sound Studio.* (London: Focal Press)

Reisz, K. and Millar, G. (1968). *The Technique of Film Editing.* (London: Focal Press)

Souto, H. (1977). *The Technique of the Motion Picture Camera.* (London: Focal Press)

Spottiswoode, R. (ed.). (1969). *The Focal Encyclopaedia of Film and Television Techniques.* (London: Focal Press)

Walter, E. (1973). *The Technique of the Film Cutting Room.* (London: Focal Press)

Wilkie, B. (1971). *The Technique of Special Effects in Television.* (London: Focal Press)

## *Practical assignments*

(1) For a real (or hypothetical) film production demonstrate the various steps involved in the planning and preparation for a single-concept or self-instructional production.

(*a*) Develop a storyboard outline of the production.
(*b*) State the purpose and the audience level of the production.
(*c*) Prepare a budget including any extra expertise, equipment hire or laboratory services you need to complete the production.
(*d*) Present the full production schedule.

(You may submit the actual finished film as supporting evidence but this assignment purely tests your skills of production *planning* and *costing*.)

(2) Produce a short motion picture or videotape record of a procedure which cannot be repeated for your convenience, e.g. a surgical operation. Finished screen time should be not less than 5 minutes. The finished production should be accompanied by notes on the planning, costing and production techniques you employed.

## *Examination questions*

Q.1 How can you identify film stock as having 'winding A' or 'winding B'? Give detailed examples of how each is used.

Q.2 How is running time determined with 16 mm motion picture footage?
What exposure compensation is necessary in changing from 24 fps, to (*a*) 64 fps, (*b*) 32 fps, (*c*) 16 fps, (*d*) 12 fps?
How may changes in running speed be useful in medical photography?

Q.3 Describe the set-up needed for conforming A and B rolls and C roll narrative sound track to a workprint (include titles and effects).

Q.4 Motion picture film production invariably involves liaison with a laboratory. Explain the meaning of the following requests:
(*a*) Timed print
(*b*) Work print
(*c*) Answer print
(*d*) Print edge numbers
(*e*) Release print
(*f*) One-light print.

(Q.5) Describe the technique of double system sound. Compare this with single systems for synchronous sound and picture and give examples of appropriate use.

(Q.6) Discuss the use of (*a*) wild, (*b*) magnetic striped and (*c*) synch-pulsed sound for medical motion picture production.

(Q.7) Give a brief description of three types of video tube which you might encounter in a medical environment. How can the tendency of a vidicon tube to 'lag' be reduced?

(Q.8) Give a definition and appropriate examples of use for the:
(*a*) Waveform monitor,
(*b*) Synch generator,
(*c*) Time-base corrector,
(*d*) Film chain,
(*e*) Vision mixer.

(Q.9) What is a 'colour burst'? Describe its relationship to the television standard.
How is a vectorscope used in television production?

(Q.10) Describe the usefulness of (*a*) studio-based, (*b*) location-based television recording to medicine. How does the technique used affect the requirements for 'post-production' facilities?

*Multiple choice questions (any of the statements may be true or false)*

(Q.11) In small scale television production:
(*a*) Vidicon tubes are useful because they are quick to respond to changes in light intensity at low illumination levels.
(*b*) The monitors are able to resolve 256 logarithmic grey steps.
(*c*) 'Buzz-track' is used where there is no signal on the sound track.
(*d*) 'Squashed' highlights are a result of excessive video record level.
(*e*) Gen-locked line and field pulses allow the use of mixed special effects.

(Q.12) In medical motion picture production:
(*a*) A 400 foot film running at normal speeds lasts approximately 10 minutes.
(*b*) On an optical sound print the sound track is 26 frames ahead of the picture.
(*c*) The 'standard' lens is 40 mm focal length.
(*d*) The use of 'A' and 'B' rolling eliminates splice marks.
(*e*) 'Work prints' are the same as 'cutting copies'.

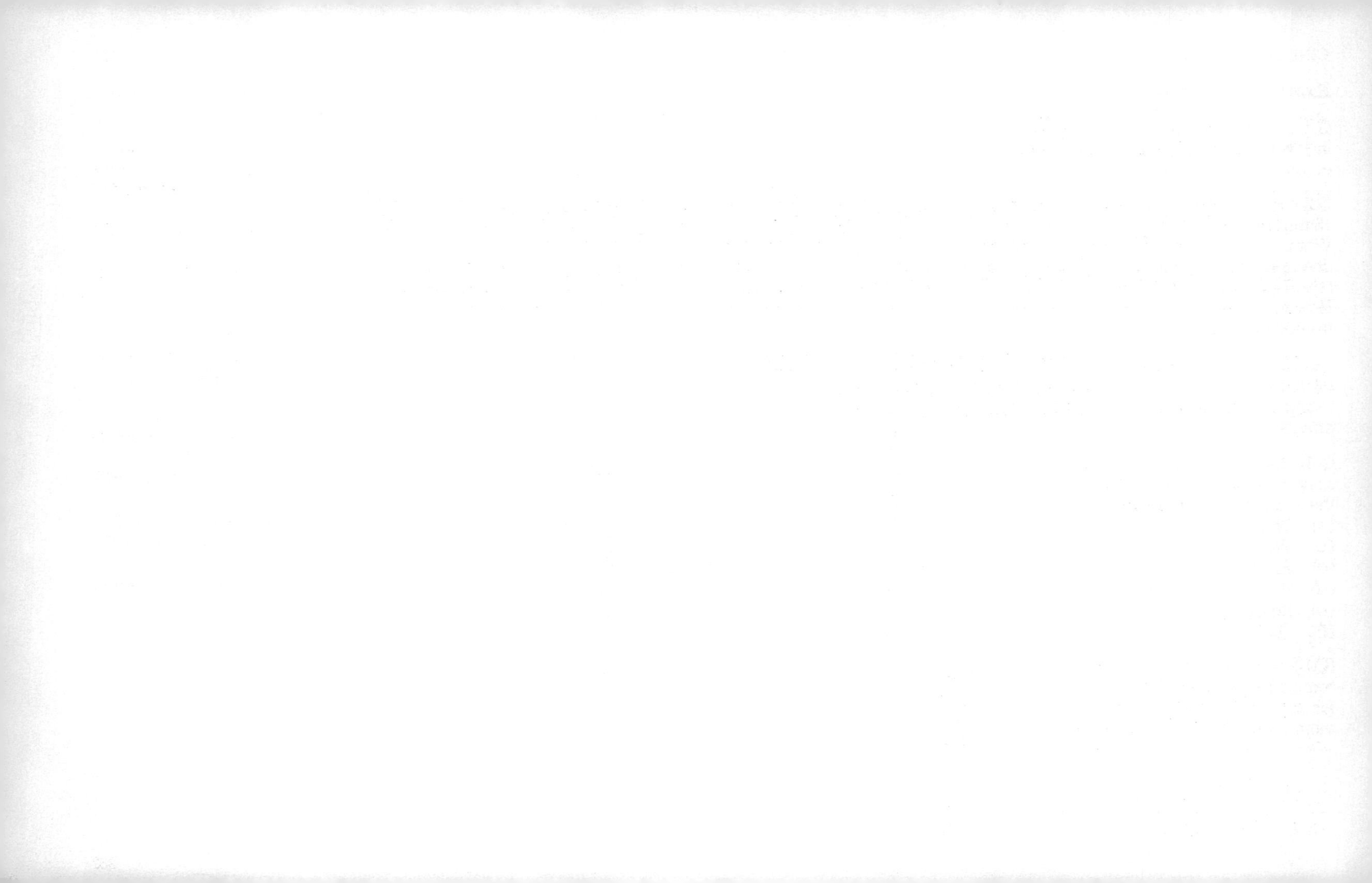

# Section 22
# Photogrammetry (incorporating perspective and somatotyping)

**A.R. Williams**, MPhil, FBIPP, FRPS, FBPA, AIMBI
Head of Medical Illustration and Teaching Services
Charing Cross Hospital and Medical School, London

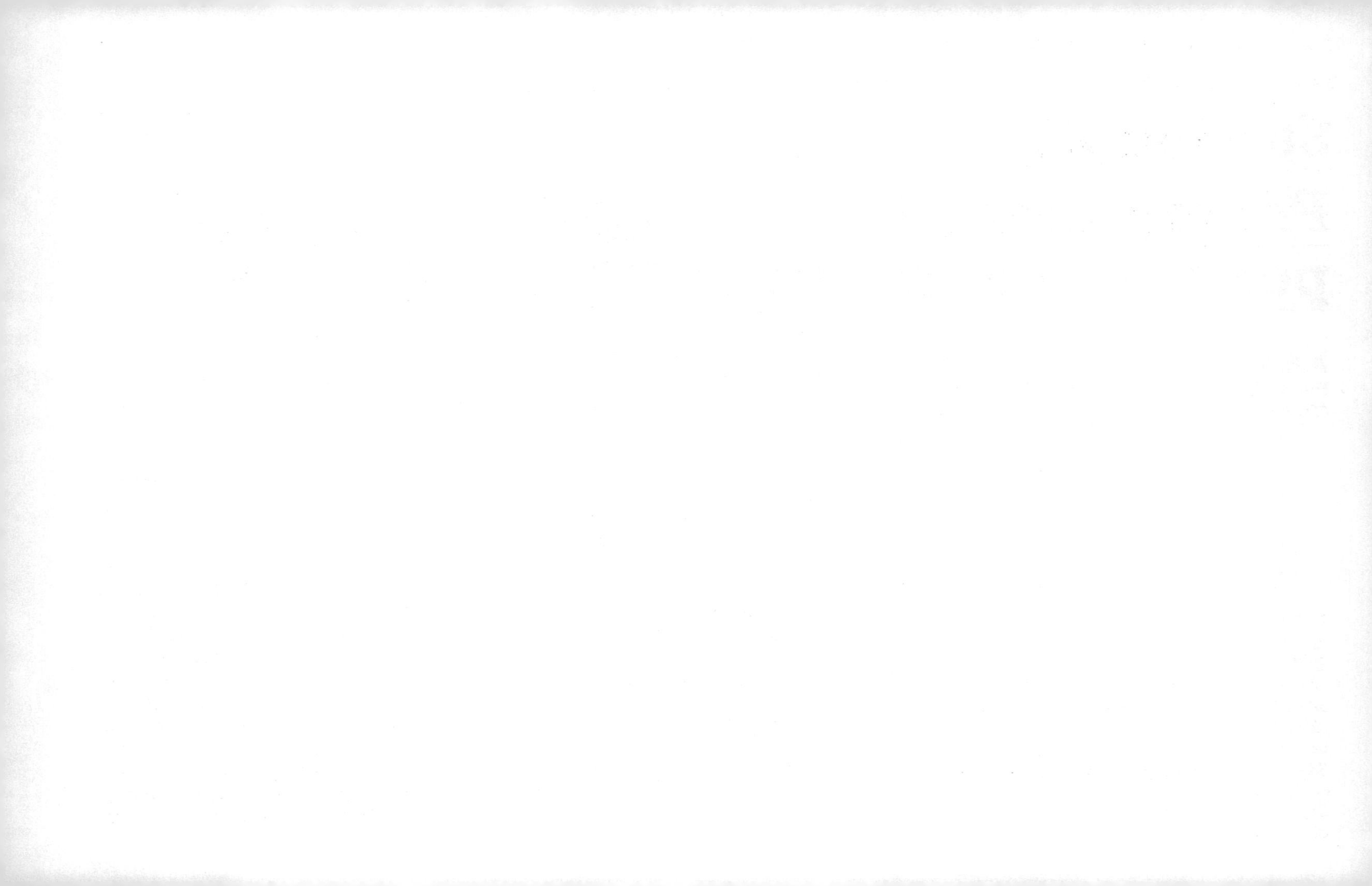

## 22.1 PERSPECTIVE

Perspective is defined as the apparent relationship between the shape, visual scale and position of visible objects. It is sometimes described as the art of delineating solid objects on a flat surface so as to convey the same impression of sizes, shapes and positions as the actual objects do when viewed from a particular point.

### 22.1.1 Theory

As one moves about when looking at any scene the apparent geometry of it changes. Also the apparent size of an object is dependent upon the distance from which we view it. For example, one object may appear from, or disappear behind another. Thus, a drawing, painting or photograph can represent a given scene from only one fixed point of view. The scale of any photograph depends solely on the position occupied by the lens in relation to the subject. Alteration of the focal length of the lens or the size of the negative will affect the area of the subject recorded on the photograph but not the perspective. Conversely, any alteration in subject-to-lens distance will affect the perspective even though a different focal length of lens is chosen to maintain the chief point of interest at the same magnification.

In order to get the same impression from a contact print of the negative, the eye of the observer must be placed at the same point relative to the picture as was the lens when the photograph was taken. For example, if a picture were taken with a 12" lens on a 10" × 8" camera it should be viewed at 12" distance (or to be more accurate, at the distance to which the lens was extended – say 13"). With the short focal length lenses used on 35 mm cameras the eye cannot of course focus, but an enlargement can be made or the image magnified through a projector. Under these conditions, the focal length (or extension) of the lens is multiplied by the magnification factor to obtain the correct viewing distance. Thus, an image taken with a 50 mm lens on a 35 mm transparency and projected to fill a 48" × 72" screen should be viewed at (2" × 48") 8 feet, if the perspective is to appear exactly as it did to the camera.

### 22.1.2 Practical implications

(1) In any system of standardization (*see Section 1.4.10*), not only must the scale be kept constant, but the subject-to-camera distance must be constant if the perspective is to remain the same in comparable pictures.

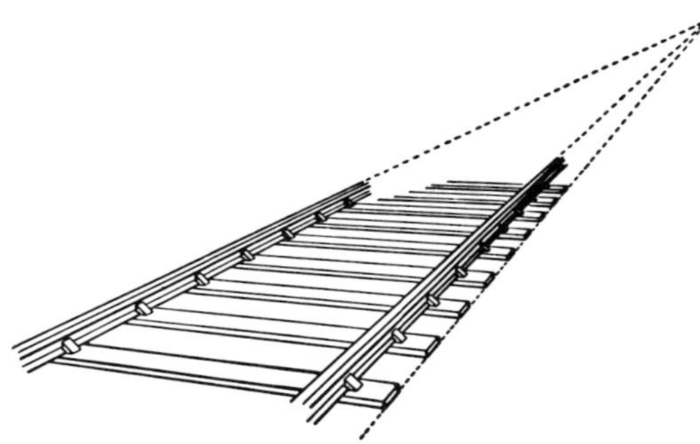

***Figure 22.1*** *The perspective effect. The parallel railway tracks appear to converge as they become more distant*

(2) There is only one viewing distance for any picture or screen image in which the apparent perspective is exactly similar to that seen by the camera. Since in practice any member of an audience in even the best designed lecture theatre may be sitting at a distance varying from 2 to 6 screen widths, it follows that most viewers will have to make a psychological adjustment to com-

pensate for the discrepancy. Luckily we are accustomed to this exercise and do it unconsciously unless the discrepancy is too marked. This occurs principally when the photographer has approached the subject too closely when using a short focal length lens. Note that even in the example quoted above, the 'correct' viewing distance from the 6' screen was only 8' while in reality the average member of the audience will be sitting some 20' from the screen. To him the discrepancy gives the appearance of 'exaggerated' perspective though this would vanish if he could approach the screen closely enough. If the photographer had used a 4" instead of a 2" lens and had adopted a viewpoint twice as distant, the correct viewing distance would become 16' and thus approximate to that of the average member of the audience.

(3) In order to avoid perspective 'distortion' it is imperative that the photographer should not approach the subject too closely, particularly when recording a subject which involves 'depth' such as a face. The viewer will be very sensitive to slight distortions in the face but where the subject presents a flat plane, such as a section of a kidney, the effect of perspective distortion is negligible. Where a scale is included alongside a specimen, however, it is imperative that it is placed exactly in the plane one wishes to measure – which should also be the plane of principal focus.

(4) Where single photographs are to be used for accurate measurement purposes, e.g. in craniofacial pre-operative planning, it is important to minimize the effects of perspective by using the most distant viewpoint that studio space will allow. This will then necessitate the use of a long focal length lens to obtain a satisfactory image size. As a rough rule of thumb to obtain an acceptable level of perspective distortion the camera should be placed at least ten subject diameters away from the subject. For example, if we require accurate photographs of the head, which can be considered as having a maximum diameter of 10", then the camera must be placed at least 100" from the subject.

## 22.2 PHOTOGRAMMETRY

Photogrammetry may be defined as the science of obtaining accurate and precise measurements from conventional photographs taken under strictly controlled conditions. Traditionally the subject is divided into monophotogrammetry, which is measurement from single photographs, and stereophotogrammetry, which is measurement from stereo-pairs of photographs. There are now, however, a number of photo-optical photogrammetric techniques, such as moiré interferometry, holographic interferometry, and light sectioning which whilst being monophotogrammetric by definition are more similar to stereophotogrammetry in that the end product they produce is a contour map – giving three-dimensional information.

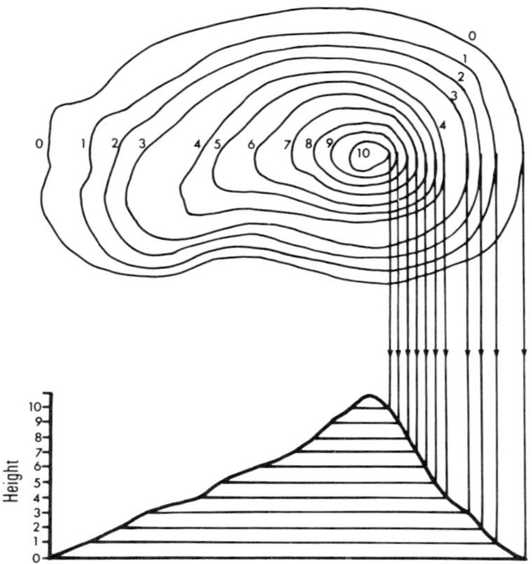


***Figure 22.2*** *The contour map is the most useful way of representing three-dimensional information. The lines of the contour map (above) delineate the edges of imaginary sections through the subject (below). The scale of the map and the contour interval can be altered to suit the subject. Volume, surface area, cross-sections, profiles and point-to-point measurements can all be taken from the map*

### 22.2.1 Monophotogrammetry

For a long time now it has been usual in medical photography to make use of standardized scale photographs for specimens and for recording characteristic facies or body shapes. It should be routine practice to include a measuring scale in the field of view, or to take the photograph at a known magnification, so that the photographs may be measured in place of the subject. All too often the photographs are not taken under sufficiently well controlled conditions and the results are unreliable. The problems of distortion and elimination of errors in the photographs are complex and many factors need to be taken into consideration. Some of the important recommendations would be as follows:

(1) Reduce perspective distortion to a minimum by using the longest lens-to-subject distance that studio space will allow. Ideally a ratio of subject diameter: lens-to-subject distance of 1:10.

(2) Use the highest possible quality optics to minimize geometric distortion caused by lens aberrations.

(3) Wherever possible use estar based film and resin coated paper, squeezed and air dried at normal room temperature.

(4) Wherever possible, measure from negatives – use a travelling microscope if necessary. (The printing process introduces some of the largest errors.)

(5) Use 'posing' aids for the subject. It is critical for accurate serial photography that the subject assumes the same body position each time they are photographed. This will require some imagination and ingenuity in devising head rests, bite-blocks, cephalostats or even plaster bandage shells to ensure accurate re-positioning of the patient.

There are several special monophotogrammetric techniques worth mentioning:

***Skiagraphic or shadowgraph***

This technique does not even require the use of a camera but instead relies on a beam of collimated light from a distant spotlight falling on the subject so that it casts a shadow onto photographic paper held behind the subject. When developed and fixed the result is an accurate and permanent record of the outline of the subject. It means, of course, that the procedure has to be undertaken

***Figure 22.3*** *The skiagraphic method*

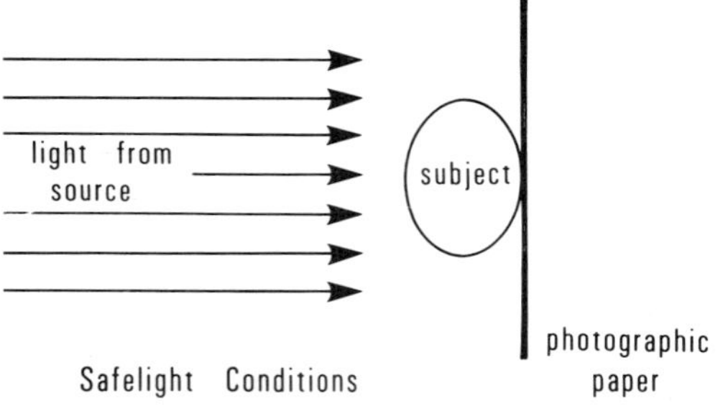


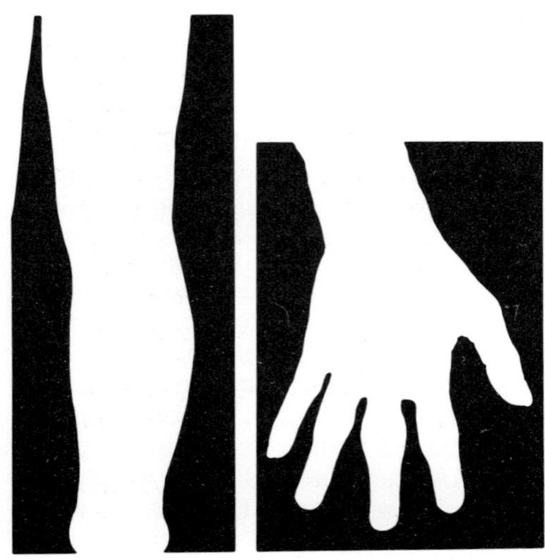

in safelight conditions. If the system is properly adjusted the image should be exactly life size – but it is advisable to check this by imaging a transparent plastic ruler in the same plane as the subject. Serial recordings of this kind can be used to monitor changes in tumour volume or oedema for example.

***Perspective reconstruction***

Where the photograph contains clear perspective, rectilinear objects and a usable reference object within the object space it is possible to reconstruct the geometry of the photograph, either analytically or by drawing. Normally a flat, square, reference frame is laid horizontally in the foreground – from which it is possible to extrapolate out lines to find the perspective centre and vanishing points of the scene. The exact dimensions of the test object must be known. Heindl was one of the first to describe the technique, but Williams gives a thorough account with examples of both graphical and analytical solutions.

***Orthographic or perspectiveless photography***

Orthographic photographs are ones which are free of perspective – that is, all points in the object space are recorded at exactly the same magnification irrespective of their position. It is possible to achieve this either with a mirror camera, similar to a schlieren system, or with a telecentric lens system. A simple telecentric system consists of a large diameter positive lens with an axial stop arranged at the principal focus of the lens so that the central image forming ray from any point on the object is initially parallel to the axis, this makes the image size independent of the object distance. The recording camera lens can be used to form the axial stop. With such a system, however, the size of the subject which can be recorded is limited by the size of the large telecentric lens.

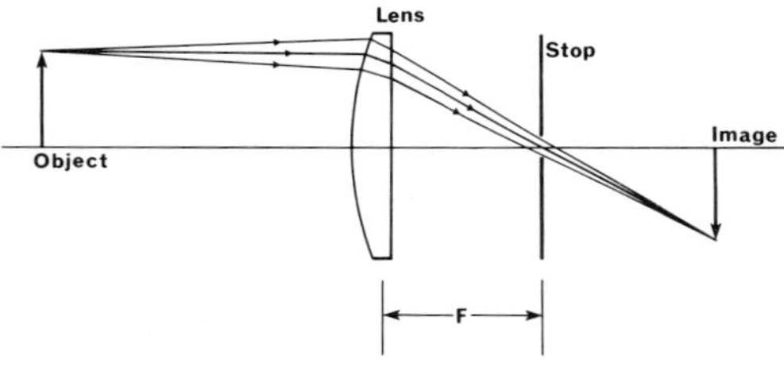


***Figure 22.4*** *A simple telecentric system for perspectiveless photography*

### 2.2.2 Stereophotogrammetry

In appreciating stereoscopic photography it is helpful to relate the conditions of the photography to those of normal binocular vision. When we view an object, it subtends an angle to each eye called the parallactic angle. Objects at different distances from the eyes subtend different parallactic angles. Thus the impression of depth is dependent upon the changes in magnitude of the parallactic angle formed in the object space. This change in parallactic angle shows itself as a change in position of an object ray on the retina of the eye. It can be shown that the central perspectives of a pair of photographs are analogous to the central perspectives on the retinae of the eyes. The stereocameras, therefore, show a permanent record of a central perspective at a chosen scale, a perspective which is only momentarily retained by the eye in normal vision. Once having recorded all the parallactic angles of all the points within the scene on the stereo-pair we can by simple geometric principles measure the co-ordinate points on the stereo-pair, and calculate the co-ordinates of the points in the object space. Alternatively, the stereo-pair can be projected in such a way that the observer sees a 'model' of the subject recreated in three dimensions, allowing this to be measured and a contour map plotted. This requires the images to be coded as left and right by coloured or polarizing filters.

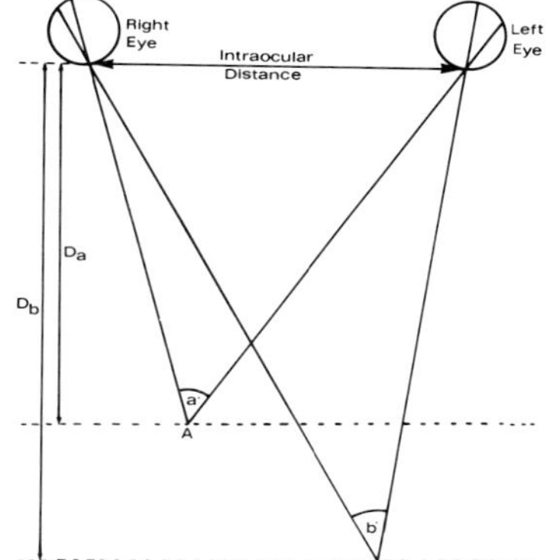


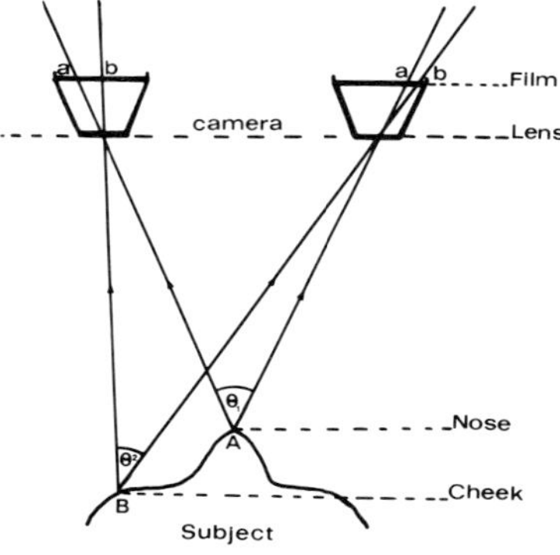


***Figure 22.5*** *The conditions of binocular vision (above) are reproduced by the cameras in stereophotogrammetry (below)*

There are several general textbooks on stereophotogrammetry, examples being Thompson and Valyus, which give full details of the principles and practices involved.

Commercially available stereophotogrammetric equipment tends to be very expensive and is usually designed for long range or aerial photogrammetry. This has led to the use in medicine of non-metric cameras or the design of purpose built equipment. The most successful of these is described by Beard who employs the simple expedient of utilizing the camera as a projector for the plotting – geometric distortions introduced by the lenses at the taking stage are eliminated during the plotting stage. Recent developments have included the use of desk top computers with 'graphic tablets' for the analysis of the differences in parallatic angles stored on the stereo-pairs.

Stereophotogrammetry is undoubtedly the most accurate and versatile of the photographic methods of measurement and is ideally suited to medical applications. It is a versatile, non-contact method of measuring patients to very high orders of accuracy. It can be used on any size of subject with convex or concave surfaces, the only photographic technique to be able to do this.

### 22.2.3 Moiré interferometry

Moiré interferometry is a method of mapping the surface contours of a subject by photographically recording the interference pattern caused by a linear grid and the shadow of that grid on the subject.

When a linear grid falls on a subject the grid becomes distorted according to the topography of the surface. If in some way we view the original grid superimposed onto the grid which has been distorted by the subject's topography, the two grid patterns interfere and the resulting moiré pattern is in the form of a contour map of the subject. Unfortunately, the contour spacing is not equal, therefore one has either to calculate the actual depth of each fringe (from a simple formula relating the distance from the light source to grid and to the camera, with the grid spacing), or make an approximation of the contour interval. The error involved with such an approximation depends upon the depth of the subject.

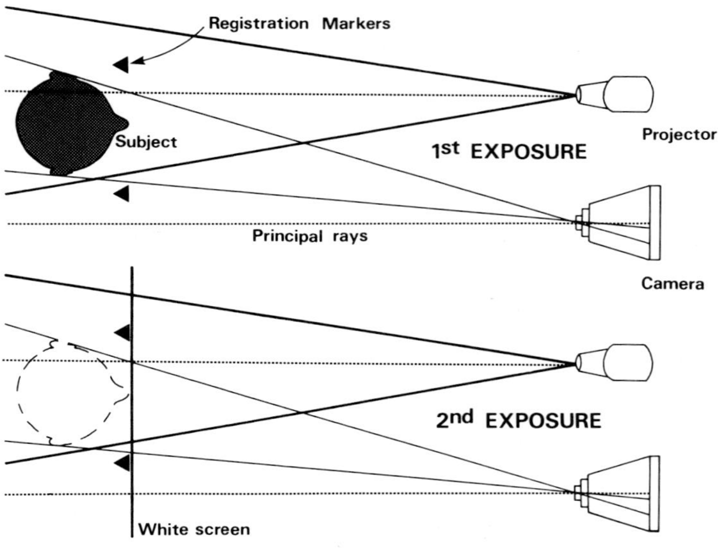


***Figure 22.6*** *The additive moiré method*

In practice there are two ways of producing the moiré interferometric contour map, which can be referred to as additive and subtractive methods. They differ only in the way the undistorted or control grid is combined with the distorted grid projected on the subject.

#### *(1) Additive moiré*

A fine line grid is projected from a conventional slide projector first onto a plane reference surface and then onto the subject, each result being recorded photographically onto a separate piece of film.

It is essential to have reference markers within the field of view so that the two photographs can be combined (either as negatives, or as a print and an overlay) to obtain the interference map. In the second exposure the subject must be placed in the same plane as the reference surface. The camera and projector axes must be parallel, and the camera displaced from the projector by a known distance. Full details of the technique can be found in the references cited. Several problems arise with additive systems in practice:

(1) Fringes are of low contrast because they only appear at those places where the brightness of the subject matches that of the reference frame.

(2) If the grid is of the usual square-wave form and the subject surface is one of steep inclination, e.g. the side of the face, a form of unwanted secondary moiré occurs as a set of confusing lines.

(3) Sandwiching the two negatives together can be difficult and great care has to be taken.

(4) Obtaining sufficient illumination to photograph living human subjects can be problematic – a typical exposure would be ¼ second at *f*/8 with 400 ASA film.

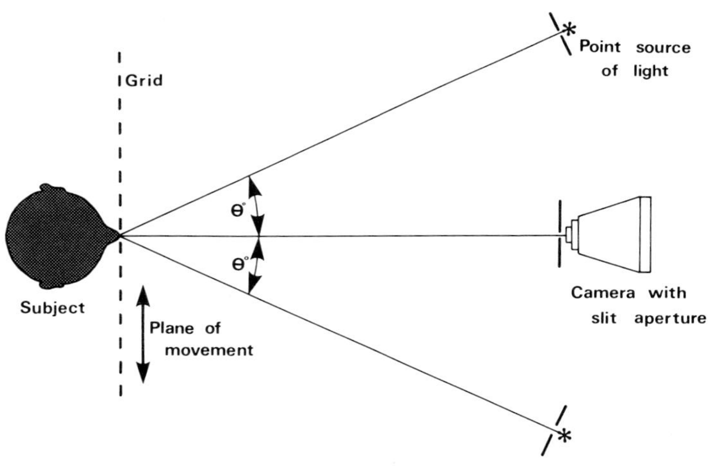


***Figure 22.7*** *The subtractive moiré method*

### *(2) Subractive moiré*

A large scale transparent grid is placed in front of the subject and shadowed onto the subject by a point source of light in the plane of the camera. The subject is then photographed through the grid. The reference grid and the shadow of that grid are therefore imaged together, and a contour map is produced instantaneously. The large grid is often constructed of black threads stretched over a frame with some kind of device to maintain spacing.

The problems of lighting level and shadowing found in the additive system can be overcome in the subtractive technique by using two light sources placed symmetrically about the camera axis – this produces bright 'shadow free' lighting. The unwanted secondary (or aliasing moiré) can be removed in this technique by moving the grid in its plane at right angles to the camera axis; only the equal depth fringes remain constant, all others being washed out by the movement. The selection of grid spacing, camera-to-grid distance and angle of illumination are critical to achieve the best contour spacing and fringe contrast. Again full details of the technique can be found in the literature.

However it is produced the moiré map is subject to perspective distortion as described above and some method of correction must be used to obtain accurate results. This can either be done by using telecentric systems or by geometric drawing or by computer manipulation of digitized co-ordinates.

Moiré topography is a non-contact method of producing a contour map of the subject instantaneously. It is quick, simple and has a low unit cost, a large range of subject sizes can be measured with very simple equipment. To achieve accurate results, however, some form of perspective correction is essential.

### 22.2.4 Light sectioning

Light sectioning is a photo-optical method of measuring three-dimensional subjects by sectioning the subject with parallel slits of light projected at a known angle to the camera axis. In the simplest system parallel slits of light are projected at a known frequency of spacing parallel to the long axis (Y) and at right angles to the depth axis (Z) causing the subject to become striped or sectioned by the lines of the grid. Viewed along the axis of the grid projector each slit of light covers an equal depth of the subject, say 2 mm. When viewed along the depth axis (camera axis) the light from each slit of the grid spills around the front of the subject and 'describes' all those parts of the subject at that particular depth co-ordinate. It then becomes a simple matter to record the resulting contour map photographically. The result will be a true record of the subject's contours provided that the grid projector and camera axes are at 90°. When using only one grid projector one side of the subject is not contoured; so for a full contour map two identical grids and projectors are placed either side of the subject. Cross-wire slides are used to align the optical centres of the projectors after the dis-

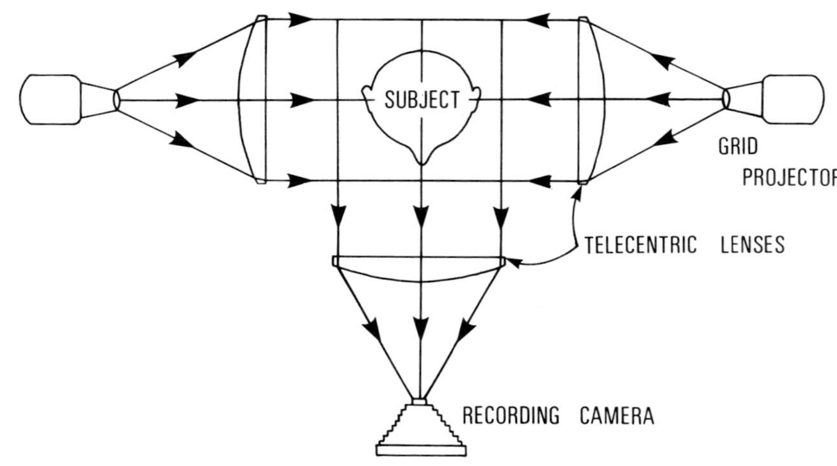


***Figure 22.8*** *The optical arrangement for double-sided geometrically corrected light sectioning*

tance to the subject, height and elevation of each projector has been carefully measured and matched. The use of a multi-coloured grid, instead of plain black and white, aids the interpretation of the finished contour map especially in steep areas of contour.

Such a simple system suffers from geometric distortion in both the projection and recording beams and depending on the accuracy required these errors must be more or less corrected. The simplest method is to use telecentric optics (as described above) for both projection and recording beams. Other methods of correction include mathematical compensation and the projection of distorted grids which become accurate on reprojection.

Various other light sectioning techniques have been described in the literature such as: utilization of a single slit with a moving subject, use of large scale grids shadowed onto the subject, projection of various types of chequerboard grids, and projection of linear grids at known angles other than 90°, particularly for contouring the optic fundus.

Light sectioning is an inexpensive non-contact method of obtaining a contour map instantly at the time of photography. A wide range of subjects can be contoured from a few millimetres up to a metre or so. Larger subjects are much more difficult and concave subjects impossible. The contour interval has to be fixed before photography, and low light levels reduce resolution and demand a degree of co-operation in the case of the living subject. It is simple to apply, quick and has a low unit cost.

### 22.2.5 Holography

Holography may be defined as the technique of recording all the light reflected from an object as an interference pattern on a photographic plate – which when processed is called a hologram. In order to achieve this, highly coherent, or laser, light is used to illuminate the object and to image a reference beam onto the plate. On subsequent viewing with coherent light the hologram reconstructs the wavefronts originally coming from the object, to give a three-dimensional image with full parallax. Holography is also known as 'wave-front reconstruction' or 'lensless photography'. Although the theory was described much earlier the first hologram was not made until 1963, this is therefore the newest of the photographic techniques of measurement. Holography relies on illumination of the subject with coherent light and splitting off some of the coherent light before it reaches the subject to act as a reference beam. Light reflected from the subject is combined with the reference beam at the surface of the photographic plate – which records the resulting interference pattern. The beam of light from the laser has to be widened by the use of a microscope objective and then made spatially coherent by the use of a pinhole. The fine hologram fringes require a high resolution emulsion – usually of the Lippmann type having enhanced red sensitivity to suit the helium–neon lasers in common use. All the components of the holographic system have to be mounted on vibration free mountings, since movement in excess of a few nanometres destroys the image. Laser light is again used to reconstruct the hologram to yield a virtual image which can be measured in the same way as the virtual stereophotogrammetric image. In order to provide a brighter reconstruction image the silver in the hologram may be bleached out of the plate to leave a gelatine relief image called a phase hologram.

There are several special features of the hologram worth mentioning:

(1) Because each point on the hologram receives light from every part of the object, any portion of

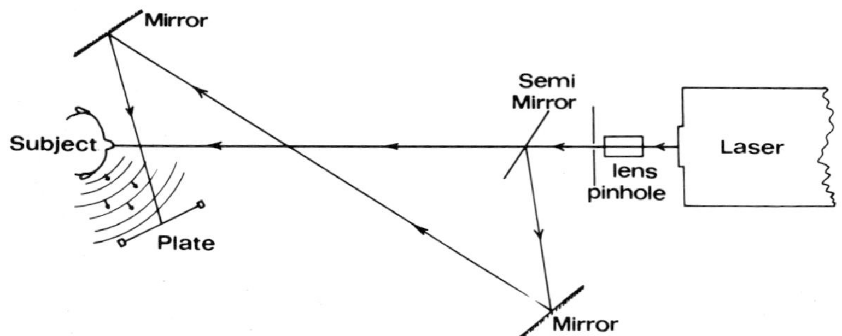


***Figure 22.9*** *Simple holographic recording arrangement*

the hologram will provide a complete reconstruction of the subject.

(2) Direct contact prints of the hologram reproduce exactly the same – there are no negatives or positives.

(3) Because no lens is used the reconstructed image has high metrical qualities – there are no aberrations to take into account – and there is infinite depth of field. Extreme magnification of the reconstruction is possible.

Apart from conventional holographic reconstructions there are a number of other specialized techniques which use holographic principles.

*Multiple frequency contouring* – two holograms are made simultaneously on one plate with two lasers of different frequency. The developed plate is then illuminated with light of a single frequency to reveal a complete photo-optical contour map.

*Multiple index contouring* – is analogous to multiple frequency holographic contouring, except that instead of changing the wavelength of light between exposures the refractive index of the medium surrounding the object is changed. Like multiple frequency contouring the technique is used to measure very small objects, e.g. the surface of teeth.

*Double pulsed holography* – a conventional exposure is given to the hologram, a short delay is allowed during which time the subject may move or alter, then a second exposure is given to the hologram which is then processed and reconstructed in the normal way. If any change takes place in the topography of the subject between exposures the reconstruction will show interference fringes which are contours of equal separation between the two surfaces.

*Holographic multiplexing* – many conventional photographs are taken of the subject at known angles, and these are then imaged onto a hologram with laser light at the same angles. When processed and reconstructed the hologram forms a kind of three-dimensional model.

The novelty of holography has precipitated a surfeit of predictions about its future implications for medicine and biology, but in the realm of stereometric analysis holography seems to have least to offer. The chief application might seem to be in micro-anatomy, where multiple index or frequency contouring can quantify minute topographic changes.

### 22.2.6 Applications of photogrammetry

Just about every conceivable part of the body has been successfully measured by photogrammetry for one medical speciality or another, and for one reason or another. Complete reviews are published elsewhere and the advanced student would do well to consult some of these publications. A few selected examples will illustrate the breadth of application.

Whole body photographic measurement has enjoyed considerable success, probably because of the difficulties of measuring whole body surface area, volume or point-to-point limb measurements on the living person, especially children. Athletes, astronauts and physically handicapped children have all been measured.

The trunk has been measured for assessment of spinal deformities, e.g. scoliosis, for studies on respiration and for measurement of breast volume. The effects of trauma, drugs and exercise on respiration have been measured, as have deformities of the chest such as pectus excavatum. Leg oedema in congestive heart failure and lymphoedema in arms have been measured. The heart, bladder and liver have all been measured photogrammetrically *in vivo.*

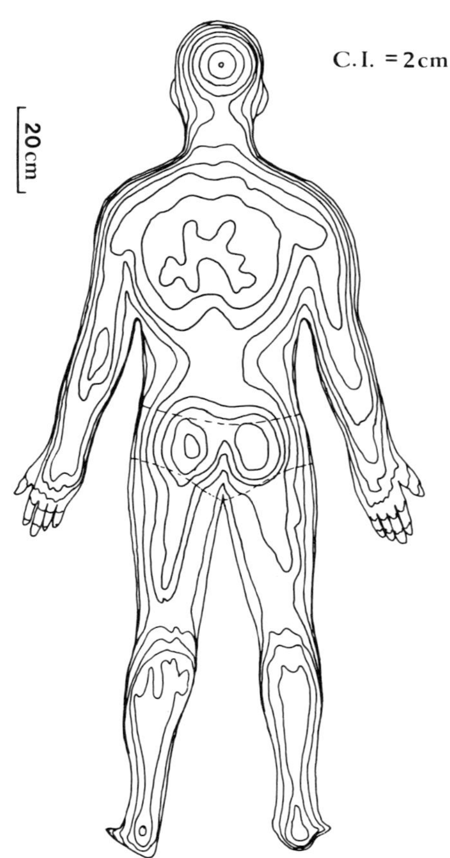


**Figure 22.10** *Contour map of an adult, full-length, male subject*

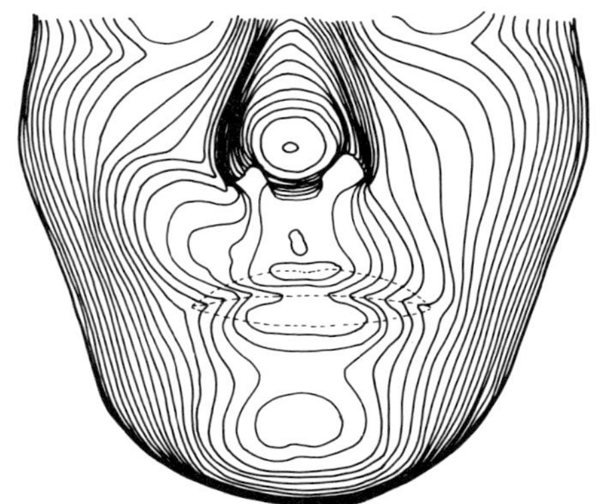

**Figure 22.11** *Post-operative swelling following extraction of the upper-right wisdom tooth*

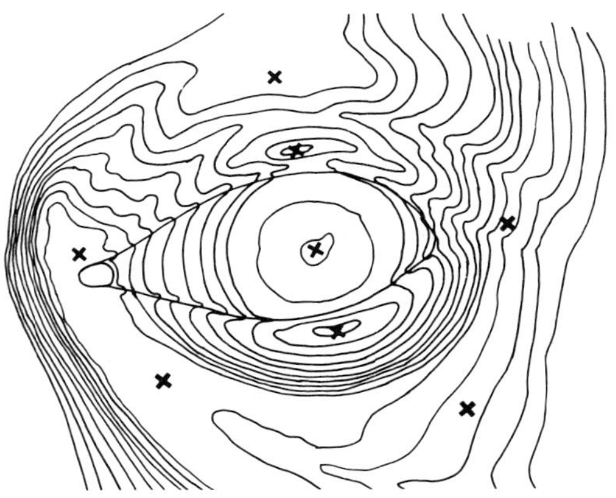

**Figure 22.12** *Exophthalmic proptosis*

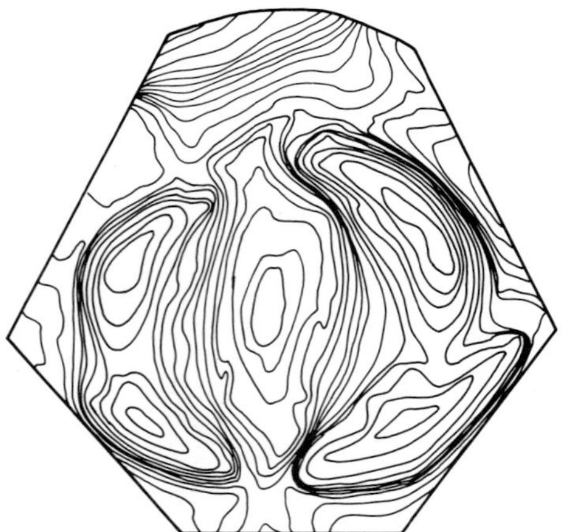

***Figure 22.13*** *The hard-palate of a child with cleft lip and palate deformity*

The head and face have been extensively studied and measured for assessment of asymmetry, prognathisms, functional structure and characteristic facies. Orthodontists and dentists have been particularly keen with studies on growth, resorption, eruption, and studies of the gingival tissues. Plastic surgeons have measured pre-and post-operatively rhinoplasty and cleft lip and palate.

Ophthalmologists have been particularly active in the use of photogrammetry, with such applications as measurement of keratoconus, optic disc morphology, proptosis, and pupillary aqueous flow.

Other applications have included measurement of tumour volume, surface area of skin lesions, thyroid swelling and fitting for prostheses.

## 22.3 SOMATOTYPING

Somatotyping is the study of the relationship of body build and configuration with disease, although it often now includes longitudinal growth studies and the general study of body build and physique. Classically there are three body types said to be derived from the three layers of the early embryo – the ectomorph, mesomorph and endomorph. Photography has been used in this area for decades with measurements of fixed parameters being taken from full length highly standardized records. Often relatively unskilled operators are employed to operate automatic cameras. To minimize errors extremely long working distances are used so special long studios are needed. The subject being photographed stands on a rotatable platform controlled by the operator so that accurate AP, PA and lateral views can be obtained. On occasions aerial survey cameras have been adapted to this role. Contemporary applications centre around child growth studies.

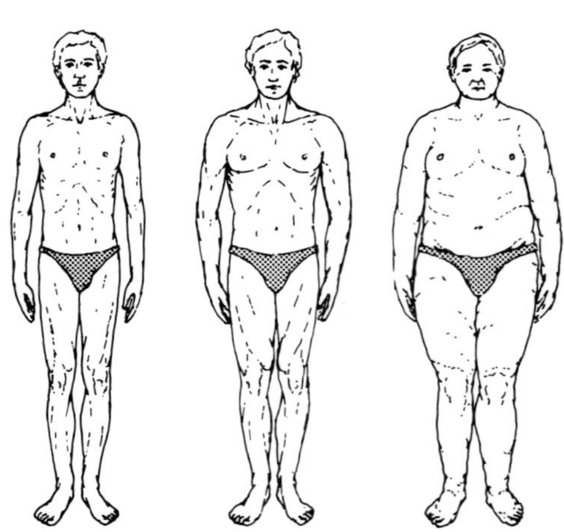

***Figure 22.14*** *The three classic body types described in somatotyping. The ectomorph (left) with lean features, the mesomorph (centre) with normal proportions but strong muscular features and the endomorph (right) with overweight 'flabby' features*

## References

Ansley, D. (1970). Techniques for pulsed laser holography of people. *Appl. Optics.*, **9**, 815-821

Beard, L. (1967). Three-dimensional contour mapping by photography. *Photogr. J.*, **107**, 315-323

Beard, L. and Burke, P. (1967). Evolution of stereophotogrammetry for the study of facial morphology. *Med. Biol. Illustr.*, **17**, 20-25

Beard, L. and Dale, P. (1976). A portable stereometric camera for clinical measurement. *Med. Biol. Illustr.*, **26**, 107-110

Berghagen, N., *et al.* (1968). Changes in the volume of the gingival tissues – a stereophotogrammetric study. *Acta. Odontol. Scand.*, **26**, 369-393

Berkowitz, S. and Cuzzi, J. (1977). Biostereometric analysis of surgically corrected faces. *Am. J. Orthodon.*, **72**, 526-538

Berkowitz, S. and Pruzansky, S. (1968). Stereophotogrammetry of serial casts of cleft palate. *Angle Orthodon.*, **38**, 136-149

Burke, P. and Beard, L. (1979). Growth of soft tissues of the face in adolescence. *Br. Dent. J.*, **146**, 239-246

Chmielewski, N. and Varner, J. (1969). An application of holographic contouring in dentistry. *Biomed. Sci. Instrum.*, **6**, 72-79

Cobb, J. (1972). A projected grid method for recording the shape of the human face. RAE *Tech. Rep.* TR 71184, Farnborough.

Cohan, B. (1978). Multiple-slit illumination of the optic disc. *Arch. Ophthalmol.*, **96**, 497-500

Dervin, E. *et al.* (1976). The photographic measurement of dental models. *Med. Biol. Illustr.*, **26**, 219-222

Donaldson, D. (1955). A stereo-camera for medical photography. *Med. Biol. Illustr.*, **5**, 209-213

Dupertuis, C. and Tanner, J. (1950). The pose of the subject for photogrammetric anthropometry with especial reference to somatotyping. *Am. J. Phys. Anthropol.*, **8**, 27-48

Elion, H. (1967). *Lasers: Systems and Applications.* (Oxford: Pergamon Press)

Engel, C. (1958). Silhouettes. *Med. Biol. Illustr.*, **8**, 214-217

Eriksson, G., *et al.* (1979). Evaluation of leg ulcer treatment with stereophotogrammetry. *Br. J. Dermatol.*, **101**, 123-131

Frobin, W. and Hierholzer, E. (1983). Rasterstereography : a photogrammetric method for measurement of body surfaces. *J. Biol. Photogr.*, **51**, 11-17

Geoghegan, B. (1953). The determination of body measurements, surface area and body volume by photography. *Am. J. Physiol. Anthropol.*, **11**, 97-119

Heflinger, L., *et al.* (1966). Holographic interferometry. *J. Appl. Phys.*, **37**, 642-649

Heindl, R. (1916). Photogrammetry without a special camera. *Arch. Crim. Anthrop. Criminol.*, **65**, 1-6

Hills, B. and Witton, J. (1951). A skiagraphic method of measuring changes in profile. *Med. Biol. Illustr.*, **1**, 201-203

Holm, O. and Krakau, C. (1965). A photogrammetric method for estimation of the volume of superficial tumours and similar objects. *Acta. Univ. Lundensis.*, **II**, No 31

Jackson, H. (1968). Minimizing perspective error in gross photography. *J. Biol. Photogr. Assoc.*, **36**, 55-57

Kanazawa, E. and Ikeda, N. (1979). Perspective correction of the moiré photograph. *J. Biol. Photogr. Assoc.*, **47**, 107-109

Karara, H. (1972). Simple cameras for close-range stereophotogrammetric application. *Photogram. Eng.*, **38**, 447-451

Kodak. (1971). *The Dimensional Stability of Photographic Films and Plates.* (Publication RF10). (London: Kodak Ltd)

Kodak. (1974). *Viewing a Print in True Perspective.* (Publication M-15). (Rochester, NY: Eastman Kodak Ltd.)

Koepfler, J. (1983). Moiré topography in medicine. *J. Biol. Photogr.*, **51**, 3-10

Leith, E. and Uptanieks, J. (1964). Wavefront reconstruction with diffused illumination and three-dimensional objects. *J. Opt. Soc. Am.*, **54**, 1295-1297

Lovesey, E. (1973). A simple photogrammetric technique for recording three-dimensional head shape. *Med. Biol. Illustr.*, **23**, 210-212

Malhotra, R. (1970). Holography as viewed by a photogrammetrist. *Photogram. Eng.*, **36**, 152-159

Martin, T. and Pongratz, M. (1974). Mathematical correction for photographic perspective error. *Res. Am. Assoc. Health Phys. Educ.*, **45**, 318-323

McGregor, A., Newton, I. and Gilder, R. (1971). A stereophotogrammetric method of investigating facial changes following the loss of teeth. *Med. Biol. Illustr.*, **21**, 75-82

McShane, R., *et al.* (1978). Quantitative optics : the control of perspective in comparative photography. *Ann. Plast. Surg.*, **1**, 466-473

Miskin, E. (1960). Simple photogrammetric methods in medicine. *Med. Biol. Illustr.*, **10**, 230-236

Pierson, W. (1961). Monophotogrammetric determination of body volume. *Ergonomics*, **4**, 213-218

Savara, B. (1965). Application of photogrammetry for quantitative study of tooth and face morphology. *Am. J. Phys. Anthropol.*, **23**, 427-434

Spetzler, R. (1980). Holographic interferometry applied to the study of the human skull. *Neurosurgery*, **52**, 825-828

Takasaki, H. (1970). Moiré topography. *Appl. Optics*, **9**, 1467-1472

Takasaki, H. (1973). Moiré topography. *Appl. Optics*, **12**, 845-850

Tanner, J. and Weiner, J. (1949). The reliability of the photogrammetric method of anthropometry. *Am. J. Phys. Anthropol.*, **7**, 145-186

Terada, H. (1974). A new apparatus for stereometry – a moiré contourgraph. *Adv. Exp. Med. Biol.*, **49**, 27-46

Tsurata, T. and Itoh, Y. (1969). Interferometric generation of contour lines in opaque objects. *Opt. Commu.*, **1**, 34-37

Williams, A.R. (1976). Orthographic photography. *Br. J. Photogr.*, **123**, 1131-1132

Williams, A.R. (1977). Control of scale in specimen photography – a look at telecentric systems. *Med. Biol. Illustr.*, **27**, 55-59

Williams, A.R. (1977). Light sectioning as a three-dimensional measurement system in medicine. *J. Photogr. Sci.*, **25**, 85-90

Williams, A.R. (1978). Medical biostereometrics. *Photogr. J.*, **118**, 104-108

Williams, A.R. (1981). A survey and assessment of photographic methods of measurement in medicine. *Mphil (medicine Thesis* University of London)

Williams, A.R. and Davis, P. (1980). Photogrammetry in anatomical research. *Br. J. Photogr.*, **127**, 875-877

Williams, J. (1969). *Simple Photogrammetry.* (London: Academic Press)

## *Practical projects*

(1) Look up Scheimpflug's rule and its application to medical photography and measurement from photographs. With a large format camera, photograph various scenes with swing front and back movements to obtain (*a*) increased depth of field and (*b*) geometrically accurate representations of specific planes.

(2) Photograph a cube from a two or three point perspective aspect using a short object distance and wide angle lens. Mount a small print onto a large sheet of paper and by geometric drawing determine the vanishing points and horizon.

(3) Practise making stereo pairs with any single-lens reflex of different sized subjects by using a camera shift to obtain the parallax. Use the simple formula S=A/50 where S= separation and A the distance to the nearest subject of interest. Present the finished results in a form suitable for viewing in a conventional stereoscope.

(4) Research the meaning of the following terms and make certain that you understand them:
Stereoscopy, stereography, stereophotography, stereophotogrammetry, orthostereoscopy, hyperstereoscopy, hypostereoscopy, pseudoscopy, autostereoscopy, binocular vision, anaglyph and parallax.

(5) Read the technique of simple depth measurement (in for example Arnold, Rolls and Stewart, 1971 London: Focal Press); then practise taking measurements from large format negatives of any static medical subject. Choose a close-up subject and wide stereobase. Be certain you understand the principles of parallax measurement.

## *Examination questions*

Q.1 Define perspective and explain its importance in standardized clinical recording.

Q.2 Explain with the aid of simple diagrams the principle of binocular vision and how the same principle is used in stereophotography.

Q.3 Describe with the aid of diagrams the optical principles involved in any two of the following techniques:
(*a*) Light sectioning,
(*b*) Subtractive moiré,
(*c*) Stereophotogrammetry,
(*d*) Holography.

Q.4 Describe three possible applications of stereophotography in medicine. Without stereo equipment, how would you set about producing and viewing a stereopair of 35 mm colour transparencies of an articulated human skeleton.

Q.5 What parts do viewpoint and focal length play in the perspective rendering of the finished photograph? Explain how to calculate the correct viewing distance for a print.

Q.6 What is 'photogrammetry' and how may it be usefully used in medicine? Illustrate your answer by reference to specific applications and techniques.

Q.7 You are required to make a series of stereoscopic pairs of colour transparencies of cleft palates. Describe in detail the technique of your choice.

Q.8 What is somatotyping? Describe fully the application of photography to this field.

*Multiple choice questions (any of the statements may be true or false)*

Q.9 The following are measurement techniques used in ophthalmology:
(*a*) Light sectioning,
(*b*) Tonometry,
(*c*) Stereophotogrammetry,
(*d*) Keratography,
(*e*) Perimetry.

Q.10 Perspective is important in medical photography:
(*a*) Camera back movements control perspective.
(*b*) Longer focal length lenses give more accurate perspective.
(*c*) The correct viewing distance for a 10" × 8" print from a 5" × 4" negative is 12".
(*d*) Orthographic systems are effectively 'perspectiveless'.
(*e*) Correct perspective for a 35 mm colour slide taken with a 100 mm lens and projected onto a 48" × 38" screen is 10' 6".

# Section 23
# Specialized techniques

**A.R. Williams**, MPhil, FBIPP, FRPS, FBPA, AIMBI
Head of Medical Illustration and Teaching Services
Charing Cross Hospital and Medical School, London

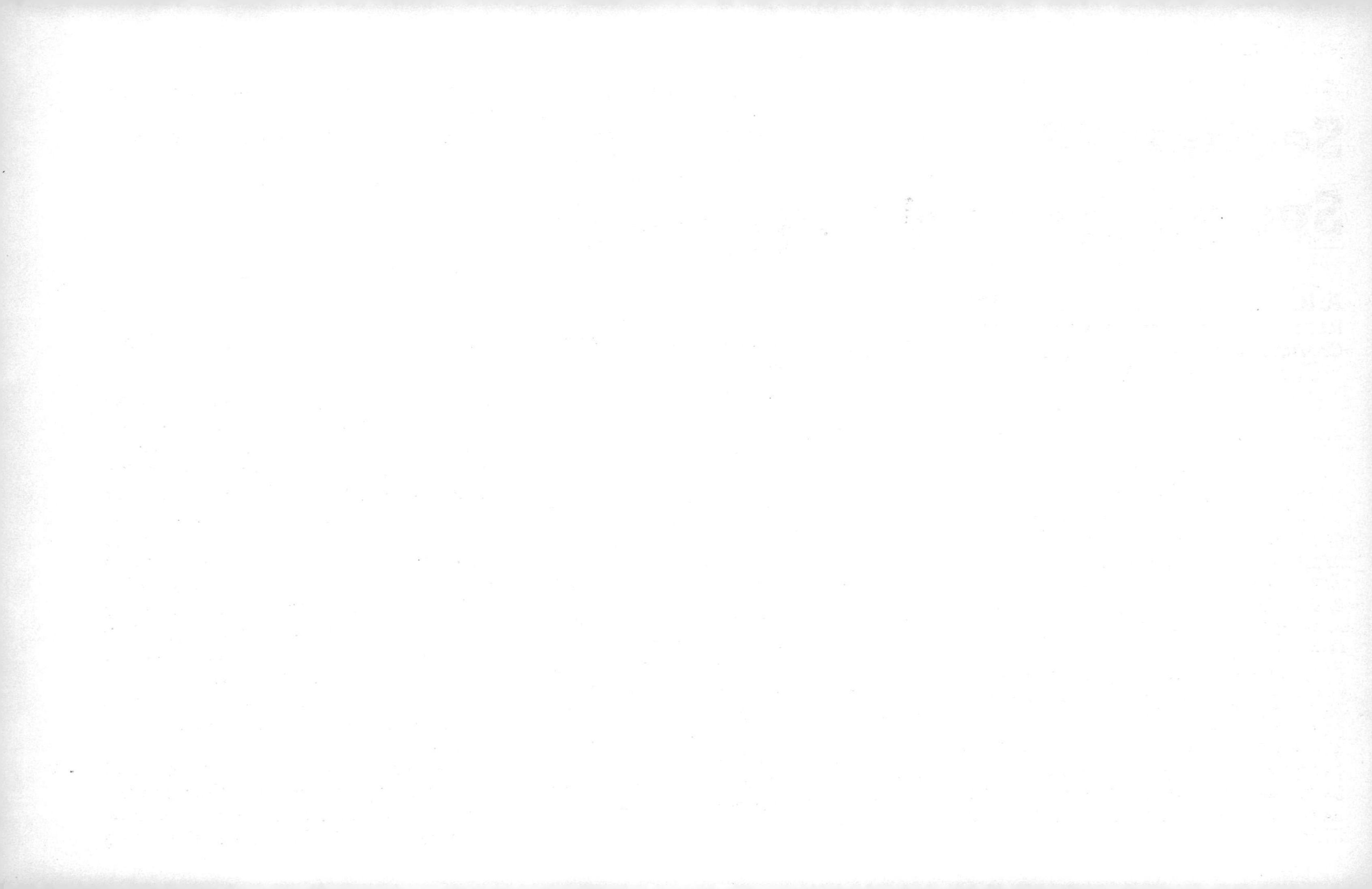

## 23.1 INTRODUCTION

The aim of this section is to remind the student of the many specialized photographic techniques, and to give an indication of their usefulness in medical research. These techniques will not be used routinely in clinical practice, but the advanced student should understand the principles so that he might be able to give sound advice to the medical researcher on the visualization and measurement techniques which scientific photography has to offer.

## 23.2 TIME-LAPSE PHOTOGRAPHY

Events which happen too slowly to appreciate, e.g. the growth of bacterial cultures, the eruption of teeth, the growth of finger nails, the movements of neonates or of adults during sleep, etc., have all been studied by condensing the time scale with time-lapse photography. Essentially a cinematographic technique, still frames are taken at relatively long intervals then re-projected at the normal speed of 24 fps. Intervals may vary between two frames a second and one frame a week depending upon the duration of the event. The framing rate is calculated by dividing the desired running time by the actual event time and multiplying by 24, all in seconds. Some cine cameras may be run continuously at speeds as low as 2 fps and some provide single shot facilities (e.g. Bolex, Beaulieu). Manual operation is practical for short periods but automatic control with a separate intervalometer is more usual. The intervalometer may control exposure duration, exposure frequency and the switching of lights. Lighting must be consistent from frame to frame – small variations in illumination are most annoying – as are small subject movements. A rigid camera mounting is essential, and some means of ensuring the subject is in the same place highly desirable. Electronic flash can be very useful as the light source. It is sometimes helpful to present the finished result as a cine loop so that the event can be viewed repeatedly.

## 23.3 HIGH-SPEED PHOTOGRAPHY

High-speed photography is of great value in studying events which occur too rapidly for the eye to follow, e.g. the movement of muscles when running, the vibration of the vocal cords, the vibration of various types of probe. Many short exposures are made in rapid sequence but are then reprojected at normal speed or even hand analysed to measure subject movement.

Typically exposure times are very short,
and can be calculated from the formula:

$$T = \frac{S}{K \times V_s \times \cos\theta},$$

where:

S = size of smallest detail
$K$ = constant (2 or 3)
Vs = subject velocity
$\theta$ = angle of motion relative to film plane

Obtaining bright enough illumination can be a serious problem with biological subjects where a continuous record is needed. Tungsten halogen lights particularly when focussed by condenser lenses can be used down to about 10 $\mu$s, but heat filters should be used to avoid burning the subject. Flash bulbs should not be ignored – the peak output of a PF60 is 2.8 megalumens (equivalent to about 100 kW of tungsten lighting) with a half peak duration of 20 ms. A number of bulbs may be fired sequentially.

High-speed cameras come in various types according to the framing rate required.

***Intermittent claw*** – the slowest class of camera using conventional claw and pin mechanism, e.g. Eclair, Mitchell, Vinten. Records 4000–16 000 frames at framing

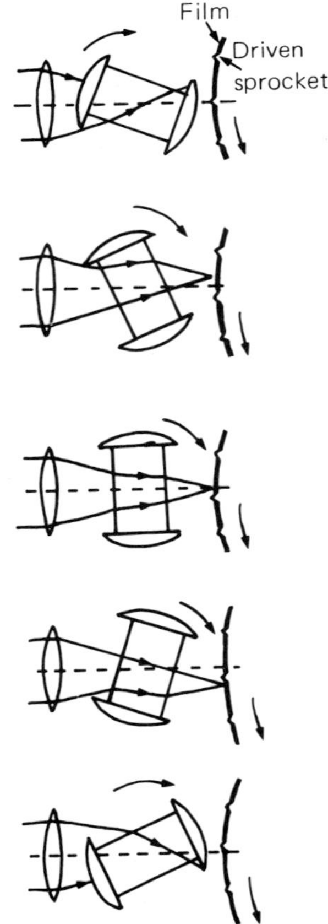


***Figure 23.1*** *The principle of the rotating prism camera*

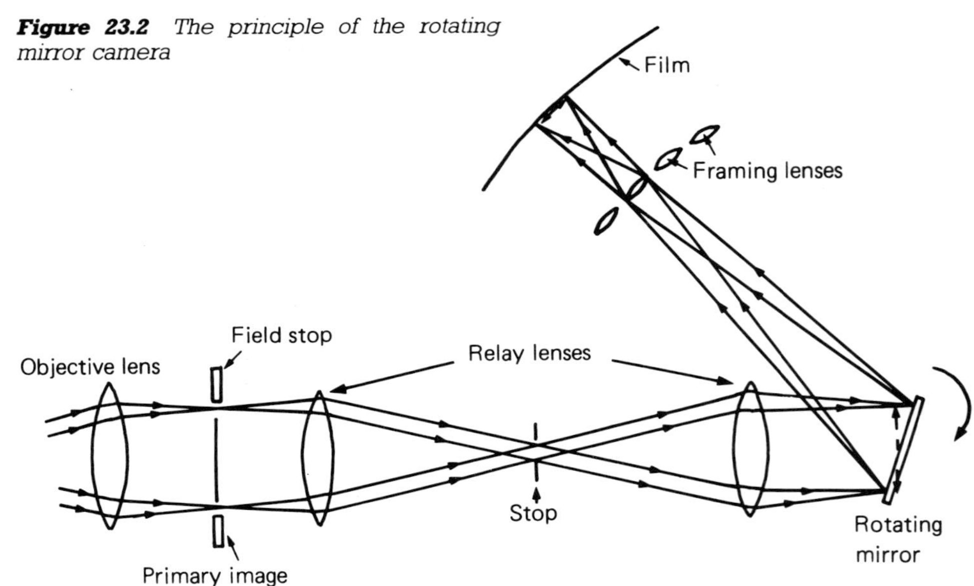


***Figure 23.2*** *The principle of the rotating mirror camera*

rates varying from 50 to 500 fps

***Rotating prism*** – the standard camera for high-speed work with optical compensation for image movement provided by a rotating prism, e.g. Fastax, Hitachi, Hycam and Photo-sonics. Records 4000–16 000 frames at framing rates up to 10 000 fps.

***Drum cameras*** – the film is located within a cylindrical drum which is rotated at high speed. Since the drum diameter is limited the number of frames rarely exceeds 300, but framing rates up to 70 000 fps are possible, e.g. Uyemura.

***Rotating mirror*** – the image is formed in the plane of a rotating mirror which

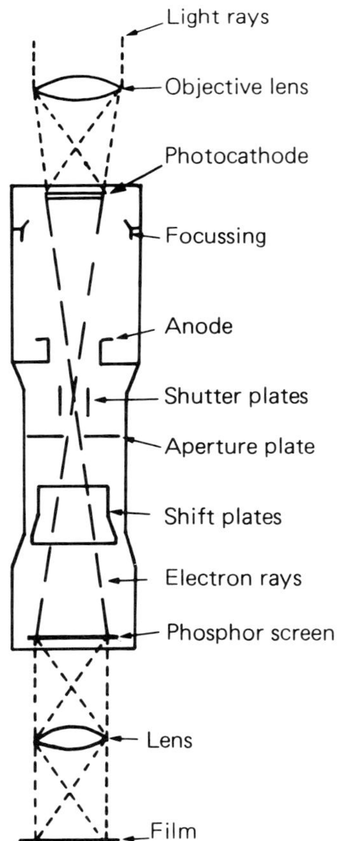


***Figure 23.3*** *An image tube camera*

passes the image on to a number of framing lenses which image each frame onto the stationary film, e.g. Barr and Stroud or Beckman and Whitley. Framing rates up to 20 × $10^6$ fps are possible over 25–120 frames.

***Image tube*** – the fastest of all cameras likely to be encountered by the medical photographer, with framing rates exceeding 3 × $10^8$ fps, and exposure times as short as one thousand millionth of a second! e.g. Hadland Imacon. Basically it is a pulsed photocathode with the image displayed on a phosphor screen which is photographed. The maximum number of frames possible is approximately 20.

Analysis of high-speed film is accomplished by projection in an analysis projector with single-frame facility or on special film analysers which allow for varying degrees of complexity, such as co-ordinate and angular measurement.

## 23.4 CHRONOCYCLOGRAPHY

In this technique multiple records of a subject are recorded onto a single sheet of film either by lighting the subject with a stroboscope or attaching a small light to parts of the subject. Applications reported have included gait analysis using reflective strips attached to the thigh, calf and foot; and measurement of jaw motion using light emitting diodes attached to the jaw by a tooth brace. The technique was originally used to assess hand movements at a work bench by attaching a red flashing light to the left hand and a green flashing light to the right hand; a time exposure in a semi-darkened room recorded all the movements. If the LEDs or lights flash at a known frequency an assessment of subject velocity can be made. Sometimes stereochronocyclography is used to accurately measure patient's gaits in three dimensions. Various types of stroboscope are commercially available (e.g. Dawe, Turner) with flash rates varying from 5 to 4000 flashes per second, with a duration of 5 $\mu$s and power output of 2–60 joules.

## 23.5 EQUIDENSITOMETRY

A technique in which a continuous tone image is converted into single iso-density lines delineating points of equal density. The original method utilized the Sabattier effect in combining high contrast positive and negative images and printing the resulting sandwich onto high contrast bromide paper. Modern applications all use Agfa's special 'Agfacontour' film which gives instantaneous results. The technique is particularly useful wherever equal densities need to be mapped, e.g.

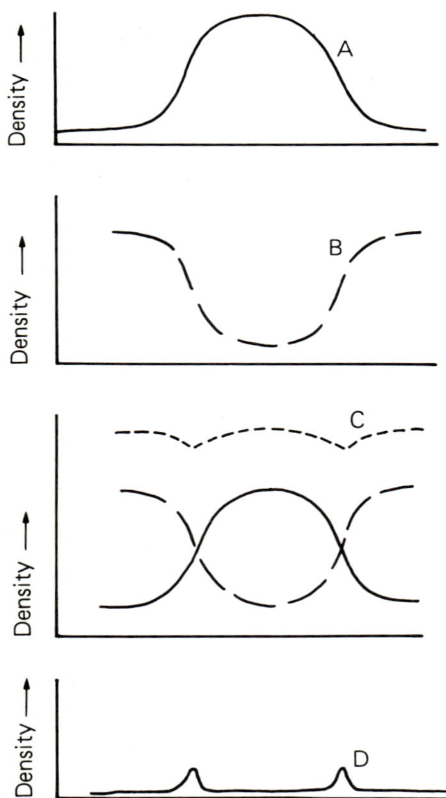


**Figure 23.4** *Equidensitometry relies on combining positive and negative images (A and B) to give a sandwich negative (C) which then prints as edge detail only (D)*

assessment of cataracts *in vitro*. Repeated applications include detailed investigation of malignant melanoma cell colonies, assessment of illumination and differentiation of chromosomes.

## 23.6 PHOTO-ELASTIC STRESS ANALYSIS

This technique uses polarized light to detect the stress distribution in objects under complex loading situations. Plane polarized light is passed through a transparent model of the object which is then photographed through the polariscope. Two types of line may be observed:

*Isochromatic lines:* which are coloured when using white light and are contours of stress.

*Isoclinic lines:* which are superimposed on the isochromatic lines, are always black and give directions of the principal stresses.

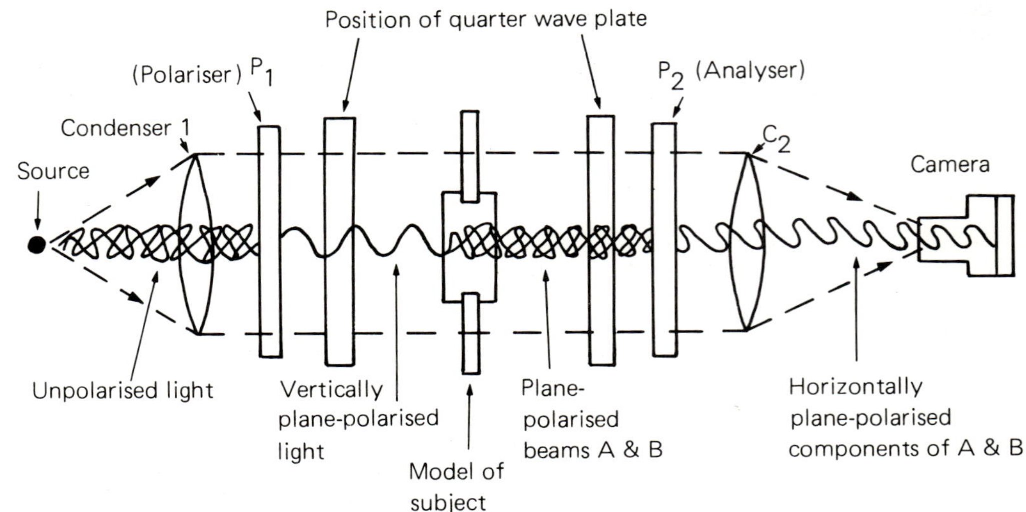


**Figure 23.5** *The photo-polariscope*

The technique depends upon the fact that an isotropic transparent material becomes doubly refracting when stressed.

The polariscope consists not only of the crossed polarizing filters but also condensers to give a parallel beam through the subject and quarter-wave plates to remove the isoclinic lines.

Transparent models of subjects are often made from epoxy resins; the sensitivity of technique increasing with model thickness. Bi-refringent surface coatings can also be applied and a reflected light technique used to study the surface strain. The surfaces of teeth, bones and joints have all been successfully studied using this technique.

## 23.7 SCHLIEREN PHOTOGRAPHY

Schlieren methods detect small changes of refractive index in transparent subjects and reveal them as light and dark or coloured bands. The name comes from the German 'Schliere' meaning streaks.

A typical system employs a parallel beam of light formed by a small source at the focus of a lens or spherical mirror. This passes through the transparent object and is brought to a focus again by a similar lens or mirror. Part of this image is obscured, or cut off, by a knife edge and the light which passes falls on a screen on which the image of the transparent object is focussed by an auxiliary lens. If any part of the light is deflected in a direction at right angles to the knife edge by refractive index gradients the image of the source at the knife will be displaced in that direction. More or less light will pass over the knife edge, and corresponding areas of the image lighten or darken in proportion to the displacement. By using a multi-coloured filter instead of a knife edge the differences in refractive index are represented as different colours. The width of the Schlieren field is limited by the diameter of the condensers or mirrors.

Medical applications have included the study of heat flow over the body, and the photography of the invisible output from ultrasonic probes used in ENT surgery.

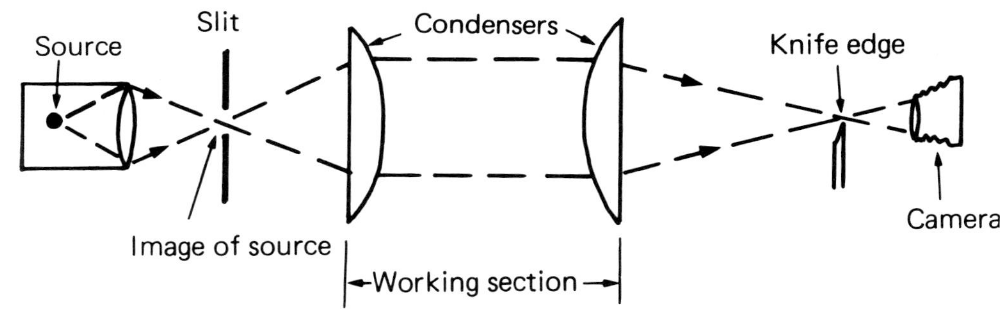


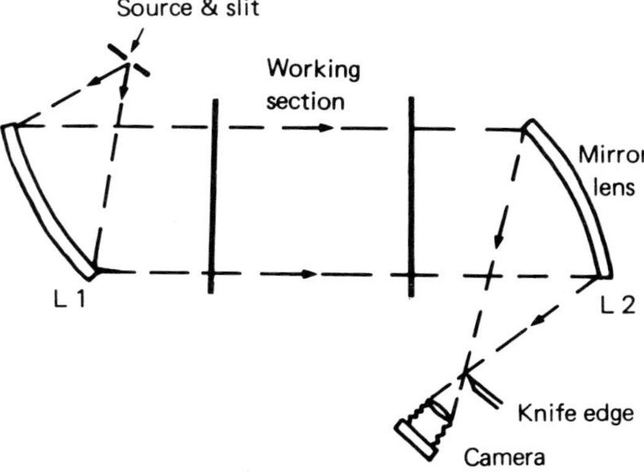


***Figure 23.6*** *(top) A double-lens Schlieren system*
***Figure 23.7*** *A double-mirror Schlieren system*

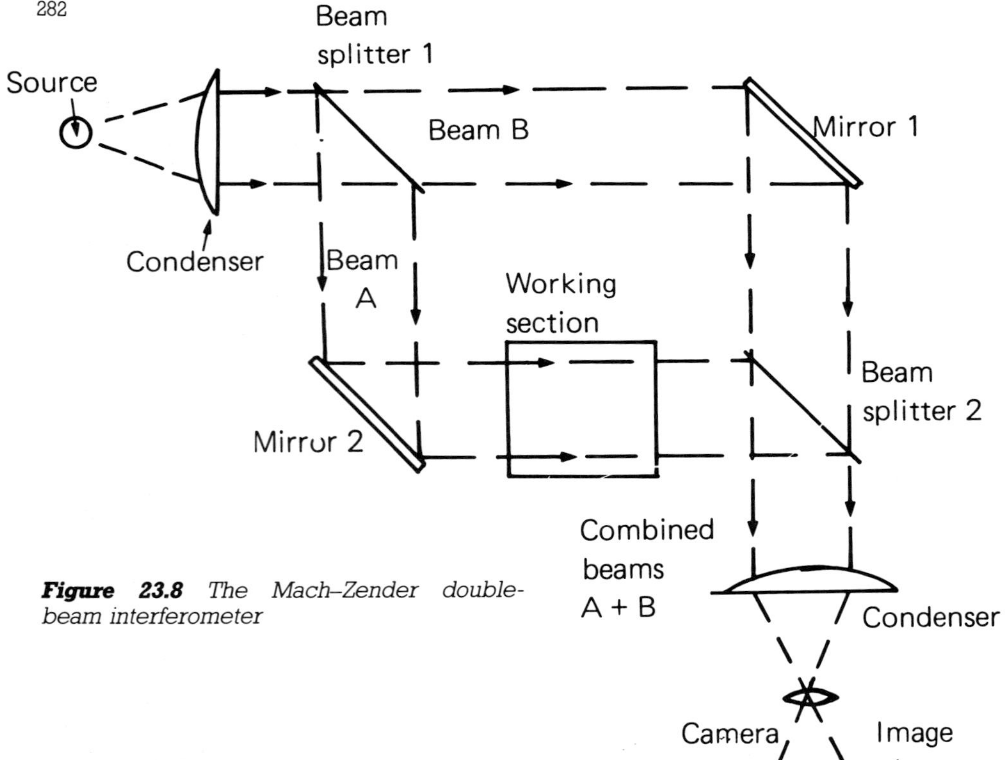


*Figure 23.8* *The Mach–Zender double-beam interferometer*

## 23.8 INTERFEROMETRY

Another technique for recording small changes in refractive index within transparent subjects (interferometry can also be used to map surface topography of very small objects – this is covered in Section 22).

If two light rays are coherent and are in the same plane of polarization, they interfere when they are superimposed. The interference may be partial or complete, constructive or destructive depending on the relative phase of the two beams at the point of combination. The technique then is to divide a collimated beam into two beams by a partial reflector; pass one through the test area and recombine it with the reference beam; the combination being focussed into the recording plane by a condenser lens. The Mach–Zender double-beam interferometer is normally used.

The interferometer can be used to obtain quantitative values of gas density from which pressure and velocity can be calculated, e.g. of anaesthetic gases.

## 23.9 KIRLIAN PHOTOGRAPHY

Also known as electrophotography or corona discharge photography. In this technique a high voltage, low current, discharge is fed to a flat copper electrode which is covered with a sheet of photographic film. The subject is placed in contact with the film and the generator switched on for a determined exposure time. The film is processed conventionally to reveal a spiky coloured halo or 'aura' around the subject. Extravagant claims have been made for the technique, e.g. that it could detect early cancer, but recent evidence shows that it reveals only the state of hydration of the skin. The most likely explanation is that it is a cold electron emission phenomenon.

## 23.10 FLOW VISUALIZATION

Apart from Schlieren photography and interferometry there are several other simple flow visualization techniques. The duration of exposure can be important – a short exposure might show individual particles or droplets, whilst a longer exposure might demonstrate the direction of flow rather better and measurement of the 'track' length against exposure would enable the velocity to be calculated.

Simple flow visualization can often be obtained from using dark ground lighting technique especially with aerosols. Smoke generators may be used to study the flow of gases – white smoke is normally preferred in combination with a black background and dark ground illumination. Coloured dyes, fluorescent solutions, polystyrene spheres and powdered aluminium have all been used to study fluid flow. A simple shadowgraph technique with a point source of light can be useful for airflow detection.

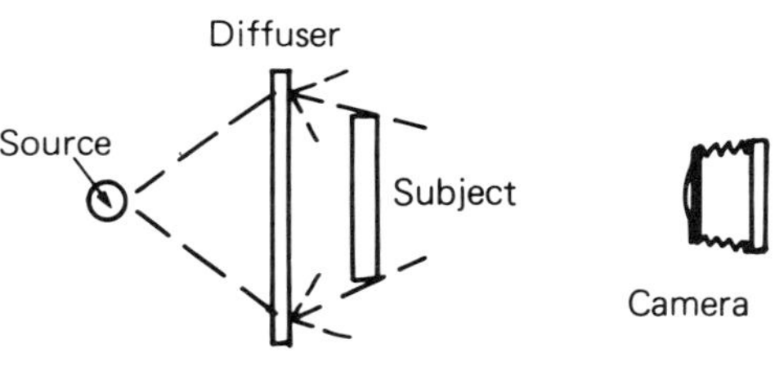


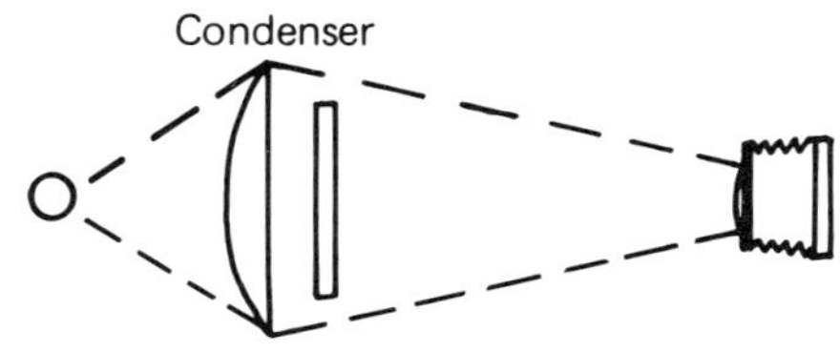


***Figure 23.9*** *Two simple shadowgraph techniques for flow visualization. The condenser system gives much sharper shadows*

## 23.11 FALSE COLOUR SYSTEMS

Various techniques exist for rendering the subject in artificial colours for greater clarity; infrared Ektachrome (*Section 18.5*) and the Land Ultraviolet microscope (*Section 19.3*) are good examples, as is colour Schlieren (discussed above).

One most useful technique is 'colour posterization'. A series of tone separation negatives are made on 'lith' film of the continuous tone subject which are then printed in combination through a series of colour filters onto colour printing paper. This can be useful in studying radiographic detail for example. Often this type of image enhancement, especially density to colour, will be performed electronically and photographed from a television screen.

In stroboscopic photography of motion, interpretation can be helped by using alternate flashes of red, blue and green.

## 23.12 PERIPHERY PHOTOGRAPHY

This is the recording in a single 'rolled out' photograph of a complete cylindrical surface. Various simple but limited methods have been described, but the best results are obtained by using a purpose built camera such as the RE Periphery Camera. The principle of the system is that the object is rotated about its vertical axis while the film in a stationary camera is driven past a vertical slit at a velocity related to the radius of the object. Medical applications have mainly been forensic, related to obtaining geometrically accurate images from curved surfaces.

## 23.13 MULTISPECTRAL ANALYSIS

In this technique cameras with multiple lenses, or multiple camera assemblies are used to obtain a variety of records of

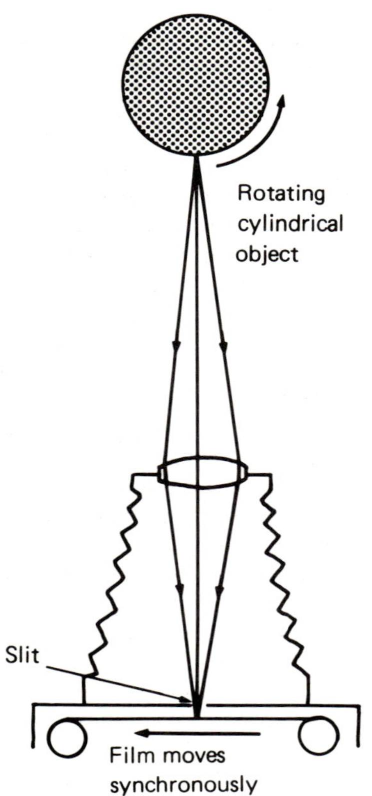


***Figure 23.10*** *The principle of the periphery camera*

the same subject using different wavelengths of light. It may be visible, ultraviolet and infrared, or red, green, blue and ultraviolet, for example. This is often using photography as a real tool for 'exploration' in medical research. Previous applications have included assessment of burns and pigmented lesions of the skin.

## 23.14 PHOTOMETRY

This is the measurement of radiation intensity by examination of a photographic image. Equal brightnesses in the subject are rendered as equal densities on the film, provided of course that a film/developer combination is chosen so that the response is linear. Thus it is possible to measure the subject reflectance (or luminance in the case of a self-luminant subject) by measuring densities on the film and relating them to the densities produced by known standards or references placed within the scene. The strictest standardization and process control are needed if the measurements taken are to be useful. For example, the image points should be positioned similarly in relation to the lens axis to avoid the effects of uneven camera image illumination ($\cos^4$ law), and the image areas must be of similar size to avoid complications due to development adjacency effects and reduced MTF in small images. Previous applications in medicine have been the quantification of ultraviolet fluorescence (intra-orally and for the dansyl chloride test for skin 'turnover time'), the quantification of skin surface roughness, and the assessment of pigmented lesions of the skin.

## 23.15 INSTRUMENTATION RECORDING

The student should be aware that virtually every piece of electronic instrumentation in the hospital outputs visual information – often onto some form of cathode ray tube – and that photographs are taken routinely of these displays for record purposes. Special CRT cameras mounted into hoods are routinely used with polaroid instant film for quick results. The student should familiarize himself with the various types of screen phosphors, cameras and emulsions used. Although there is nothing complicated about this type of photography the medical photographer's advice is frequently sought when purchasing new equipment or when things go wrong.

## References


Anselmo, V., *et al* (1977). Multispectral photographic analysis. A new quantitative tool to assist in the early diagnosis of thermal burn depth. *Ann. Biomed. Eng.*, **5**, 179-193

Arnold, C., Rolls, P. and Steward, J. (1971). *Applied Photography.* (London: Focal Press)

Babcock, M. (1954). Method for measuring fingernail growth rates in nutritional studies. *J. Nutr.*, **55**, 323-330

Benjamin, A. (1968). Liquid crystal photography. *Vis. Sonic Med.*, **3**, 10-14

Boxler, C. and Paulson, M. (1977). Kirlian photography: a new tool in biological research? *J. Biol. Photogr. Assoc.*, **45**, 51-60

Burke, P. and Newell, D. (1958). A photographic method of measuring eruption of human teeth. *Am. J. Orthodon.*, **44**, 590-602

Croot, C. and Robins, R. (1967). Schlieren photography of an ultrasonic beam. *Med. Biol. Illustr.*, **17**, 202-207

Ebrahim, H. and Williams, A.R. (1982). Kirlian photography – an appraisal. *J. Audiovis. Media Med.*, **5**, 84-91

Ernford, L. (1981). A fracture study of the diametral compression test by means of high-speed photography. *Acta Odontol. Scand.*, **39**, 71-77

Fraser, R. and Dombrowski, N. (1962). The selection of a photographic technique for the study of movement. *J. Photogr. Sci.*, **10**, 155-169

Gurjian, E. and Lisner, H. (1961). Photoelastic confirmation of the presence of shear strains at the cerebrospinal junction in closed head injury. *J. Neurosurg.*, **18**, 58-59

Haboush, E. (1952). Photoelastic stress and strain analysis in cervical fractures of the femur. *Bull. Hosp. Jt. Dis. N.Y.*, **8**, 252-257

Hansell, P. (1962). Growth of the human finger nail – a time lapse study. *Res. Film.*, **4**, 219-223

Hollinger, H. (1958). Photography in photoelastic stress analysis of restorations. *Dent. Radiogr. Photogr.*, **31**, 31-36

Holwill, M. (1967). High-speed kinematography of flagellated micro-organisms. *J. Photogr. Sci.*, **15**, 229-302

Kent, J. (1969). Multiple spark photography with image separation by colour coding. *Appl. Optics*, **8**, 1023-1026

Kodak. (1981). *High-speed Photography.* (Publication G-44) (Rochester, NY: Eastman Kodak Ltd)

Kodak. (1977). *Schlieren Photography* (Publication P-11) (Rochester, NY: Eastman Kodak Ltd.)

Kodak. (1977). *Films for Cathode Ray Tube Recording.* (Publication P-37.) (Rochester, NY: Eastman Kodak Ltd.)

Konikiewicz, L. (1977). Kirlian photography in theory and clinical application. *J. Biol. Photogr. Assoc.*, **45**, 115-134

Krippner, S. (1979). Biological applications of Kirlian photography. *J. Am. Soc. Psychosom. Dent. Med.*, **26**, 122-128

Lau, E. and Krug, W. (1968). *Equidensitometry.* (London: Focal Press)

Lester, J. (1975). Kirlian effect, cancer coronas and questions. *J. Kansas Med. Soc.*, **76**, 194-202

Makler, A. (1980). Use of a microcomputer in combination with the multiple exposure photography technique for human sperm motility determination. *J. Urol.*, **124**, 372-374

Marshall, R. (1980). Evaluation of a diagnostic test based on photographic photometry of infrared and ultraviolet radiation reflected by pigmented lesions of the skin. *J. Audiovis. Media Med.*, **3**, 94-98

Marshall, R. (1982). Photographic photometry of ultraviolet fluorescence. *Br. J. Photogr.*, **129**, 958-960

Marshall, R. and Marks, R. (1983). Assessment of skin surface by scanning densitometry of macrophotographs. *Clin. Exp. Dermatol.*, **8**, 121-127

Marshall, R.J. and Marshall, R.W. (1983). Quantification of skin surface roughness by macrophotography and computer aided scanning densitometry. *J. Audiovis. Media Med.*, **6**, 98-103

Moore, G. (1975). Ultra high speed photography in laryngeal research. *Can. J. Otolaryngol.*, **4**, 793-799

Murray, W. (1967). The sensitivity of a black and white single mirror schlieren apparatus. *J. Photogr.*, **15**, 191-196

Nelson, M. (1980). Image enhancement using equidensitometry. *Br. J. Photogr.*, **127**, 868-871

Nelson, M. (1981). Simple multispectral photography of patients. *Br. J. Photogr.*, **128**, 927-928

Pehek, J., *et al.* (1976). Image modulation in corona discharge photography. *Science*, **194**, 263-270

Stanford, B. (1961). Petri-dishes, lighting and time-lapse. *Med. Biol. Illustr.*, **11**, 224-227

Stephens, D., *et al.* (1972). Schlieren photography of microenvironment. *Cornell Vet.*, **62**, 20-26

Tyson, J., *et al.* (1981). Analysis of newborn intensive care by time-lapse photography. *Crit. Care Med.*, **9**, 780-784

Window, A. (1963). Photostress. *J. Photogr. Sci.*, **11**, 186-193

## *Practical projects*

(1) Advanced students only should read the references cited on the various scientific techniques.

(2) Produce a time lapse sequence of a subject of your own choice, e.g. the growth of a bacterial colony. Indicate in some way on the film the timescale. Submit notes on your technique with the film.

(3) Make a short cine loop of a patient's gait with a conventional cine camera running at its fastest speed. Note any problems or difficulties you encounter.

(4) Use a stroboscope (or computerized electronic flashgun very close to the subject) to record any fast moving action, e.g. a drop of milk into a saucer of milk. Describe fully the method you choose to synchronize the action, camera and flashgun. Submit an exhibition quality 10" × 8" print.

(5) Using simple crossed polarizers photograph some transparent plastic object under stress (e.g. a plastic ruler). Submit an exhibition quality 10" x 8" colour print.

(6) Produce a 10" × 8" colour print to demonstrate the technique of colour posterization. Work from a continuous tone black-and-white print of any medical subject. Submit the original print, tone separation and finished colour print.

## *Examination questions*

Q.1 Discuss the important factors involved in reflection photometry and describe fully at least one application to medical photography.

Q.2 What is 'multispectral analysis' and how might it be applied to clinical recording? Cite specific examples.

Q.3 Describe at least two different types of high speed camera, their relative merits and applications.

Q.4 Write short notes on the following:
(*a*) Time lapse photography,
(*b*) Chronocyclography,
(*c*) Kirlian photography,
(*d*) Instrumentation recording.

Q.5 What is equidensitometry and how might it be used in medical photography? Describe the process of colour posterization.

Q.6 Discuss the techniques of stroboscopic photography and high-speed photography as applied to the recording of gaits. Include equipment, methods and merits of each.

Q.7 With the aid of simple diagrams explain the principle of the polariscope. How may the isoclinic lines be removed from the image? Describe briefly one application of photoelastic stress analysis to medical photography.

Q.8 Describe fully the technique of Schlieren photography and its application to assessment of heat flow over the body surface.

*Multiple choice questions (any of the statements may be true or false)*

Q.9 In scientific photography
(*a*) Interferometry may be used to record small changes in refractive index.
(*b*) Equidensitometry utilizes the Sabattier effect.
(*c*) Photometry is used to measure the spectral response of emulsions.
(*d*) Image tube cameras are used for framing rates up to $3 \times 10^8$ fps.
(*e*) Electrophotography records cold electron emission phenomena.

Q.10 In photo-elastic stress analysis:
(*a*) Isoclinic lines are shown as colours.
(*b*) Quarter-wave plates are used to remove isoclinics.
(*c*) Bi-refringement surface coatings may be used.
(*d*) Isotropic transparent materials become doubly refracting when stressed.
(*e*) Isochromatic lines depict the magnitude of stress.

# Section 24
# Photography of instruments and apparatus

**A.R. Williams**, MPhil, FBIPP, FRPS, FBPA, AIMBI
Head of Medical Illustration and Teaching Services
Charing Cross Hospital and Medical School, London

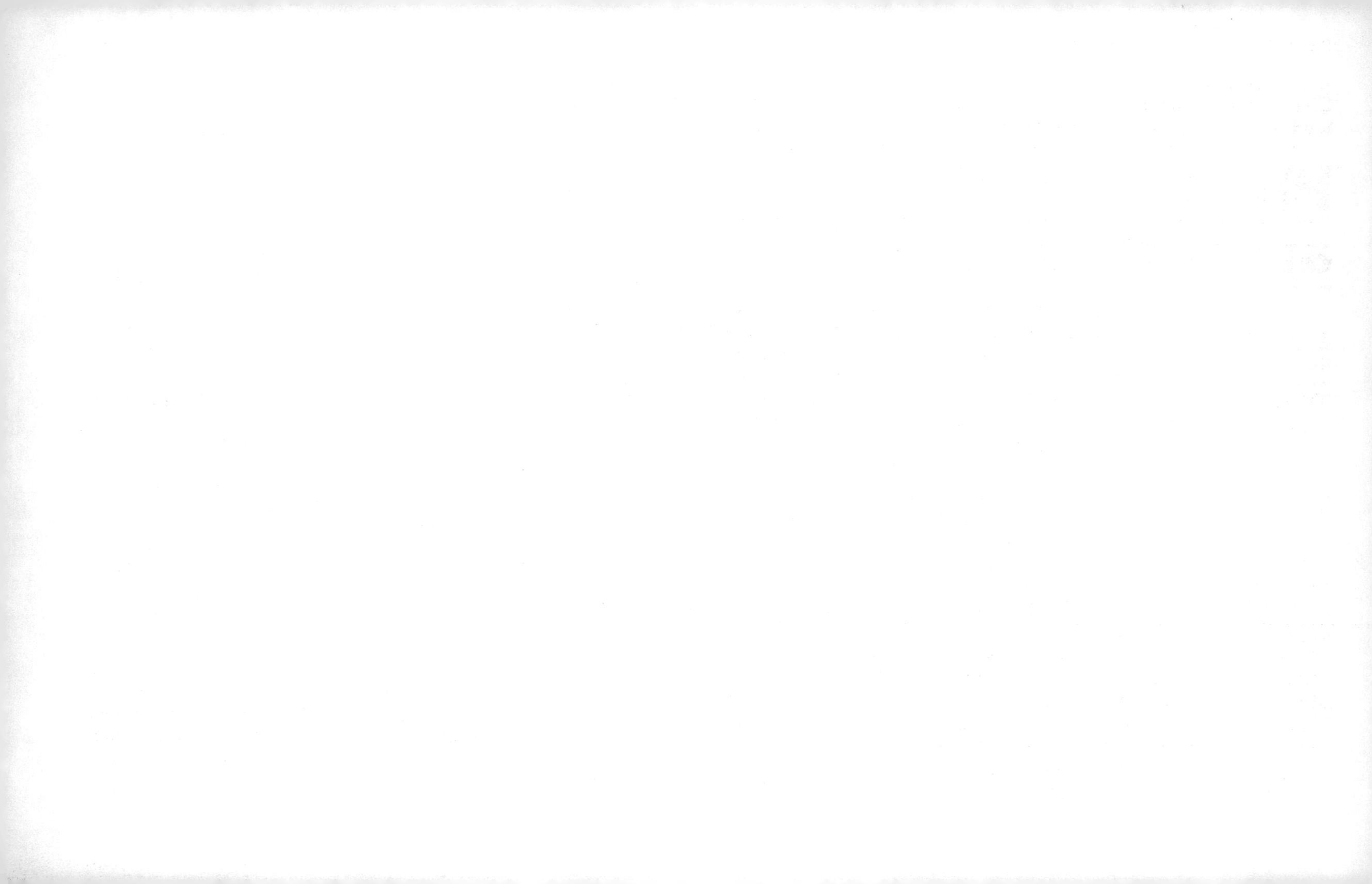

## 24.1 INTRODUCTION

The medical photographer is often requested to take photographs of surgical instruments, apparatus and equipment, laboratory glassware, dental models, etc., to illustrate clearly their form and function. This type of photography calls on the skills of the advertising photographer rather than the clinical photographer. Special problems occur, for example, with highly polished surgical instruments, with confusing backgrounds to apparatus, and with all-white plaster dental models. The key to success in this area of work is almost always good lighting. It is most important that the photographer obtains complete instructions from the client; note any special features, understand the apparatus, then consider how best to illustrate it. Will plan, elevation or three-quarter views work best? Or should you consider a magnified inset of some detail? Or perhaps an 'exploded' view photograph? Will the scale of the object be apparent in the finished photograph? Or should a rule or other familiar object be included in the field of view? Intelligent choice of viewpoint will also affect the perspective – remember to use the camera back movements to compensate for perspective changes and camera front movements to increase depth of field according to Scheimpflug's rule. The student should revise thoroughly the principles of still life photography learnt during the years of basic photographic training.

## 24.2 LIGHTING AND BACKGROUNDS

Medical instruments and apparatus present the greatest challenge to the photographer's skills of lighting. The aim is to present in the photograph a 'natural' appearance. This can be difficult in the case of surgical instruments, for example, which are usually made of polished chrome, glass or Perspex, sometimes in combination with dark rubber tubing or black vulcanite. The viewer of such instruments builds up a mental impression, ignoring specular and black reflections and comes to the conclusion that he is looking at uniformly shiny, chrome objects. The camera, however, will record the instruments as black with the exception of some stark highlights representing images of the windows, studio lights, camera tripod and photographer!

There are three possible solutions to this problem:

(1) To surround the instruments with

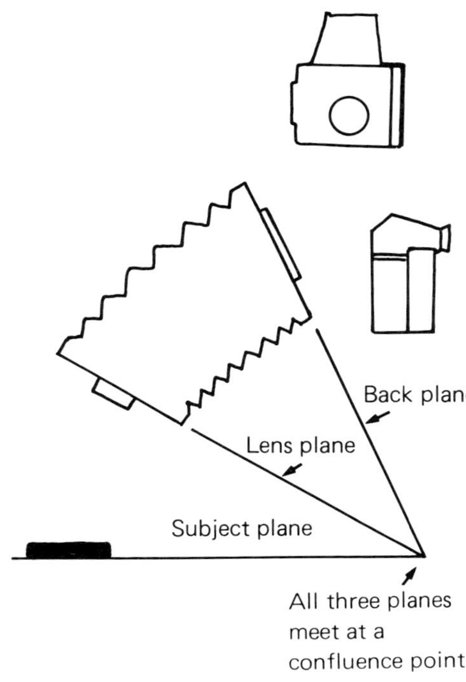


***Figure 24.1*** *Scheimpflug's rule states that the subject plane will be rendered in sharp focus when the subject plane, lens plane and film plane all coincide at a point. Camera front swings control depth of field, camera back movements control perspective*

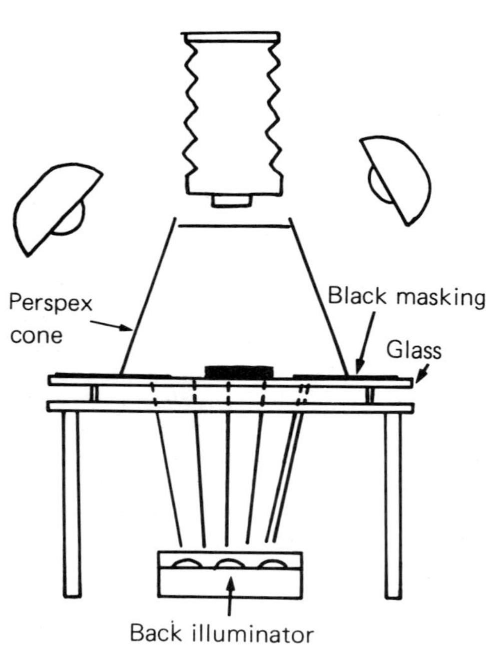


*Figure 24.2* *Lighting arrangement for polished surgical instruments*

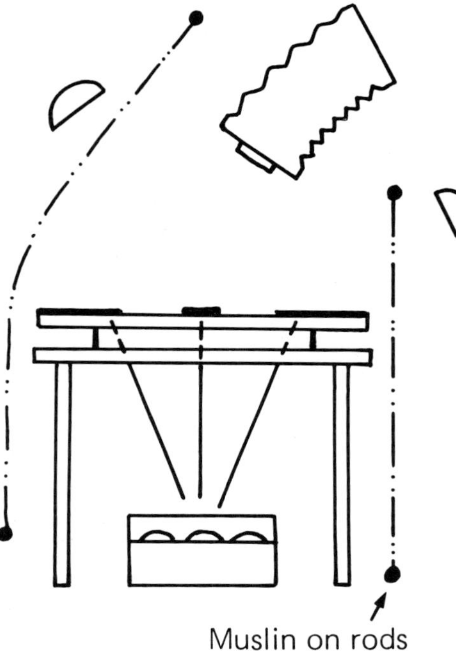


*Figure 24.3* *Large sets of instruments may be lit by utilizing pieces of muslin stretched over rods*

light-coloured reflectors so that the natural reflections are all even and light in tone.

(2) To treat the surfaces of the instruments so that they become diffuse reflectors.

(3) To use a source of illumination which moves continuously during the exposure.

### 24.2.1 Diffuse lighting

Diffuse lighting is the technique of choice for all polished instruments and apparatus. The simplest method is to surround the instrument to be photographed with a cone of white paper (or opalescent Perspex) leaving just a small opening for the camera lens at the top. This cone is then illuminated as evenly as possible with the exact lighting effect being assessed on the ground glass screen. For large sets of instruments an alternative to the cone is to drape sheets of white muslin attached to long rods on either side of the camera and light these. Alternatively, always remember you can use daylight which on a dull day can be remarkably successful. This diffuse lighting technique can produce a dull pewter-like effect, so consider the introduction of pieces of black card to the inside of the cone to give crisp edges and an additional light to provide an odd highlight – this will give sparkle and shine to the photograph.

### 24.2.2 Surface treatment

An alternative to diffuse lighting is to make the instrument a diffuse reflector. There are several ways of achieving this. There are a number of commercially available sprays which put a dull finish to the object – or alternatively milk can be sprayed with a very fine airbrush jet. Other workers advocate dabbing the surfaces with putty or plasticine, or alternatively getting the instrument very cold by refrigeration then breathing on it before photography. Great care needs to be exercised with any of these techniques as one is altering the actual reflection characteristics of the subject and the final picture may give a completely false impression. Of these techniques spraying milk with an airbrush is the most effective; though care should be taken to ensure that the metal surfaces are completely free from grease, that the finest spray at highest pressure is used, and that the final effect is built up from several light applications – each of which is allowed to dry. This gives a pleasant satin finish which often escapes detection in the final print.

### 24.2.3 Moving light source

The technique of 'painting' with a single light is well known in commercial photography and the objective here is to cover the instrument with adjoining reflections of the moving source, and to avoid burnt-out images of some reflections and gaps elsewhere. To facilitate even coverage a low powered tungsten lamp is used with the lens well stopped down so that the lengthened exposure time allows for a greater number of 'circuits' with the light. The single light is moved up and down, left and right and around in a systematic manner throughout the whole of the exposure time. This technique can be particularly useful for large sets of surgical instruments which need to be photographed *in situ* in their trays or as layouts on the theatre trolley. Such a large group of instruments may make the construction of a paper tent impractical and surface treatment unduly time consuming: the moving light source is therefore a useful alternative. In such cases inter-reflection between the instruments is bound to produce a result different in character from the small group where each reflection is carefully controlled. Luckily the large group forces the individual instruments to appear small in size and undesirable reflections become less noticeable.

### 24.2.4 Background control

As with specimen photography, the most satisfactory background for instrument photography is a transilluminated one, giving a shadowless background without unwanted detail. The light source may be either direct, as with an X-ray illuminator, or indirect, where lights are aimed at a sheet of white or coloured card. The instruments are placed on a sheet of plate glass at least 2 feet from the illuminated surface. As with the photography of morbid specimens it is critical that the area around the instruments is masked off to avoid excessive flare and that the background level of illumination is adjusted to the minimum level that will produce the required density on the negative. Excessive background illumination causes the edges of the instruments to be lost, particularly where they are curved.

Backgrounds for larger pieces of equipment and apparatus should be clean and uncluttered. A large gently curving piece of 'Colorama' or similar paper is most suitable – white being particularly good as this can be reproduced as any tone from white to dark grey by judicious use of background lighting. The overall aim is to reduce confusing shadows to a minimum. 'Confusing' is the operative word here, as controlled shadows may be eliminated by:

(1) Keeping the background well back and the lights high.
(2) Photographing the apparatus against black – but this is not good for reproduction in books and journals.
(3) Throwing the shadows out of the picture area by using plate glass support above a white background.
(4) Using a transilluminated background.
(5) Using separate 'soft' lighting to kill the shadows.
(6) Utilizing the moving light technique described above.
(7) Using large umbrellas, softlights or bounced lighting off white walls and ceilings.

When background control is not possible it will become necessary to work on the negative and/or print to block out the background. This may be done partially with photo-opaque on a large format negative then completed by airbrushing with process white on a print specially made for copying, i.e. slightly soft. A copy negative and final print complete the process.

### 24.2.5 Glass and plastic appliances

It is very difficult to photograph glassware so that it looks like glass. Essentially there are two techniques: (1) brightfield and (2) darkfield.

In brightfield illumination the glassware is placed some distance from a transilluminated background and masked carefully with black card. The details of edges within the subject are revealed by black edges. A slightly enhanced result can be obtained by using well diffused reflected light off a white background. The angle of the lamps is adjusted so that the majority of light reaches the subject by diffuse reflection from the background but some light is allowed to spill onto the glassware to give the occasional highlight.

The darkfield technique is basically the same as that used for immunoelectrophoresis plates where the subject is placed in front of a black background and lit from behind by directional beams of light at an angle such that only light dispersed and diffused by the glass surfaces enters the lenses. Diffuse directional lighting from above and below ensures that all the edges are recorded adequately, and a single spotlight to one side may add just enough frontal detail.

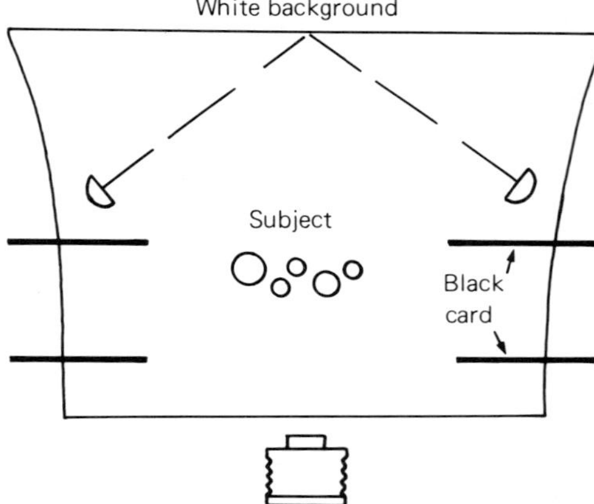

***Figure 24.4*** *Brightfield glassware technique*

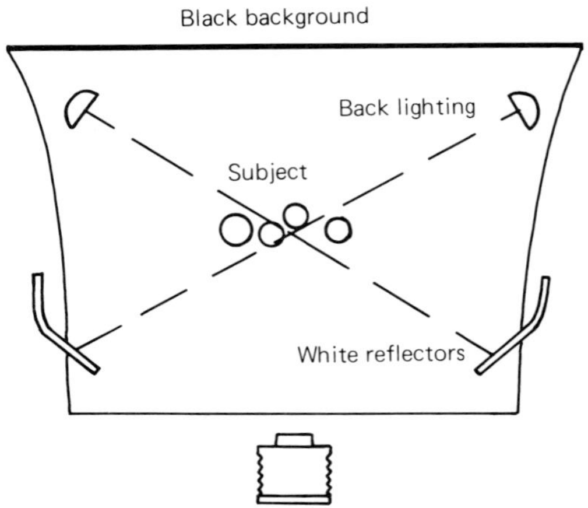

***Figure 24.5*** *Darkfield glassware technique*

Either of the two techniques above, with appropriate modifications can be used for all laboratory glassware, transparent and translucent plastic objects such as syringes, and other similar items, such as contact lenses. Considerable time, however, may have to be spent adjusting the lighting to obtain good results.

### 24.2.6 Dental models

The lighting of white, pink or yellow dental casts can be particularly difficult, and even worse when shiny metal bridges are included. Opinions vary widely as to the most suitable technique. Some have maintained that a single axial source of light gives accurate rendition of overbites and malocclusions with good detail in the plaster. Others find this illumination too stark and prefer softer illumination. The two most satisfactory methods are:

(1) Ringflash – especially when combined with two 45° mirror reflectors placed on either side of the dental model.
(2) Two large light sources placed at 45° to the camera axis aimed at the canines.

With acrylic dental models probably the only way to eliminate confusing reflections is to use the technique (2) above, in combination with polarizing filters. Complete highlight control is achieved by using polarizing filters over both light sources and camera lens.

## 24.3 SPECIAL TECHNIQUES

Two specialized techniques for the photography of polished chrome instruments are worth mentioning:

### 24.3.1 Combination of line and tone images

When polished instruments are photographed with diffuse light and transilluminated white background there is a tendency to lose the curved edges of instruments. One technique of overcoming this problem is to superimpose a line negative of the edge of the instrument over a continuous tone image produced by conventional technique. The line negative is produced by solarization of the silhouette image of the instrument. The finished combination has a good range of tones, but retains the edge detail normally lost because of specular reflection. The principal difficulty with this technique is that of registering the two images at the printing stage. One may either use pin registration darkslides and enlarger, include registration markers in the original scene, or simply expose the continuous tone bromide, develop and stop it – then re-expose the paper to the line image adjusted to fit exactly. Whichever method is adopted, the technique is time-consuming but it does produce spectacularly good results.

### 24.3.2 Photomontage

When large sets of instruments are to be photographed it can be very difficult to produce consistent illumination across the whole set which shows all the required detail. An alternative is to photograph the instruments in small groups, or individually, then assemble them into a montage which is re-photographed and retouched. It is helpful to lay all the instruments on a piece of paper and sketch the final layout before you attempt any photography – this helps in assembling the final montage and in choosing the scale and angle of view, which must remain the same throughout the series of individual photographs. If the finished assembly is to go to the block-maker then it is only necessary to request a 'free-standing mask' which will eliminate the paste-up marks and obviate the need for a photographic copying process.

## References


Bullock, P. (1957). Partial line reversal photography. *Med. Biol. Illustr.*, **7**, 210-216

Hopkins, W. (1975). Illuminating plastic appliances for photography. *Med. Biol. Illustr.*, **25**, 170-171

Le Beau, L. (1982). Photography of tiny reflective biomedical objects. *J. Biol. Photogr.*, **50**, 101-120

Williams, A.R. (1977). The photography of contact lenses. *Br. J. Photogr.*, **124**, 807-809

Williams, A.R. (1977). Revised technique for instrument photography. *Med. Biol. Illustr.*, **27**, 186-187


## *Practical projects*

(1) Produce a mounted set of black-and-white prints of a plaster cast of a patient's dentition; anteriorly, left and right laterals and occlusal surfaces. Make notes on the technique which you adopted and on any other method you tried.

(2) Photograph either an individual, or small set of (<5) polished chrome surgical instruments. Experiment with different lighting techniques and produce three mounted 10″ x 8″ black-and-white prints to demonstrate the variations you were able to achieve.

(3) Photograph in a medium of your choice a large set of polished surgical instruments (i.e. >15), using two different lighting techniques, e.g. moving light and white umbrellas. Submit lighting diagrams along with your finished photographs.

(4) Make a colour transparency of a set of either:
(*a*) Plastic syringes,
(*b*) Contact lenses,
(*c*) Plastic tracheostomy tubes.

(5) Photograph a Boyle's anaesthetic apparatus (or similar large piece of equipment) and produce a 10″ x 12″ exhibition quality print with all the relevant parts of the equipment labelled (it is not sufficient to submit the finished print with dry-transfer lettering on it. Pay particular attention to lighting and background control.

(6) Demonstrate the control of specular reflections by photographing in colour a pink and white plastic model of human dentition, using polarizing filters. Submit colour prints to show the effect of (*a*)no filtration, (*b*) lens only filtration, (*c*) lens and light source filtration.

## *Examination questions*

Q.1 You are asked to photograph some 30 sets of instruments as they appear to the surgeon on the gowned theatre trolley for an instructional tape–slide programme for operating room nurses. The photography must be done on location and either colour or black-and-white prints will be required. Describe in detail the equipment and method you would select for this assignment giving reasons for your choice.

Q.2 Describe with the aid of diagrams two different lighting techniques suitable for laboratory glassware; one against a black background, one against a white background.

Q.3 Discuss under the following headings the photography of polished chrome instruments:
(*a*) Camera controls
(*b*) Lighting
(*c*) Background control
(*d*) Surface treatment.

Q.4 How may the 'Sabattier effect' be useful in the photography of surgical instruments? Describe in detail the practical use of the technique.

Q.5 Discuss the photography of plaster dental models, illustrating your answer with diagrams where necessary. What special precautions would you take if these photographs were eventually to replace the stored dental models?

*Multiple choice questions (any of the statements may be true or false)*

Q.6 When photographing polished chrome surgical instruments you could:
(*a*) Use a dark-ground technique to retain edge detail.
(*b*) Place the instruments directly onto a light box to obtain a white background without loss of image quality.
(*c*) Utilize the Sabattier effect and combination printing to put a fine line around the instruments.
(*d*) Lower the view camera's rising and falling lens panel to alter the plane of the depth of field.
(*e*) Use a polarizing filter over the camera lens to eliminate all the reflections from the instruments.

Q.7 When photographing plaster dental models you would
(*a*) Use a panchromatic film with a long 'toe' to the characteristic curve.
(*b*) Use a yellow filter to help to differentiate between the yellow stone support and the white plaster teeth.
(*c*) Select a long focal length lens to reduce perspective distortion.
(*d*) Place the incisors in carefully matched occlusion.
(*e*) Expect to see the molar cusps in an occlusal view.

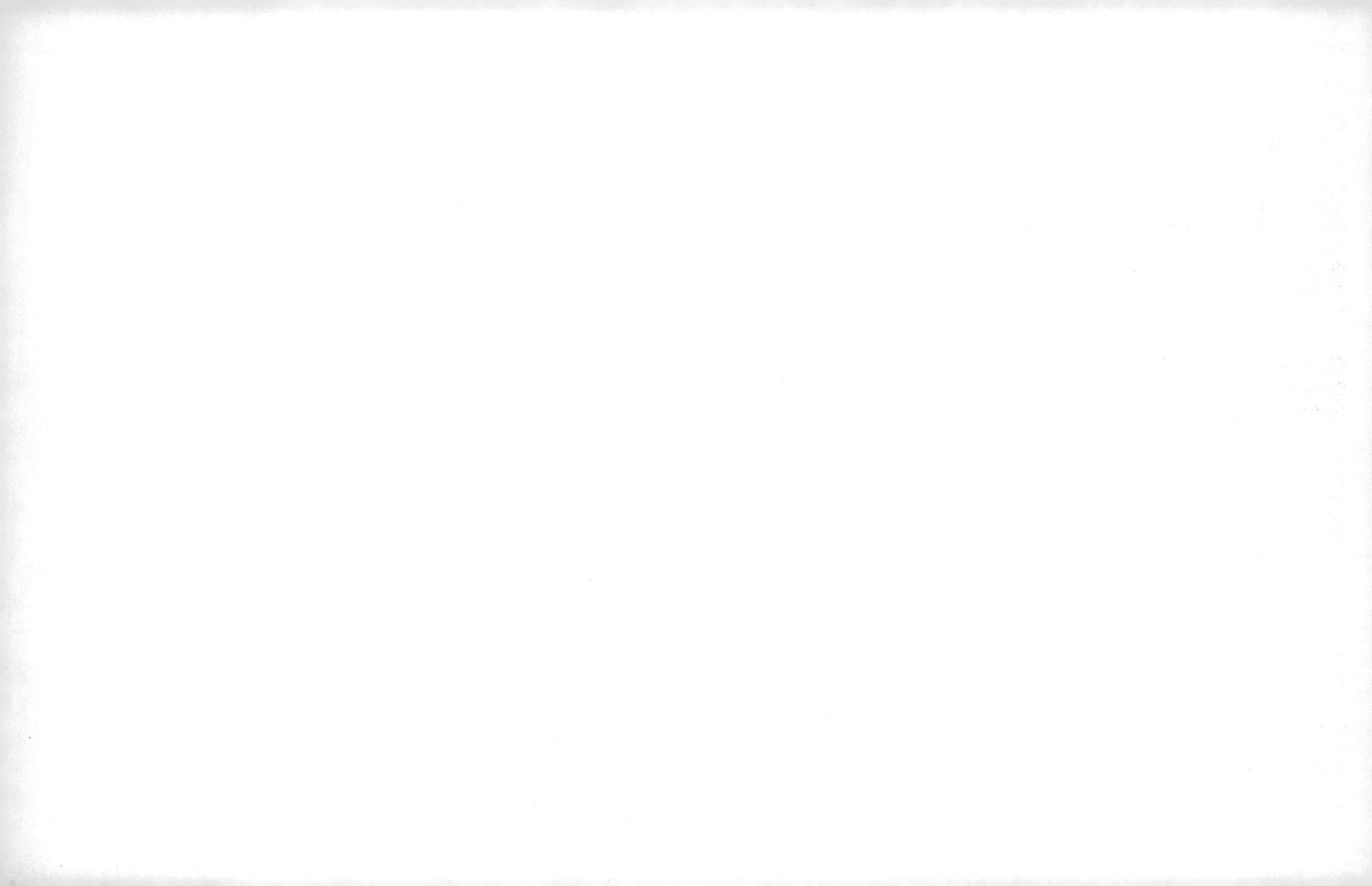

# Section 25
# Photoreprographics for medical teaching

**C. Reeves**, FIMBI, ABIPP
Senior Photographer
Institute of Child Health and Hospitals for Sick Children, London

## 25.1 INTRODUCTION

A great part of the medical photographer's day will be taken up with the reproduction of artwork, graphics, transparencies and published material for use both within his own establishment and outside – for teaching, research and publication. This is the so-called 'routine' work – the constant outflow of reprography so vital to an academic unit where information exchange provides a continuous need for media resources. This work may be routine but it does not have to be boring or monotonous even though the work may often be familiar. This section aims to gives the medical photographer an idea of the type of work likely to be encountered in this field and the type of consumer it will be attempting to reach. Hopefully, it also gives a few guidelines for producing the best possible results and perhaps gives thought for further experimentation. A survey of many of the general areas of reprography undertaken in most departments is included, together with some hints and advice within each area. Some specialist units may undertake highly individual reprographic work as a matter of routine, but an analysis of these has not been included, neither have the mechanics of flat copying, duplication or other photographic processes, a good working knowledge of which is assumed.

The medical photographer acts as the communicating link between the purveyor of information and the consumer. The ability to transform an abstract concept into a tangible product capable of imparting the desired information on its own merits is essential. The work will involve the production of material covering all aspects of medical education and for all areas of medical teaching and publication, where the consumers will cover the entire range of medical, para-medical and non-medical personnel. The ultimate success of the transference of information from progenitor to recipient may well depend upon the medical photographer's ability to act as a communicator.

In order to facilitate this ability, it is essential to maintain an awareness of the range of audio-visual aids available and to possess a good working knowledge of graphic, photographic and reprographic processes so that the best tools for the job are as far as possible, always used. It is equally essential that if a project requires 'team effort', that the whole team should be involved from the planning stage – it is bad management and a sheer waste of time and effort to embark on an ambitious project only to find that it comes to a halt half-way through due to the technical impossibility of reproduction, or because the concept has to be reorientated through lack of all round consultation.

## 25.2 ADVISING THE CLIENT

Whilst the medical photographer will naturally be audio-visually orientated through close association with sound and image making, he should be aware that most of his clients will not automatically be able to discuss their requirements or to translate their thoughts into audio-visual language, and indeed, may not even know what they require until they see a finished or half-finished product. They will almost certainly not be aware of the total range of the medical photographer's skills and it is the latter's job to use as much of his skill in extracting all possible information from his client before undertaking a project as he does in executing the work itself.

The following questions and points are set out as guidelines for gleaning information relevant to the intended use, market and purpose of a projected teaching package.

### (1) *Where is the information to be used?*

In a book, a lecture, an informal seminar, an international congress, a tape–slide programme, a teaching manual, a scientific paper, a poster demonstration or an exhibition?

The answer to this question will decide the form of the finished product and will also determine the amount of information capable of being assimilated by the recipient. A book illustration, designed to be perused at leisure can, by its very nature, be more comprehensive than a transparency which is designed for rapid assimilation by a larger audience. A transparency intended for inclusion in a tape–slide programme may well have to be planned utilizing only the horizontal format of 35 mm projection, depending upon the method of projection. A print for an exhibition or poster demonstration will need to be considerably larger size than that required for publication which may well have to correspond with the column width of the journal or paper for which it is intended. The facilities available to the user are an important consideration. It would be unfortunate to prepare a set of excellent 35 mm transparencies, only to discover that the user's sole means of projection is via an overhead projector, or that the department's video recording equipment is incompatible with the equipment on which the finished tape is to be played.

**(2) *Who is the information aimed at?***
Specialists in the field, non-specialists, a general mixed audience, a non-medical audience, the general public, a young audience or a foreign audience? The answer to this question will determine the content of the finished product and the level of understanding it aims to reach. A dissertation on the relationship of DNA to the formation of cancer cells would necessarily be simplified in content as the level of the audience's existing knowledge is decreased. If the intended recipients of the information are of an ethnic group not akin to the producer of the information, and he imparts his information in a way which is alien to their experience, it will be rejected. Similarly, if information becomes outdated by perhaps showing equipment no longer in use it will lose its impact, particularly if the audience is familiar with the subject matter.

**(3) *What information does the user wish to impart and what does he wish the recipients to assimilate?***
Is it step-by-step instruction, part of a series, a complete topic, an introduction to a major topic, a subject intended to stimulate audience participation, a presentation of a written paper? The answer to this question will not only determine the content of the finished product but also decide how best the information may be conveyed, whether it be by film, video, sound recording, slide or overhead transparencies, booklets or handouts. A good teacher should be guiding his student in the direction *he* wishes them to take and good teaching material ought to complement this guidance. It should be considered an aid to the student and not his teacher, although it is generally true to say that good teaching material assists in boosting the confidence of the teacher and his ability to put across his subject in a well-constructed and vital manner. Good teaching material may be defined as the best choice of learning aid needed to accomplish the learning process and, whilst high quality is always desirable, it is not always essential to the achievement of this aim. For example, a 15 s sound recording of the distinctive sound of whooping cough may well be more valuable and dynamic than a perfectly composed transparency of a child in bed.

Three other important factors will also determine the type of teaching aid produced – the *time* available to complete the project, the overall *cost* of the project and the *availability* of materials. In the area of reprography, time is not usually on the medical photographer's side and it may often be

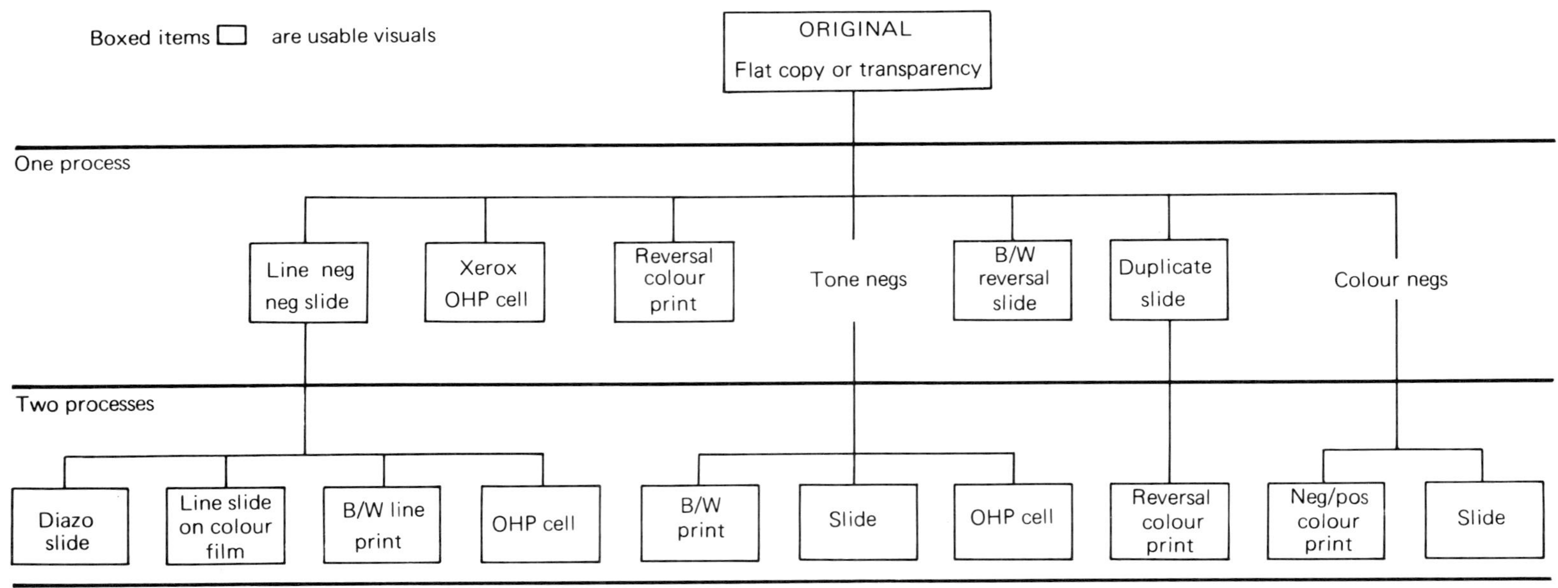


**Figure 25.1** *Just some of the possible types of visual which can be produced photographically from an original transparency*

Ratio of 2:3

A maximum of
twenty-five characters to a line
including spaces
and not more
than seven lines of type
makes the ideal
transparency

Ratio of 3:4

For film and
television visuals
this is the
correct format required
to utilize
total picture area

***Figure 25.2*** *Format ratios for original artwork*

necessary to produce the best possible aid in the shortest possible time. Coupled with this is the cost-effectiveness of the project. It would be uneconomical to produce an expensive time-consuming item which may be classed as disposable material, i.e. relevant for use only once, or obsolete within a very short period of time. The availability of materials and equipment will determine the working range of the photographer's skills and therefore the ability to provide the required teaching package. The diagram in Figure 25.1 sets out the type of reproducible item possible from an original piece of artwork or transparency. Each item is given a time/process status so that cost-effectiveness may be balanced against a usable teaching aid.

## 25.3 PLANNING THE TEACHING MATERIAL

The following presents a list of simple but desirable rules to adhere to when planning and preparing teaching material in order to achieve the best possible results.

The best typed material is made on a typewriter with a carbon ribbon rather than a cloth ribbon. The former produces black unbroken letters whilst the latter usually produces grey letters with the imprint of the 'weave' of the cloth. Similarly, computer printout and word processors used with a matrix dot printer produce 'prick point' grey lettering which is made up of dots and is equally unsuitable for photography on line film. Lettering stencils used with Indian ink and rub-down instant lettering are very effective but time-consuming.

A good teaching slide is one which contains a maximum of seven lines of writing and not more than 25 characters (including spaces, per line.)

When planning or producing graphics or photographs to fit into a 35 mm format, the working ratio is 2:3; it is 3:4 when preparing for television and 3:4 for 16 mm filming.

Tables and lists of statistical figures make bad slides; most can be converted to graphs, histograms, or pie charts quite easily and are more readily assimilated by the viewer.

Axis lines, curves, lettering, symbols, grid lines and toning should be bold to ensure instant impact and allow accurate exposures to be made if using lith type film. Underexposure to retain thin, weak lines results in a background which does not achieve $D_{max}$, and lines and lettering which spread and make unsatisfactory positives.

Complicated charts and diagrams for use as overhead projection transparencies can be divided into areas of discussion by overlaying and building up a picture. This is more successful than attempting to show everything at once.

Do not be afraid to use colour. It is tempting to 'play safe' and produce only black-and-white or blue diazo transparencies in the belief that colour distracts from subject matter but, if used well and intelligently, it can enhance and enliven a topic, perhaps separating its component parts into areas of colour may aid the audience's understanding of a difficult subject.

Do not be browbeaten into producing material which is obviously not going to do its job but, on the other hand, do not be too dogmatic about refusing to reproduce anything but first class originals. Usually, a compromise is possible if the medical photographer is respected as being able to advise and discuss alternatives in an expert and articulate manner.

If it is suspected that an illustration or typescript will be unintelligible when made into a 35 mm transparency, a simple test will confirm this suspicion. Measure the greatest dimension of the illustration and view it at a distance equal to eight times this amount. This is the equivalent of viewing the transparency projected at a size of 1.2 × 1.8 m from a distance of 14 m. If it cannot be seen

Expenditure of a small hospital over a six-month period

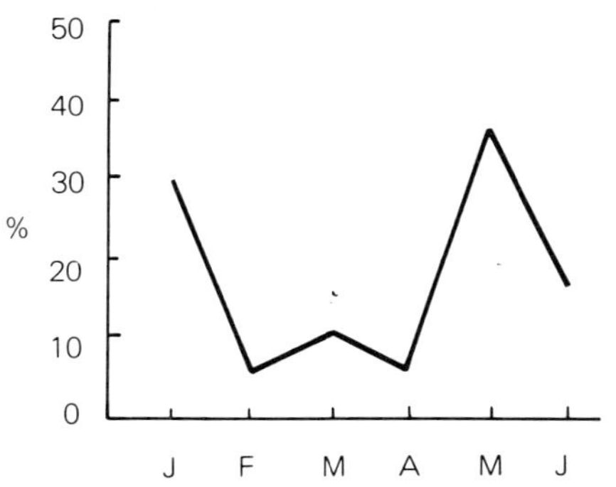


Total expenditure £1,000,000

Expenditure of a small hospital over a six-month period

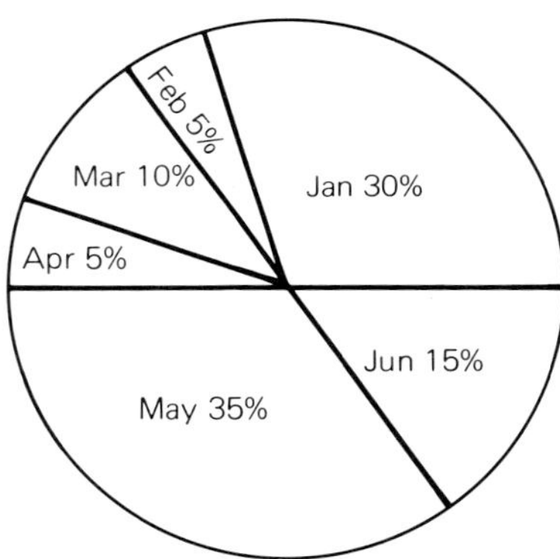


Total expenditure £1,000,000

Expenditure of a small hospital over a six-month period

| Month | Amount £ | % |
|---|---|---|
| Jan | 300,000 | 30 |
| Feb | 50,000 | 5 |
| Mar | 100,000 | 10 |
| Apr | 50,000 | 5 |
| May | 350,000 | 35 |
| Jun | 150,000 | 15 |
| Total | 1,000,000 | 100 |

Expenditure of a small hospital over a six-month period

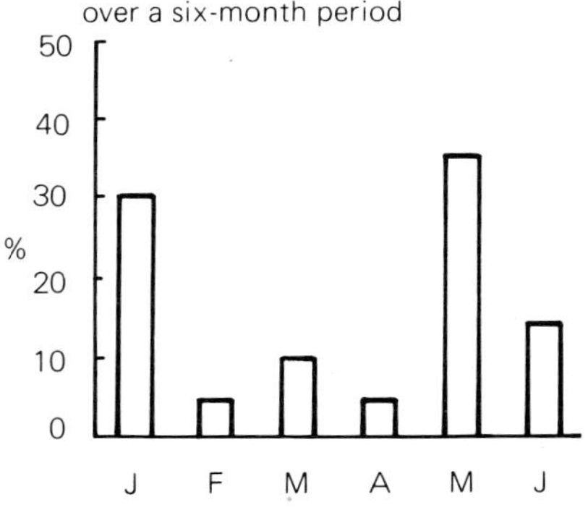


Total expenditure £1,000,000

***Figure 25.3*** *Four different ways of presenting the same statistical data – a graph, pie-chart, table and histogram*

clearly, it will be useless as a transparency.

## 25.4 COPYRIGHT (SEE ALSO SECTION 2.3)

The medical photographer, producing other people's work, i.e., figures, tables, diagrams and photographs from papers, books and journals must *always* be aware of the infringement of copyright. Generally speaking, it is accepted practice to use another person's material in slide form for discussion amongst immediate colleagues and within your own medical school. It is bad practice to do this without the copyright owner's permission outside your own teaching establishment although, if permission may be difficult or time-consuming to obtain, the name of the original author of the work with publication and dates, should be included within the image area. A generally accepted policy, whilst not strictly within the aegis of the copyright act, allows for one copy only to be made for the person requesting the reproduction. If more than one copy is made then copyright problems could certainly ensue.

It is an infringement of copyright to copy another person's material for re-publication in a new work without the written permission of the holder to the original copyright and no medical photographer should undertake to do this unless he has satisfied himself that this permission has been obtained by the new author. This also applies when duplicating transparencies made in other hospitals and institutions. The copyright of a photograph belongs to the commissioner of the photograph, whilst the negative is the property of the photographer, or institution employing the photographer, unless specifically contracted otherwise. The photographic copyright of artwork belongs to the original artist or the employer of the artist. This means in practice that the person who photographs copyright material is the infringer of the copyright, not the person requesting the photograph, or the person re-using it.

## 25.5 GENERAL PHOTOGRAPHIC CONSIDERATIONS

The medical photographer using a large format copying set-up has the advantage of a wider choice of film materials than the photographer confined to 35 mm, although the sheer volume of copy work passing through most medical illustration units makes 35 mm the more viable proposition both in terms of economy of labour and economy of cost.

It is worthwhile buying film stock in bulk rather than a few boxes at a time, and this should be kept refrigerated in a household refrigerator until required. It is particularly important to batch-buy colour film stock as any necessary filtration will remain constant for a longer period of time and change in effective speeds of some professional reversal films may vary from batch to batch.

The inclusion of a grey scale within the image area is useful when reproducing black-and-white copy, particularly when the original cannot be available for reference during the printing stage. It is essential to accurate reproduction where a colour print is required from a colour negative, particularly where the printer is not familiar with the subject matter. To ensure stringent processing quality control, a grey scale must be photographed at the beginning of each colour reversal film. This enables a tight control to be kept over the processing, either within the department or the outside laboratory, as any slight deviation from neutral will be noted.

If glass is employed to flatten the original artwork, it should be colourless. Any green tint inherent in the manufacture of the glass will affect the colour reproduction of the original and this looks particularly objectionable on a colour transparency. It may be necessary to filter out this tint when making the copy.

When reproducing black-and-white tone and all colour images, a black background should be used behind the original, and large areas of white on light surround should be masked with black paper. When making colour transparencies from flat copy, the use of a piece of black velvet, recording as maximum black, as a background to a complete illustration which does not fill the image area, obviates the need for masking the finished transparency. The use of black paper placed behind a book page or illustration prevents an image showing through from the reverse.

## 25.6 SPECIAL PHOTO-REPRODUCTION PROCESSES

Methods of slide production abound and space does not allow them all to be reproduced here; but the following is a brief resumé of the most commonly used processes. The student should familiarize himself with the practical details of the processes by referring to the references.

### 25.6.1 Line copying

***Negative***. Probably the most widely used film is the orthochromatic lith type film such as Kodalith, which is available in a variety of sizes including 5" × 4" and 35 mm. The latitude of this very high contrast line film is not great – overexposure produces distortion and disappearance of fine lines and an unevenness of dot and grid tones, whilst underexposure allows lines and lettering to 'spread' and produces a background which does not achieve $D_{max}$. Lith type films are usually processed in lith developers, but a PQ type developer may be used to produce a 'soft' line negative. This is particularly suitable for the reproduction of iodine isotope radiographic tissue scans which have a tonal range hardly much higher in many cases than the base plus fog level of the radiographic film.

Where the original may be essentially a line illustration but may contain fine lines and hatching, a high contrast blue-sensitive film such as Ilford Line Film may give more satisfactory reproduction. Although classed as a line film, the characteristic curve shows a longer toe section than lith film, and therefore has a greater tonal range across the shorter exposure range. It is also an excellent

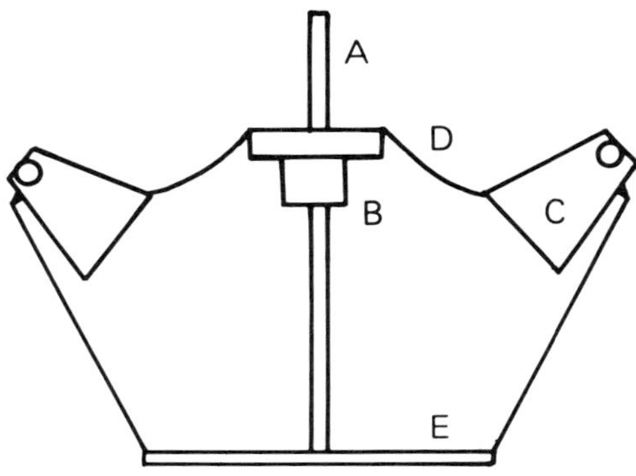


***Figure 25.4*** *A typical 35 mm reprographic camera (B) mounted on a rigid vertical column (A) at right-angles to a baseboard (E). The lights (C) are masked by black cloth (D)*

film for making positive slides from line and tone negatives. It is not available in 35 mm.

***Positive***. Lith type films may be reversed to produce positive line transparencies of good quality but, of course, without retaining a negative. The film is exposed conventionally then developed in a highly active PQ developer, the developed silver is bleached out and the remaining silver fogged and developed, the film is then cleared, hardened and washed. Alternatively one of the 'pre-fogged' direct reversal materials such as Kodak's LPD4, S80–185, or MP5360, may be used to obtain good quality positive line slides. These films are particularly quick to process and eminently suitable for copying E.C.G., E.E.G. and other traces.

Electrophotography is becoming more popular for positive line slide production with at least two semi-automatic slide copier/processors on the market. These both use a type of 'Xerox' process to obtain ready mounted positive slides in less than one minute. Running costs are, however, extremely high.

Vesiculation films (e.g. Kalvartone) are still available and comprise a thermo-plastic resin impregnated by diazo salts which produce small bubbles of nitrogen gas on exposure. The image is 'developed' by heating the film to produce a high resolution line image. These films are very slow and little used in professional practice.

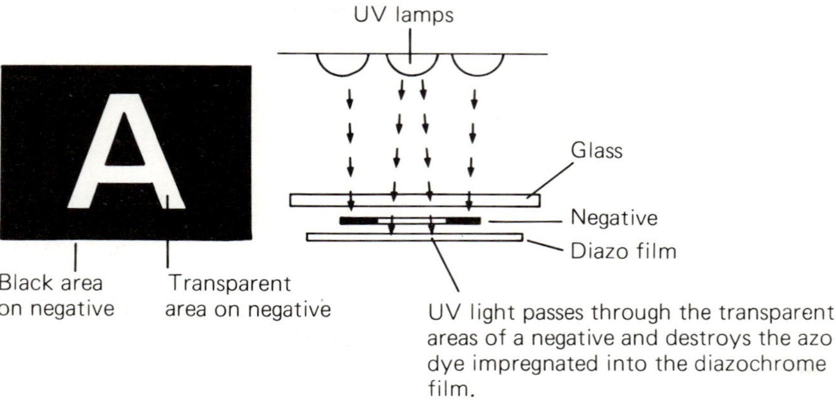


***Figure 25.5*** *The diazochrome process*

### 25.6.2 Transparencies from lith negatives

**(1) *Lith positives.***
Lith negatives may be contact printed or printed through the enlarger onto lith or other high contrast film to produce transparent positive slides. When contact printing onto film it is useful to place several sheets of translucent draughtsman's tracing paper over the glass of the contact printer. This diffuses the light source and reduces the likelihood of dust spots spoiling the transparency.

**(2) *Diazochromes.***
The most common form of transparency made from a lith neg is the diazochrome. Diazochrome film material is impregnated with an azo dye which is sensitive to UV and reacts with ammonia vapour to produce a colour. A lith negative placed in contact with a sheet of diazochrome film and exposed to UV allows UV to pass through its transparent areas, i.e., the image area where the dye has been

destroyed. Diazochrome is available in various colours, but the blue variety is no doubt the most popular. This is a relatively quick and inexpensive process, although the major disadvantage is that diazochrome material retains its sensitivity to UV which means that such transparencies fade after a period of time. The manufacture of diazochrome slides involves the handling of ammonia solution which is toxic, and a suitable fume cupboard should be constructed for its use so that adequate extraction of the ammonia vapour may be effected.

**(3) *Tinted slides.***
Negatives may be hand-coloured, although this can be time consuming particularly when working directly on to 35 mm film. Very fine spirit based felt tip pens, or liquid dyes, are often used to accomplish this. These have a high luminosity but on larger areas it can be difficult to obtain any degree of even distribution of colour. If possible, the use of a transparent self adhesive film such as Letraset's 'Project-a-film' is recommended. It is advisable not to use more than four colours on a transparency, and better to choose complementary tones rather than primaries together. For example, green and red on a black background cannot be focussed at the same time and produce visual confusion to the viewer.

**(4) *Duplicating onto colour film.***
Colour transparencies may be made from line negatives using colour filters, colour film and a slide duplicator which incorporates a contrast control mechanism such as the Bowens Illumitran. A colour filter is placed in the filter holder of the contrast control unit which is switched to maximum light intensity and maximum contrast control. The line negative is placed ready for copying, the light source transilluminating the negative turned to minimum intensity and the exposure made. The result is a transparency with a white image on a coloured background. A coloured image may be obtained by placing a filter in the filter drawer beneath the negative

The principle of contrast control works by means of a pre-fogging exposure which bounces off a glass held at 45° between the lens and transparency or negative, then directly back through the lens onto the film thus reducing the inherent increase in contrast so noticeable in duplicated transparencies. The greater the contrast control, the greater is the intensity of pre-fogging. However, the intensity of transilluminated light through the image area of the negative is too great

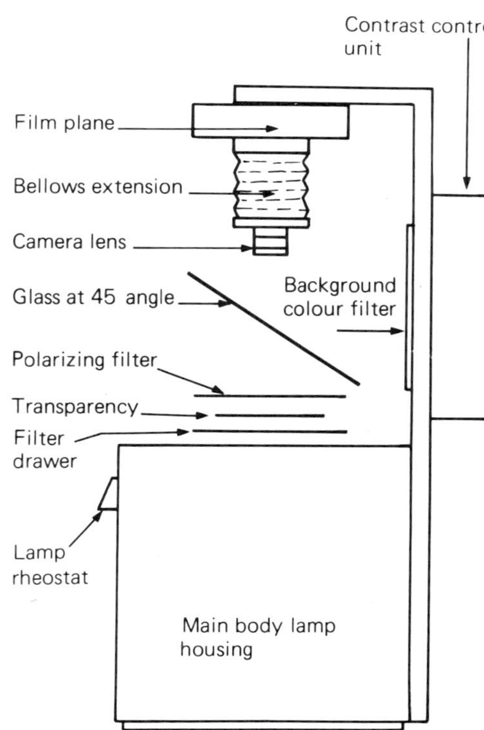


**Figure 25.6** *A modified slide duplicator*

to be affected by this pre-fogging, so a light image on a darker background is achieved. Because of this principle, it is not possible to achieve a dark image on a light background. Further colour modifications may be achieved by varying the lens aperture and the colour balance of the reversal film. It is essential to place a polarizing filter between the 45° angle glass and the negative in order to prevent the appearances of a 'double image' on the finished transparency. The following Kodak Wratten filters make a useful set for producing these coloured slides: 44a, 47b, 16, 22, 12, 25, 58, 32.

**(5) *Pre-fogged colour film.***
Another technique using colour reversal film and a slide duplicator is to 'fog' the whole length of a colour film in a darkroom to a low level coloured light, e.g. blue, green or red, then rewind the film into the cassette. Line negatives are placed in the duplicator and coloured filters, e.g. pale blue or yellow placed in the filter drawer. The pre-fogged film is then loaded into the duplicator and used in the ordinary manner. This technique yields coloured letters on a different coloured background, but has the disadvantage of having to produce a whole roll of slides of one background colour.

**(6) *Dye-coupling (chromogenic development).***
In this technique conventional colour photography dyes are coupled to the silver image of the Kodalith ortho negative by mordanting the film to convert the silver image to a silver–copper–thiocyanate complex. A range of very saturated and stable colours can be produced by this method which yields white letters on a coloured ground. A one-step chromogen process has been developed but this process has ever assumed any level of popularity.

### 25.6.3 Colour transparencies from positive slides

There are three ways to make colour transparencies from positive slides to produce black lettering on a coloured background. (1) Positive slides may be dyed with a cold water fabric dye, although evenness of tone is not always satisfactorily obtained – a better alternative is the use of 'Project–a–film' overlay. (2) A good result can be achieved by sandwiching with the positive either a piece of evenly exposed and processed diazochrome film or colour transparency made by photographing a plain piece of coloured paper. Variations of hue may be obtained by varying the exposure. (3) If the original is blemish free, it may be photographed directly onto colour reversal film with a coloured filter placed directly over the lens. This works particularly well with a yellow filter.

### 25.6.4 Black-and-white half-tone copying

As with line copying, the user of the large format copying apparatus has the advantage of being able to choose from a fairly wide range of half-tone films available, most of which will give excellent quality reproduction on large format. The 35 mm user is faced with the often formidable task of producing good quality exhibition sized prints. This makes the use of a slow film of high resolution and processed for maximum acutance absolutely essential to ensure the highest quality reproduction over all the tonal range. It is useful to bear in mind that it may be necessary to reproduce a colour original in black-and-white which has relied upon its colour to convey information and which does not do the same when converted to monochrome. It may, therefore, be advisable or even necessary to employ a colour filter of contrasting hue to the original in order to reproduce accurately the information portrayed. Black-and-white half-tone films may also be reversed to give a direct positive transparency or negatives may be printed through the enlarger or in contact with a suitable film of good tonal range.

### 25.6.5 Copying onto colour Negative film

Much of what has been said for monochrome copying also holds true for colour copying onto negative film, with the addition that particular attention be paid to the colour temperature of the light source in relation to film stock used. Whilst it is accepted practice to use colour films which are not balanced to the light source in use and therefore necessitate the employment of colour conversion filters to render film and colour temperature compatible, the best colour reproduction is not obtained this way. Conversion filters are reliable only when the existing colour temperature is reasonably accurate.

Mention has been made of the importance of the inclusion of a grey scale in colour copying and this is particularly essential when an original may contain only shades of one or two colours. An automated colour printer integrates to grey, and this works completly efficiently if the negative contains a mix of red, blue and green, as most negatives do. The system breaks down if this mix is deficient in two out of the three colours, but this may be rectified with accuracy by printing the grey scale correctly. It is worth noting here that for colour block making reproduction, a transparency will be required by the publishing company and not a colour print.

### 25.6.6 Colour reversal copying

Good colour reversal copying may be accomplished using either artificial light (tungsten or photoflood) or daylight balanced flash provided the correct film or conversion filters are used with the relevant light source, although the best reproduction is achieved with matched film/light source. All light sources have a useful life which is rather shorter than their actual life – colour balance shift may be noticed on transparencies as lamps start to blacken. If one lamp fails, it is advisable to change the set as uneven lighting and colour imbalance may result.

### 25.6.7 Duplicating transparencies

Most departments of medical illustration will have some sort of slide duplicator such as the Bowens Illumitran with or without contrast control and these are extremely versatile. The important word here is 'duplicating' rather than 'copying' transparencies; it is easy to copy a slide but rather more of an exacting task to produce a duplicate matching the original, or colour corrected to improve on the original. It is extremely difficult to produce a first class result without some ability to control the contrast of the duplicate, so equipment with this built-in mechanism is recommended for the best results. Again, it is advisable to buy a batch of colour reversal film in order to standardize filtration as most batches will require a basic filter pack to correct to neutral before any colour corrections are made. When colour correcting, it is often helpful to place colour correction filters in front of the transparency until the desired degree of correction is obtained visually – usually about two thirds the final filtration is required when actually photographing the transparency. On duplicators with dial-in filtration, this visual interpretation is made much easier.

### 25.6.8 Black-and-white tone negatives from colour transparencies

A slow speed film with high resolution should be used for making black-and-white negatives from colour transparencies. The transparencies should be dirt and dust free and, if mounted in glass, care should be taken to ensure that no 'Newton's rings' are visible which will appear on the final reproduction. As with black-and-white tone flat copying, it is sometimes necessary, when reproducing colour transparencies to monochrome, to use a contrasting filter to enhance detail in black-and-white. This may be employed for example, when making negatives from retinal images which generally rely on gradation of red to show deviations from normal. Photographed straight onto panchromatic film, these produce flat and disappointing prints, a green filter gives the contrast necessary to produce a reproduction with detail corresponding to the original transparency. Filtering also works well for photomicrographs which may have a predominance of one colour. If using a slide duplicator which has the facility of contrast control to make negatives from transparencies, the contrast control should be switched off. Good quality negatives may be made using a lightbox which does not need to be colour balanced.

### 25.6.9 Line negatives from line positive transparencies

It is possible to make line negatives from transparencies by contact onto line film, but better results are obtained either through the enlarger, through a slide duplicator or by photographing the transparency on a lightbox. It is advisable to use a time exposure with lith film rather than a flash exposure when using a slide duplicator with the light source turned to minimum intensity to ensure even illumination over the whole negative area.

### 25.6.10 Colour negatives from colour transparencies

Here a lightbox or slide duplicator may be used, although it is advisable to match film with light source for good results. Batch film buying again is useful to maintain consistency of filtration and the inclusion of a grey scale is essential at the beginning of each film. It is more difficult to colour correct with colour negative film as excess filtration produces a decrease in contrast with a resultant unacceptable print. If heavy filtration is necessary as much as possible should be done at the printing stage. As with the reproduction of black-and-white negatives, when using a slide duplicator which incorporates a contrast control mechanism, this should be switched off.

### 25.6.11 Lettering on slides, double exposures, composite transparencies

The easiest way to put lettering on a transparency is to make a positive transparency of the lettering and sandwich this with the existing slide. The advantage here is that the original may be used, although the sandwich could cause a shift of image focus. An alternative is to duplicate the transparency, and then re-expose this image to a line negative positioned in place of the original transparency. The result is white lettering on the slide although this may be altered by the use of coloured filters placed in the filter drawer beneath the negative. This, of course, may only be accomplished if the camera has the facility for double exposure.

For flat copy work, lettering may be worked directly onto the original, but the disadvantage here is that this spoils the original for further use. White or coloured instant lettering is translucent when placed directly onto tone and if a print is desired, this leaves no facility for double printing where a line and tone negative may be required. Lettering on to transparent acetate sheets is very satisfactory, although good contact must be maintained during exposure to avoid shadowing between lettering and original. Both acetate with lettering and original may be photographed separately for double printing.

It is worth remembering that slide mounts are available in various designs to incorporate the size of image required within the 5 cm$^2$ format. It is therefore possible to mount two, three or four images on one slide without the difficulty of complicated masking which may be impossible to accomplish neatly. Image size, of course, must be predetermined in the camera.

## 25.7 PRINTING FOR EXHIBITIONS AND POSTER DEMONSTRATIONS

Exhibitions and poster demonstrations are becoming an increasingly popular medium for information exchange, because it is possible for a greater number of people attending a conference to participate than would otherwise be the case if the programme only contains lectures and seminars.

These demonstrations need to be planned carefully bearing in mind that a defined area of space will have been allocated to each presenter and that the finished product may have to be carried halfway across the world. If the area designated is 200 cm × 120 cm, it is a sensible idea to plan for four boards measuring 100 cm × 60 cm each, which can be carried separately and mounted together on site. It is desirable that any exhibition be immediately eye-catching, but not essential, nor even possible that the boards be covered with colour prints. There is a range of tinted photographic papers on the market extremely suitable for use with line negatives. These range from pastel blue and pink to vibrant amber and green, through to copper, silver and gold. An additional method of colouring black-and-white prints is by toning and tones available include red, blue and sepia. Here the image is toned leaving the background white. Photographic papers can also be dyed using cold water fabric dyes but resin-coated papers do not accept dye as readily as bromide papers and this may result in an uneven distribution of colour. A subtle combination of coloured background paper or lettering mounted on boards of contrasting or complementary tone, including black-and-white or colour prints as the subject dictates, can be definitely more eye-catching than a demonstration full of black-and-white half-tones, charts and lettering.

## 25.8 AUTOMATED EQUIPMENT

Whilst most departments of medical illustration do not operate a great deal of automated equipment because of the enormous capital expenditure involved and the unjustified through-put of work, it is becoming increasingly clear that carefully chosen automation is extremely cost-effective in a depleted labour market. Many departments employ the use of word-processor and computer units, which greatly assist in the production of typographical layouts. Repetitive labelling is accomplished speedily and efficiently and graphs and diagrams may be formulated with ease.

Automated film and paper processors obviate the need for dishes, bottles and sinks and enable darkroom time to be cut to a minimum.

Automated slide mounters, available with or without a labelling printer, cut, mount and label 36 transparencies in a minute and stack them ready for sorting. In a single-handed department, this alone could save an hour or more a day.

Available on a more commercial level are rostrum cameras, bulk film duplicators and daylight printers. These may seem irrelevant to the adequate functioning of many medical illustration departments, but with the increasing need for such departments to become financially independent, it would seem obvious that the manufacture of commercial audio–visual aids for medical teaching is best undertaken where the highly trained skills and knowledge are available.

## 25.9 PHOTOGRAPHY FOR REPRODUCTION

The student should be familiar with the major printing processes, i.e. offset lithography with metal and paper plates, gravure, silk screen, and letterpress; be able to recognize the method of production by examination of the printed page; and have an appreciation of the uses and costs of each. If this has not been learnt as part of a more general photographic training the student should refer to the many excellent Kodak publications on graphic arts photography. Similarly, a knowledge of what makes an illustration suitable for reproduction will be expected and again the references will provide the information which space does not allow to be reproduced here.

## References


Atkinson, D. (1976). An alternative to diazo slides. *J. Biol. Photogr. Assoc.*, **44**, 135

Baldwin, E. (1976). Notes on photographs for reproduction. *J. Biol. Photogr. Assoc.*, **44**, 133-134

Brown, S. (1983). Tone reproduction on monochrome transparency. *J. Audiovis. Media Med.*, **6**, 51-56

Bunker, W. (1975). Custom line copying for journal reproduction. (Part 1 – Standards, materials and exposure.) *J. Biol. Photogr. Assoc.*, **43**, 103-109

Bunker, W. (1975). Custom line copying for journal reproduction. (Part 2 – Procedures and refinements.) *J. Biol. Photogr. Assoc.*, **43**, 150-156

Canto, J. and Spencer, R. (1980). Slides of fluorescein angiograms with an illumitran copy unit. *J. Biol. Photogr.*, **48**, 175-178

Delorey, F. (1975). An inventive method for the production of educational transparencies. *J. Biol. Photogr.*, **43**, 83-84

Duguid, K. (1975). Line slides by colour coupling. *Med. Biol. Illustr.*, **25**, 17-19

Duguid, K. (1978). A brief review of the monochrome process. *Br. J. Photogr.*, **125**, 772-773

Dwyer, F.M. (1970. Exploratory studies in the effectiveness of visual illustrations. *Audiovis. Commun. Rev.*, **18**, 235-249

Edkins, S. and Hoag, M. (1982). Eastman direct MP 5360. *J. Biol. Photogr.*, **50**, 135

Fletcher, R. (1967). Line slides by colour coupling. *Med. Biol. Illustr.*, **17**, 10-11

Gaskins, L. (1973). Colouring of transparencies copied onto line film. *J. Biol. Photogr. Assoc.*, **31**, 112-114

Gray, D. (1980). Planning visual media for self-instruction. *J. Biol. Photogr.*, **48**, 117-137

Hill, T. (1975). An alternative method of producing colour line slides. *Med. Biol. Illustr.*, **25**, 151

Kenshole, G. (1968). Determining the teaching efficiency of audiovisual material and procedures. *Educ. Tech. Contin. Med. Educ.*, **38**, 41-47

Kodak. (1976). *Basic Printing Methods.* (Publication GA-11.1) (Rochester, NY: Eastman Kodak Ltd.)

Kodak. (1976). *Graphic Design.* (Publication GA-11.2.) (Rochester, NY: Eastman Kodak Ltd.)

Kodak. (1976). *Photoreproduction.* (Publication GA-11.5.) (Rochester, NY: Eastman Kodak Ltd.)

Kodak. (1976). *Film Assembly and Offset Platemaking.* (Publication GA-11.6.) (Rochester, NY: Eastman Kodak Ltd.)

Kodak. (1976). *Offset Presswork.* (Publication GA-11.7.) (Rochester, NY: Eastman Kodak Ltd.)

Kodak. (1978). *Photography for Layout and Reproduction.* (Publication Q-74.) (Rochester, NY: Eastman Kodak Ltd.)

Kodak. (1979). *Copy Preparation.* (Publication GA-11.4.) (Rochester, NY: Eastman Kodak Ltd.)

Kodak. (1982). *Finishing.* (Publication GA-11.8.) (Rochester, NY: Eastman Kodak Ltd.)

Kodak. (1982). *Basic Photography for the Graphic Arts.* (Publication Q-1) (Rochester, NY: Eastman Kodak Ltd.)

Manuel, W. (1980). Supercolour title and line art slides. *J. Biol. Photogr.*, **48**, 186-187

Michaels, K. (1977). Whole-roll flash technique for false colour title slides. *J. Biol. Photogr. Assoc.*, **45**, 33

Morton, R. and Duguid, K. (1968). Rapid reversal techniques for the production of line and tone positive monochrome slides. *Br. J. Photogr.*, **115**, 417-419

Munday, P. and Tempest, H. (1976). Illustration preparation and reproduction techniques – the publisher's needs. *Med. Biol. Illustr.*, **26**, 111-114

Murgio, M. (1969). *Communication Graphics.* (New York: Van Nostrand Reinhold)

Ollerenshaw, R. (1962). Design for projection (The Renwick Memorial Lecture.) *Photogr. J.*, **102**, 41-47

Olson, K. (1979). Preparation of multicoloured slides from black and white light and electron micrographs. *J. Biol. Photogr.*, **47**, 49-51

O'Neill. J. (1978). 101 ways to make copy and title slides – some of them good! *J. Biol. Photogr. Assoc.*, **46**, 141-152

Puzas, J., *et al* (1982). Adding selected areas of colour to black and white slides by colour coupling. *J. Biol. Photogr.*, **50**, 69-70

Rapp, J. (1974). A rapid, simple and inexpensive technique for black and white positive slides. *J. Biol. Photogr. Assoc.*, **42**, 55

Salmons, N. (1967). Standards for effective slides. *Vis. Sonic Med.*, **2**, 20-25

Siwek, R. and Chessell, G. (1981). In-house colour offset lithography for medical education: developments and applications. *J. Audiovis. Media Med.*, **4**, 40-44

Wells, R. (1973). Effectiveness of three visual media and two study formats in teaching concepts involving time, space and motion. *Audiovis. Comm. Rev.*, **21**, 233-241

Wolfe, P. (1975). Special problems of medical colour photography intended for reproduction. *Med. Biol. Illustr.*, **25**, 235-238

## *Practical projects*

(1) Photograph a mechanical trace such as an E.E.G. or E.G.G. output, or a specially prepared graph on paper with grid lines to produce two matched black-and-white prints (*a*) retaining the grid lines and (*b*) removing the grid lines. (Experiment with different film and filter combinations and make notes on your results).

(2) Produce a continuous tone copy of an original photograph which has been labelled with black letters in a light area or in the white border. Submit the original, a black-and-white print and a black-and-white transparency.

(3) Duplicate a 35 mm camera-original transparency then produce a second copy somewhat 'cropped' to improve in some way the original composition. Submit the original with both copies.

(4) Produce a 10″ × 8″ colour print of, say a Boyles apparatus, leaving space around the apparatus for annotation. Make a transparent overlay with arrows and lettering to label the various parts of the machine and produce two transparencies (*a*) without the overlay and (*b*) with the overlay. Photograph both under identical conditions and mount them such that they could be used in a 'dissolving' tape–slide presentation.

(5) From a good black-and-white line original, e.g. a graph or chart drawn by an artist, produce as many different types of teaching transparency as you can. For example; diazo, positive, negative, hand tinted negative, dye-coupled, colour duped, etc. If you do not do these processes regularly in your department read the references cited and try out the processes for yourself. Submit the original, the transparencies produced and short notes relating to the method of production for each. Present the results in a form which would be convenient for demonstrating to clients the range of slides available. (Attempt not less than six processes.)

(6) Use two methods to add a title to an existing colour transparency. Submit the original and the two 'labelled' versions with brief details of the methods used.

## Examination questions

Q.1 Distinguish between line copy, continuous tone copy and half-tone copy; and describe the photographic processes involved.

Q.2 Describe at least two simple ways of deciding how much material belongs on one slide. Outline the theorectical basis behind the methods and any 'qualifications' you would add to the use of these methods.

Q.3 Describe two methods of producing colour prints from clinical transparencies suitable for use as part of a 'poster session'. Comment on the quality of the finished result and any economic factors involved.

Q.4 You decide to produce a 15 minute audio–visual presentation on some aspect of the photography of pathological specimens as part of your staff training programme. Select objectives and describe the sequence of illustrations you would use to achieve your aim.

Q.5 Compare two methods of producing 'coloured' slides from black-and-white line artwork, under such headings as cost, time to produce, permanency, etc.

Q.6 List and define all audio–visual aids likely to be encountered in a present-day medical school.

Q.7 State what method of copying you would choose to provide up to 10 copies of:

(*a*) A continuous tone print,
(*b*) A radiograph,
(*c*) A set of committee minutes comprising 20 pages,
(*d*) An architect s line drawing.

State briefly the reasons for your choice.

Q.8 Discuss all the factors that you would consider when advising a client on the best way to present some statistical information.

Q.9 What criteria determine which of the following would be the most appropriate medium?

(*a*) Prints,
(*b*) An illustrated work book,
(*c*) Slides with tape,
(*d*) Audio tape,
(*e*) Motion picture film,
(*f*) Videotape

Q.10 What type of data are best presented graphically as a bar graph, line graph, diagram, table, or pie chart?

# Section 26
# Copying radiographs and electronic images

**Dr P.N. Cardew**, MRCS, LRCP, FRPS, FBPA, AIMBI
Director of Audio-visual Communications
St Mary's Hospital and Medical School, London

## 26.1 INTRODUCTION

Modern medical practice relies heavily on radiographic, radio-isotope and allied imaging systems and because of this importance it is imperative that the medical photographer is able to faithfully reproduce these images. Applications might be summarized as:

(1) Continuous tone prints for display, distribution and publication,
(2) Reduced transparencies for projection as lecture slides,
(3) Full size transparencies as duplicate copies (Facsimiles) and
(4) Microfilm copies for filing or bulk storage.

## 26.2 DEFINITIONS

*Facsimile* or duplicate reproduction. One having the same size and tonal relationships as the original; bones, for example, will be depicted as light tones in the radiograph. Sometimes the phrase 'reduced facsimile' may be used for the projection transparency.

*Positive reproduction*. There is much confusion in the use of this term. Some use it to describe a reproduction having tones opposite to the original (the original radiograph being used as a negative). The facsimile or duplicate is generally preferred since it takes the form which most medical staff are accustomed to viewing. Most photographers now use the term 'positive reproduction' to describe the facsimile or reduced facsimile, since they regard the radiograph as the subject (irrespective of whether it is a negative or positive) and any reproduction which has opposite tonal values as a negative and any reproduction which has similar tonal values as a positive.

*The intermediate* (positive if one regards the radiograph as a negative) is made by contact printing or photographing the original on to film and is the first step to producing the facsimile.

## 26.3 GENERAL CONSIDERATIONS

Radiographic film is double coated, having an emulsion both sides of the base. This imparts high inherent contrast and a density range extended to about 1000 : 1. Normal photographic negative material has a density range of about 100 : 1 and a good bromide print only 15 : 1.

| *Radiograph* | *Negative* | *Print* |
|---|---|---|
| 1000 : 1 | 100 : 1 | 15 : 1 |

Thus it is evident that in the reproduction of any radiograph some tonal compression is inevitable and even then it will be necessary to limit good reproduction to the upper, middle, or lower tone ranges only. No film is available which will deal with the wide contrast and density ranges necessary – selective shading and dodging may help, as will masking and electronic printing – but in the final analysis the photographer must select the most important area of the radiograph and base his exposure and processing on that area.

## 26.4 PRODUCTION OF THE INTERMEDIATE POSITIVE

### 26.4.1 Choice of emulsion

A film with good exposure latitude, fine grain and the capability of development to a low gamma (0.6) should be chosen. Film speed is not important, but it is useful to have an exposure time long enough to allow dodging or shading to be carried out if necessary. Fine grain films of medium speed and contrast with a long straight line/tone region to the characteristic curve are satisfactory. 35 mm film is preferable for quantity production but cut film allows for individual treatment of the negative.

### 26.4.2 Technique

The radiograph is placed on an evenly lit illuminator, the camera being centred and the film plane parallel to that of the

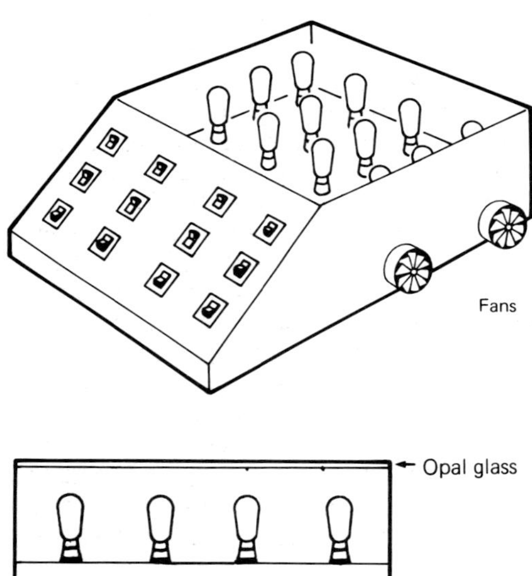


***Figure 26.1*** *A multiple-lamp illuminator for radiographic copying*

radiograph. Shading of the original by hand with a black card or cloth can be carried out at this stage if desired. Special multiple-lamp illuminators having a dozen or more individually controlled bulbs arranged in egg box form are sometimes used to allow variable intensity lighting of the radiograph. Carefully used these can often obviate the need for manual dodging methods which are difficult to repeat with accuracy. Development should be such as to give a soft-looking appearance, but full of detail. It is most important to mask down the radiograph to the minimum area required at the intermediate production stage; this prevents flare from the light-box degrading the image. The facsimile print or transparency is made by normal photographic methods. Transparencies will show more detail than prints due to their wider density range and conditions of viewing. Local control methods, such as shading and dodging, can again be employed while printing the facsimile but care must be taken to avoid over-shading.

## 26.5 CONTRAST CONTROL

The above procedure will deal satisfactorily with most radiographs, but where fine detail prevents local shading or there is a particularly wide density range, other techniques may be employed.

### 26.5.1 Unsharp masking

This will compress the overall density range without affecting the detail in small areas. It is a reverse tone image. The procedure is to print the radiograph on a contact printer separating it from the film by a sheet of clear glass of about 3 mm thickness. Exposure and development are arranged to give a density range of about one third the original, and an intermediate is made. Because the mask is unsharp it is easy to register with the original, and edge effects due to slight inaccuracies are not noticeable. The sandwich of radiograph and weak mask is then regarded as the original and copied in a conventional manner.

### 26.5.2 Highlight masking

An added refinement to the unsharp masking method is that of first producing a *sharp* highlight mask. This is a sharp film image made in proper contact with the original and having just enough exposure to record the highlight detail only. This is processed, placed in contact and in register with the radiograph when making the unsharp area mask. The purpose of the highlight mask is to exaggerate the highlight detail and offset the poor contrast otherwise obtained in those tones of the paper print which come within the toe of the characteristic curve.

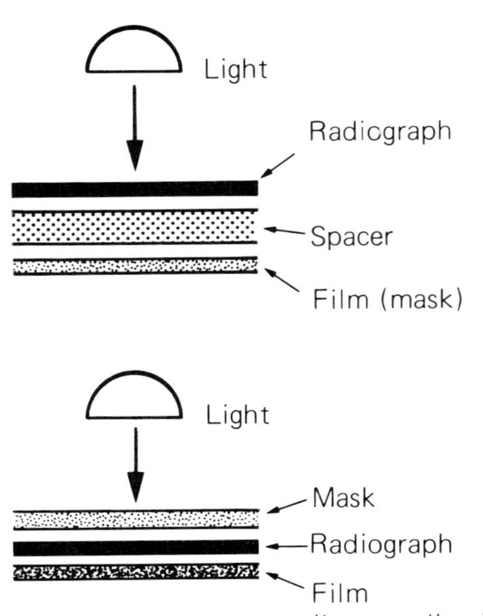


***Figure 26.2*** *The production and use of an unsharp mask*

#### 26.5.3 Electronic printing

Electronic printers, such as the 'Log E Tronics' system, scan the radiograph with a 'spot' of light, the intensity of which is automatically controlled by a feed-back system and will provide accurate and detailed 'dodging' of difficult radiographs. The degree of contrast compensation can be adjusted from no compensation through five steps of compression. Electronic printers are made as enlargers or contact printers but they are very expensive to purchase. Commercial electronic printing services are available.

*N.B.* It should be noted that the above methods of contrast control may produce facsimiles which, although showing the maximum possible detail, may well lose the characteristics of the original radiograph, and thus be unacceptable to the viewer. However, used with discretion they can be a great help in reproducing difficult radiographs for publication.

## 26.6 DIRECT REVERSAL PROCESSES

Copying without an intermediate onto monochrome or colour direct reversal films is a quick, effective method of producing projection transparencies 12.1. Exposure estimation must be accurate since reversal materials have a restricted latitude. The normal reversal technique of exposing for the brightest highlight and 'letting the shadows take care of themselves' will not suffice for radiographs. It is necessary to take exposure meter readings of the highest and lowest densities where detail is essential, and calculate the required exposure from these. Various monochrome films are available for direct reversal, or it is possible to use a conventional monochrome negative film and process it in reversal chemistry. This typically involves a first developer, stop, wash, bleach and cleaning baths, followed by second exposure, development, stop, fix/harden and wash. Most acceptable results can be obtained by using this method and full details can be found in the literature.

## 26.7 SPECIAL TECHNIQUES

### 26.7.1 Reflected light

Exceptionally 'thin' radiographs having very little density (i.e. underexposed) can often be successfully copied by using a system of reflected rather than transmitted light. The technique is to treat the radiograph not as a transparency but as flat copy. The original is laid on white paper, under glass, and evenly lit with 45° lighting. By this means the light passes twice through the emulsion of the radiograph, and therefore double the density is achieved. Film and development should be chosen to give a high contrast negative. This technique is capable of producing acceptable copies from otherwise seemingly useless radiographs.

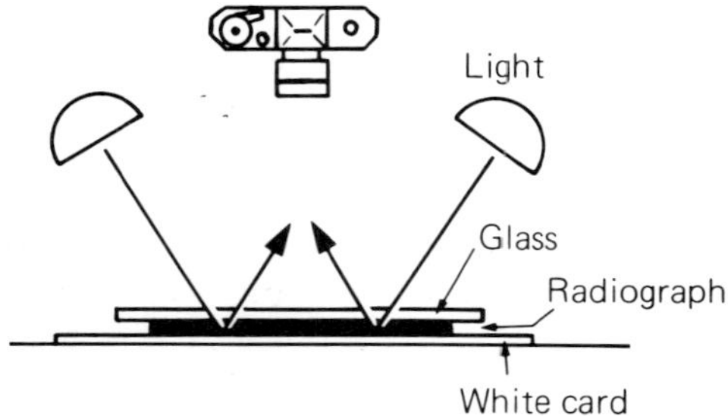


***Figure 26.3*** *Reflection copying for thin radiographs*

### 26.7.2 Bas-relief

This technique is sometimes useful for enhancing fine detail such as bone structure, by artificially introducing a low 'relief' to the image. The technique is to produce a rather soft intermediate negative and then contact print this to obtain a slightly soft positive. The two are then combined slightly out of register and re-printed to give the finished bas-relief. The result is a picture with the main outlines indicated by dark or light contours. Some experimentation is necessary with the direction and degree of displacement to obtain the best effects.

### 26.7.3 Colour coding

It is sometimes helpful to the radiologist to see the tone of the radiograph represented as different colours and it can certainly be helpful in the teaching photograph to see specific details such as arteries coloured, say, red. This may be achieved either by hand colouring a monochrome print with dyes or by using a colour posterization technique as described in Section 23.11

### 26.7.4 Combination copying

A good teaching picture may sometimes be obtained by copying a specimen in contact with the radiograph, e.g. gall-stone, foreign body, etc., The technique here is to expose the radiograph conventionally with the specimen in place, then to re-expose the negative with the light-box turned off and using modelling lighting for the specimen. Such photographs can be dramatic instructional aids.

## 26.8 ELEMENTARY RADIOGRAPHIC INTERPRETATION

In order to produce the best reproduction the medical photographer must know what the radiograph is intended to show. This will also prevent time wasted in reproducing tones which may be of little interest, at the expense of more important areas.

Conventionally small lead indicator letters are included in the radiograph to indicate *the patient's* right and left sides. Thus a small 'R' should appear on the left of the photograph and vice versa. Hands should be reproduced with the phalanges pointing upwards, feet with the phalanges downwards.

Radiographs are often given names derived from the areas of organs of the body concerned and from the methods employed in their production, e.g. pyelogram, cholecystogram, angiogram, etc.

The medical photographer must acquire a good knowledge of radiographic anatomy, the uses of the various radiographic techniques and the photographic aspects of radiography. He should be aware of the various specialized methods used to reveal detail in the major organs and vessels.

Without such a background it will be impossible to understand the radiographs and advise the radiologists on the reproduction of them. Such advice is very necessary in view of.

(1) The impossibility of faithfully reproducing all the tones of the original.
(2) The difficulty in ensuring that detail remains visible on the printed page of a publication or on the projection screen of the lecture theatre.

## 26.9 ELECTRONIC IMAGING TECHNIQUES

During recent years various imaging techniques involving electronic processing have been developed, the results of which are presented on some form of visual display unit. Most types of apparatus are also equipped with some means of making permanent records of the display, usually on film or as a Polaroid print. From a photographer's point of view these records tend to be crude in comparison with conventional radiographs but share with them the high contrast characteristic. Some of these images may be impossible to interpret without a knowledge of the parameters employed to create them so that where some densities need to be sacrificed in making prints it is essential that the photographer ensures that he is aware of the salient features to be retained.

### 26.9.1 CAT Scanning (computerized axial tomography)

A 360° rotating scan by an X-ray source supplies information to the computer which produces sectional views of the body. The computer recordings are stored on magnetic tape or disc which can then be manipulated to produce a range of pictures on X-ray film. The technique is of particular value in revealing soft tissue organs which are poorly seen on conventional radiography.

### 26.9.2 Ultrasonography

A beam of very high frequency sound pulses is directed into the body and a detector picks up reflections from tissues. The interval between the moment of delivery of the pulse and detection of the reflected signal indicates the depth of the tissue. Ultrasonography in various forms is used in many parts of the body, e.g. echo-encephalography, echo-cardiography, foetal heart monitoring. The results in some cases are displayed as a trace, in others as a scan which may need to be photographed.

### 26.9.3 Radio-isotope scanning

This technique makes use of the ability of certain body tissues to concentrate selected chemicals. If these are labelled with a radioactive tracer and administered to the patient their presence can be detected by means of a scintillation counter, and their location revealed in the form of a 'scan'. Particular applications occur in the location of tumours of endocrine glands and organs concerned with metabolism such as the liver. Scans may be either monochrome or colour, the latter indicating the intensity of radiation.

### 26.9.4 Thermography

Heat radiated from the body can be focussed by mirrors on an infrared detector, and by using a scanning technique a picture is created on a video display unit in which colours are coded to indicate temperature variations.

## 26.10 PHOTOGRAPHY OF VIDEO DISPLAY UNITS

Although most sophisticated modern apparatus incorporates an integral camera, occasions arise, particularly in developmental work, when the photographer is asked to take pictures of the oscilloscope, TV monitor or cathode ray display unit. The brightness of such displays can vary over a great range but an exposure of ¼ s at *f*/5.6 on ASA 64 film would be about correct when photographing an 18 inch screen. If the image is produced by scanning, the exposure time must be at least as long as the time taken for the flying spot to cover the whole field, e.g. in the case of a television image 1/25 s.

## References


Bodenhamer, D., *et al.* (1979). Producing slides of radiographs. *J. Biol. Photogr.*, **47**, 117-121

Brown, S. (1983). Tone reproduction on monochrome transparency. *J. Audiovis. Media Med.*, **6**, 51-56

Burnard, J. (1975). Copying radiographs. Part 1. *Br. J. Photogr.*, **122**, 834-839

Burnard, J. (1975). Copying radiographs. Part 2. *Br. J. Photogr.*, **122**, 857-859

Burnard, J. (1975). Copying radiographs. Part 3. *Br. J. Photogr.*, **122**, 886-889

Burnard, J. (1975). Copying radiographs. Part 4. *Br. J. Photogr.*, **122**, 913-915

Burnard, J. (1975). Copying radiographs. Part 5. *Br. J. Photogr.*, **122**, 932-934

Cardew, P. and Rytina, J. (1965). A standard technique for copying radiographs. *Med. Biol. Illustr.*, **15**, 82-85

Craig, D. (1955). LogEtronics. *Med. Biol. Illustr.*, **7**, 166-170

De Veer, W. (1973). Enhancement of radiographs by dodged masking. *J. Biol. Photogr. Assoc.*, **41**, 20-22

Gauthier, G. (1981). Selective illuminator for radiographs. *J. Biol. Photogr.*, **49**, 115-118

Gibson, H. (1951). Black-and-white and Kodachrome copying of radiographs. *J. Biol. Photogr. Assoc.*, **19**, 51-55

Gilliam, C., *et al.* (1979). Photography of nuclear medicine images. *J. Biol. Photogr. Assoc.*, **47**, 103-106

Gramiak, R. (1966). Contrast enhancement in photographic copies of under exposed radiographs. *Radiology*, **86**, 548-550

Harding, F. (1960). Radiographic reproduction. *J. Biol. Photogr. Assoc.*, **28**, 71-75

Harding, F. (1967). Reproducing the difficult radiograph. *J. Biol. Photogr. Assoc.*, **35**, 109-113

Harrison, N. (1951). A multiple light-box for radiographic reproduction. *Br. J. Photogr.*, **98**, 431

Hills, T. and Rytina, J. (1972). X-ray film reduction to 100 mm and 35 mm through a T.V. system. *Med. Bicl. Illustr.*, **22**, 30-33

Morton, R. and Duguid, K. (1968). Rapid reversal techniques for the reproduction of line and tone positive slides. *Br. J. Photogr.*, **115**, 417-419

Oldendorf, W. (1966). Auto-subtraction: a photographic technique for enhancement of detail in radiographic reproduction. *Acta Radiol. Diagn.*, **4**, 97-99

Seidler, B. (1970). Duplicating and dodging in copying radiographs. *Dent. Radiogr. Photogr.*, **43**, 12-16

Staub, P. (1962). Relief method of copying X-rays. *J. Biol. Photogr. Assoc.*, **30**, 113-115

Thompson, T. *et al.* (1973). A radiographic reproduction system for medical teaching files. *J. Biol. Photogr. Assoc.*, **41**, 139-141

Walters, K. (1973). Universal X-ray copying macro bench. *Med. Biol. Illustr.*, **23**, 217-220

## Practical projects

(1) Visit your department of radiography. See the production of radiographs, loading of cassettes, use of intensifying screens, development, replenishment of solutions, silver recovery, etc. Be sure you understand the effects of more or less exposure on the finished radiograph.

(2) In a textbook of radiography look up the following terms and be sure you understand the technique and its purpose. Angiocardiogram, angiogram, barium enema, barium meal, bronchogram, cholecystogram, cystogram, encephalogram, hysterosalpingogram, lymphogram, myelogram, pyelogram (both intravenous and retrograde)., tomogram and ventriculogram.

(3) Produce a 7" × 5" publication quality print of a normally exposed PA radiograph of the chest. Submit original, negative and print along with short notes on your technique.

(4) Make a 10" × 8" exhibition print of any radiograph you choose. Present three versions (*a*) unmasked (*b*) unsharp masked (*c*) highlight and unsharp masked. Make notes on your technique and comment on the results. Submit original, negative and masks in addition to the print.

(5) Use (*a*) colour reversal film (*b*) monochrome reversal film and (*c*) monochrome negative film with reversal processing, to produce 35 mm projection transparencies of any normally exposed radiograph. Write notes on the techniques used and comment on the results.

(6) Produce a 10" × 8" exhibition print of any radiograph you choose in combination with a specimen, e.g. a cholecystogram with superimposed gallstones.

(7) Choose a radiograph with fine bone detail and produce a 10" × 8" print to demonstrate how the 'bas-relief' technique may be used to enhance the detail.

(8) From any underexposed radiograph (thin) produce two 7" × 5" prints for publication; one by conventional transillumination, the other by reflection copying. Make notes on the results obtained.

## Examination questions

Q.1 Describe three different radiographic techniques used to obtain detail in abdominal or thoracic organs.

Q2 Discuss the need for density range compression in radiographic reproduction.

Q.3 Describe the techniques of unsharp masking and electronic printing as applied to copying radiographs. What are the advantages of each?

Q.4 Describe fully one technique for producing 35 mm projection transparencies of radiographs. Outline two other techniques which could be used for the same purpose.

Q.5 What equipment and techniques would you select for the regular production of publication quality prints from normal radiographs?
How would you modify this technique to deal with
(a) under-exposed radiographs?
(b) over-exposed radiographs?

Q.6 Write short notes on the following:
(*a*) Computerized axial tomography
(*b*) Angiocardiography
(*c*) Radio-isotope scanning
(*d*) Pyelography

Q.7 Discuss fully the concept of 'image enhancement' in the context of radiographic reproduction.

Q.8 With the aid of simple diagrams explain the principles of
(b) highlight masking,
when making photographic prints from radiographs.

Q.9 What factors are particularly important when photographing images on television screens? Describe the characteristics of the films you would choose for this task.

*Multiple choice (any of the statements may be true or false)*

Q.10 When producing publication prints of radiographs:
(*a*) Films with long straight line characteristic curves are ideal.
(*b*) Copying by reflected light will enhance over-exposed X-rays.
(*c*) Bas relief technique will improve the thin radiograph.
(*d*) Unsharp masking will improve fine detail.
(*e*) Sharp masking may improve shadow detail.

# Section 27
# The history of medical photography

**A.R. Williams**, MPhil, FBIPP, FRPS, FBPA, AIMBI
Head of Medical Illustration and Teaching Services
Charing Cross Hospital and Medical School, London

## 27.1 INTRODUCTION

Organized medical photography started with the inception of the National Health Service in Britain after the Second World War, so until very recently there were many people in charge of departments who remembered the pioneering days of the 1940s. Most of these early workers also made a point of learning about the history of the beginnings of medical photography. Today the new entrant to the profession knows little of the origins of clinical photography – despite the current interest generally in early photographs and photographic equipment. In order to give the student an historical perspective a brief review is presented here which may inspire further research.

## 27.2 ARTISTIC ORIGINS

The student medical photographer will do well to remember that medical illustration has been in existence for many hundreds of years – the earliest Arab manuscripts are heavily illustrated with medical artwork. The scientific accuracy of these illustrations was very dubious with some honourable Renaissance exceptions such as da Vinci, Dürer and, of course, John Stephen of Calcar, the artist who illustrated Versalius's famous anatomical text *De Humani Corporis Fabrica*. Although the camera obscura was described fully by Giovanni della Porta as early as 1589, the first description of its use in medicine does not appear until 1733 in William Cheselden's volume *Osteographia* – where the artist Van der Gucht is depicted at work with the instrument. Medical authors used every process available to them to illustrate their work and wood engraving was followed by copper engraving, aquatint and lithography. Indeed some of the finest early dermatological illustrations were lithographs in Von Hebra's *Hautkrankheiten* (1860). In 1826 Nicephore Niépce succeeded in recording the optical image of the camera obscura by chemical means and on August 19th 1839 Francois Arago made known the details of Daguerre's process, which was partly based on the work of his partner Niépce. Within 6 months the photographic process was being used to record medical images.

## 27.3 THE EARLIEST MEDICAL PHOTOGRAPHS

The first application reported was on February 24th 1840, just 6 months after the publication of the Daguerrotype process, by a Frenchman Alfred Donné. He was head of the Charité Clinic in Paris and showed several photomicrographs of bone and teeth to a meeting of the Academie des Sciences. Indeed in 1845 he published his book *Cours de Microscopie* which was illustrated with 86 beautiful engravings from original Daguerrotype photomicrographs. Donné used a solar microscope to give exposures of four to twenty seconds over a range of magnifications from ×20 to ×400.

The author of the first clinical photograph is a matter of some uncertainty. Hill and Adamson produced a paper calotype of a woman with a large goitre in Edinburgh, possibly for a Dr James Inglis, in 1847. Thompson in America published several Daguerrotypes (as engravings) in the *American Journal of Dental Science* in 1850. These depicted a resection of the left superior maxillary bone and had been taken in Columbus, Ohio in 1848.

The first attempt at surgical photography was made in October 1846, when a photographer, Josiah Hawkes, was present to record a demonstration of the use of sulphuric ether as an anaesthetic. Unfortunately, the sights and smells of the operating room were too much for the photographer and the event was never recorded! The following year, however, Southworth and Hawes successfully captured the event on Daguerrotypes.

1851 saw the publication of several engravings in medical journals taken straight from Daguerrotypes. Charles Gilbert published several clinical photographs in the *Philadelphia Medical Examiner* taken in the previous years by Laughlin. Subjects included facial plastic surgery following lupus infection and gunshot wounds. Carnochan published Daguerrotypes of 'amputation of the jaw' by P. Haas in the *New York State Journal of Medicine*, whilst Phillip Buckner describes in the *Transactions of the Ohio State Medical Society* how he took a Daguerrotypist 220 miles to photograph a woman with a truly massive abdominal tumour weighing 275 pounds.

Reports from various American journals indicate that the presentation of Daguerrotypes of patients had become common practice at medical meetings by the late 1850s. Unfortunately, most of these early medical photographs have been lost or destroyed. Often the Daguerrotypes were destroyed after the engraver had prepared a plate for publication; or they were looted in subsequent years to obtain the valuable leather frames.

The first two really consistent users of medical photographs came on the scene in 1852. In Berlin, Hermann Wolff Berend, an orthopaedic surgeon first used pre- and post-operative pictures of all his patients to assess progress. He used the wet plate process with paper prints, and presented his results at an orthopaedic conference on December 9th, 1853. Berend also reported receiving photographs of a patient with scoliosis from the University of Kiev in 1852, so the Russians were clearly taking medical pictures very early on. In England, Hugh Welch Diamond took many photographs of his patients in the Surrey County Asylum in Twickenham, to evaluate the physiognomy of the insane and to show progress of treatment. He also used the wet collodion process, and was in fact one of the founder members of the Royal Photographic Society in 1853, and its secretary from 1858 to 1868. He actually established a studio and darkroom in the asylum for his routine photography.

By 1861 stereoscopic medical pictures were being produced by J. Cranz for a Professor Billroth at the Chirurgical clinic in Zurich and some of these were published in 1867. In 1866 A.B. Squire, a London surgeon, published hand coloured photographs of various dermatological conditions – the fine surface texture was enhanced by the emulsions they worked with which were sensitive only to blue.

In America the Civil War of 1861–1865 produced literally thousands of photographs of wounds and injuries, photomicrographs, specimens, surgery, and post-operative scarring; many of them taken for the office of the Surgeon General at the Army Medical Museum by William Bell, the chief photographer or Edward J. Ward his successor. Many of these are preserved at the National Library of Medicine in Washington and form the world's largest single collection of medical photographs.

G.B. Duchenne the famous French neurologist was also an active photographer and in 1862 published a set of 17 photographs mostly of fatty degeneration to accompany his book *De l' Electrisation Localiśee*. Similarly his book *Mecanisme de la Physionomie Humaine* had an accompanying album of 73 photographs this was also published in 1862.

## 27.4 THE FIRST PUBLICATIONS ON MEDICAL PHOTOGRAPHY

In 1855 Hermann Berend wrote the first paper on medical photography *Ueber Benutzung der Lichtbilder für Heilwissenschaftliche Zweke*, in which he described the value of the photographs and also gave some advice on technique. Ransford E. Van Gieson of New York City wrote the first known article to be published in America entitled The application of photography to medical science. This appeared in 1860 and recommended the establishment of medical photography departments in all hospitals, although it largely concerned photomicrography.

In 1882, at the age of just twenty three, Albert Londe was appointed as Director of the photographic Service Laboratory of the Clinic for Diseases of the Nervous System at Salpêtrière Hospital Paris. He was appointed by J.M. Charcot the famous neurologist who had established photographic services in 1878. Great advances in medical photography were made by Londe at the Salpêtrière and when he published *La Photographie Moderne* in 1888 he included a chapter on medical photography. Probably the most famous book ever on the subject was published by Londe in 1893 – *La Photographie Medicale*. Much of the advice given in this text is still relevant today. He described and gave plans for the ideal department, discussed various techniques and novel equipment and described the photography of specimens using a vertical camera. He even mentions the effects of perspective and standardization in clinical photography and medico-legal considerations are also covered.

The first journal devoted to medical photography appeared in Leipzig in 1894 entitled *Internationale Medizinisch – Photographische Monatschrift*.

## 27.5 CONSOLIDATION AND SPECIALIZATION

By the 1880s medical photography was well established; in France the majority of hospitals had staff photographers, whereas in America and England medical photography remained mostly in the hands of individuals for several decades. Many specialist applications were developed towards the end of the nineteenth century. The first good photographs of the larynx were taken by J.N. Germak in 1882, and these were improved on by Lennox Browne, in 1883 who used a 10 000 candle power carbon arc lamp with reflectors and a lens system. In 1885 the living human retina was photographed by William Thomas Jackman and J.D. Webster, although the first truly successful photography is attributed to Gerloff in 1891. He used an immersion system which gave way to the more complex apparatus of Dimmer who actually described his results in 1889 but did not publish until 1899. His work remains the basis of the Zeiss–Nordensen retinal camera on which all modern retinal cameras are modelled.

Stereoscopy became popular and the well known *Edinburgh Stereoscopic Atlas of Anatomy* first published in 1890 can still be found in anatomy departments. Neisser (1894) also produced a stereoscopic atlas. Marey and Muybridge pioneered the study of motion and developed medical cinematography. Muybridge published many plates of abnormal gaits in his book on locomotion published in 1887. Max Nitze, inventor of the modern cystoscope, took and published the first endoscopic pictures of the inside of the bladder in 1894, whilst 4 years earlier Walter Woodbury had described and illustrated an endoscope for photographing inside the stomach.

## 27.6 THE TWENTIETH CENTURY

The first half of the twentieth century is probably the least well researched period of all. Certainly the turn of the century and the First World War brought technical innovations such as the introduction of roll film cameras, sound synchronization with cine film, photogravure process for printing, anastigmatic lenses, compound shutters, MQ developers, panchromatic sensitizing dyes, daylight developing tanks, Autochrome plates for colour photography, Dufaycolor and Kodachrome film. How these developments affected medical photography is not clear. It is certain that medical photographs were being produced in great numbers and many remain today in our hospitals' archives, but it would seem equally true that in England at any rate, most of these pictures were produced by the local commercial photographer hired for the occasion. For the student interested in historical research the period between the wars would be a most profitable area.

From the end of the Second World War medical photography became a routine and accepted part of modern medical practice, and the history of the period from the 1940s is a matter of record in the *Journal of the Biological Photographic Association* and *Medical and Biological Illustration*. The student would do well to read early volumes of these two journals, not just for the historical aspect, but it will also give ideas for new avenues of research and development to keep the profession on the established path of innovation and service to medicine.

## References

Berend, H. (1855). Ueber benutzung der lichtbilder fur heilwissenschaftliche zwecke. *Wein. Med. Wochenschr.*, **19**, 291-292

Billroth, T. (1867). *Stereskopische Photographien Chirurigischer Kranken*. (Erlangen: Enke)

Brown, L. (1883). *Voice, Song and Speech*. (London: Samson Low, Marston Seale and Rivington)

Buckner, P. (1851). anomalous case of abdominal tumour. *Ohio State Med. Soc. Trans.*, June, p55

Burns, S. (1979). Early medical photography in America (1839–1883). *N.Y.S.J. Med.*, **79**, 788-795

Burns, S. (1979). Early medical photography in America (1839–1883). (Part 2 – Physicians and early photography.) *N.Y.S. J. Med.*, **79**, 943-947

Burns, S. (1979). Early medical photography in America (1839–1883). (Part 3 – The Daguerrean era.) *N.Y.S.J. Med.*, **79**, 1256-1268

Burns, S. (1979). Early medical photography in America (1839–1883). (Part 4 – Early wet-plate era.) *N.Y.S.J. Med.*, **79**, 1931-1938

Burns, S. (1980). Early medical photography in America (1839–1883). (Part 5 – Beginnings of psychiatric photography.) *N.Y.S.J. Med.*, **80**, 270-282

Burns, S. (1980). Early medical photography in America (1839–1883). (Part 6 – Civil War medical photography.) *N.Y.S.J. Med.*, **80**, 1444-1469

Burns, S. (1981). Early medical photography in America (1839–1883). (Part 7 – American publications with photographs.) *N.Y.S.J. Med.*, **81**, 1226-1264

Carnochan, J. (1852). Amputation of the entire lower jaw with disarticulation of both condyles. *N.Y.S.J. Med.*, January, p2.

Cheselden, W. (1733). *Oestographia*. (London:)

Coe, B. (1973). *Pioneers of Science and Discovery – George Eastman and the Early Photographers*. ( :Priory Press)

Cuthbertson, A. (1978). The first published clinical photographs? *Practitioner*, **221**, 276-278

Diamond, H. (1854). *Physiognomy of Insanity*. (London: private publication)

Diamond, H. (1856). On the application of photography to the physiognomic and mental phenomena of insanity. *J. Photogr. Soc.* (Lond.)., No. 44, July 21, p88

Dimmer, W. (1899). *Ztschr. Augenh.*, **2**, 15-19

Donne, A. and Foucault, L. (1845). *Cours de microscopie complementaire des etudes medicales; Anatomie microscopie et physiologie des fluides de l'economie, au microscope-daguerreotype*. (Paris: Baillierd)

Duchenne, G.B. (1862). *Album de photographies pathologiques complementaire du livre intidule. De L 'Electrisation Localisee.* (Paris: Bailliere)

Duchenne, G.B. (1862). *Mechanisme de la physionomie humaine: ou analyse electrophysiologique de L'Expression des Passions.* (Paris: Rounouard)

Gerloff, O. (1891). *Klin. Monatsbl. Augenh.*, **29**, 397-399

Gernsheim, A. (1961). Medical photography in the nineteenth century. Part 1. *Med. Biol. Illustr.*, **11**, 85-92

Gernsheim, A. (1961). Medical photography in the nineteenth century. Part 2. *Med. Biol. Illustr.*, **11**, 147-156

Gernsheim, H. (1968). *L.J.M. Daguerre, the History of the Diorama and the Daguerrotype.* (New York: Dover Publications)

Gernsheim, H. (1969). *The History of Photography.* (London: Thames and Hudson)

Gibson, H.L. (1978). The BPA, its half century. Part 1 – The era of formation. *J. Biol. Photogr. Assoc.*, **46**, 171-191

Gibson,. H.L. (1979). The BPA, its half century, Part 2 – The era of formation (cont) *J. Biol. Photogr. Assoc.*, **47**, 82-100

Gibson, H.L. (1979. The BPA, its half century. Part 3 – The era of transition. *J. Biol. Photogr. Assoc.*, **47**, 157-192

Gibson, H.L. (1980). The BPA, its half century. Part 4 – The era of maturation. *J. Biol. Photogr. Assoc.*, **48**, 41-85

Gilbert, C. (1851). Some cases of plastic surgery. *Philadelphia Med. Exam.* April 1, p238

Gillman, S. (1979). *The Face of Madness. Hugh Welch Diamond and the Origins of Psychiatric Photography.* (Secaucus, N.J.: Citadel Press)

Graver, N. (1975). Photographie Medicale – Albert Londe's 1893 book. *J. Biol. Photogr. Assoc.*, **43**, 95–102

Hansell, P. (1959). Victorian clinical photography. *Med. Biol. Illustr.*, **9**, 70-77

Hansell, P. (1977). A backward glance. *Med. Biol. Illustr.*, **27**, 137-139

Hansell, P. (1979). A backward glance – 2. *J. Audiovis. Media Med.*, **2**, 107-111

Jackman, W. and Webster, J. (1885). Photography of the living human retina by aid of gaslight. *Photogr. News*, July 21

Julin, L. (1971). A history of still photography in the operating room. *J. Biol. Photogr. Assoc.*, **39**, 129-143

Londe, A. (1888). *La Photographie Moderne* (Paris: Masson)

Londe, A. (1893). *La Photographie Medicale.* (Paris: Gautherier-Villars et Fils)

Lyons, A. and Petrucelli, R. (1979). *Medicine – an Illustrated History.* (New York: Henry Abrams Inc)

Muybridge, E. (1887). *Animal Locomotion: an Electro-Photographic Investigation on Consecutive Phases of Animal Movements.* Univ. Pennsylvania. U.S.A.

Nitze, M. (1894). *Kystophotographischer Atlas.* (Eiesbaden: Bergman)

Ollerenshaw, R. (1961). Medical Illustration in the past. In Linssen. E. (ed.). *Medical Photography in Practice – a symposium.* (London: Fountain Press) pp1-17

Ollerenshaw, R. (1968). Medical illustration – the impact of photography on its history. *J. Biol. Photgr. Assoc.*, **36**, 3-7

Squire, A.B. (1866). *Photographs Coloured from Life of the Diseases of the Skin.* (London: Churchill)

Taft, B. (1964). *Photography and the American Scene.* (First published by Macmillan in 1938). (USA: Dover Publications)

Terry, J., *et al* (1980). Photographs tell more than meets the eye. (On the value of keeping old medical photographs.) *J. Biol. Photogr.*, **48**, 111-115

Thornton, J. and Reeves, C. (1983). *Medical Book Illustration.* (*A Short History*) (Cambridge: Oleander Press)

Williams, A.R. (1982). Victorian clinical photography. *J. Audiovis. Media Med.*, **5**, 100-103

Wilson, G. (1973). Early photography, goitre and James Inglis. *Br. Med. J.*, **2**, 104

Woodbury, W. (1890). *Encylopaedia of Photography* pp. 509-510. (London: Iliffe)

## Practical projects

(1) Make enquiries with your institution's library and/or pathology museum to see if there is a collection of old photographs. If there is, ask to photograph them, and produce either a short illustrated lecture or a small exhibition on early medical photography.

(2) Read some of the more accessible references cited, e.g. Gernsheim on *'Medical Photography in the Nineteenth Century'* and Graver on *'Photographie Medicale'*.

(3) If you have the opportunity visit one of the major centres of photographic history such as the Eastman Collection, or the museum of the Royal Photographic Society in Bath, England.

## Examination questions

Q.1 Many regard Albert Londe (1858–1917) as the father of medical photography – why is this? Write a brief description of his contribution to photography in general and medical photography in particular.

Q.2 Write short notes on the contribution of each of the following to early medical photography:

(*a*) Alfred Donné
(*b*) Hermann Wolff Berend
(*c*) Hugh Welch Diamond
(*d*) G.B. Duchenne

Q.3 Give brief descriptions of the Calotype, Daguerrotype and wet collodion processes, and their inventors.

Q.4 Write an essay on 'The earliest applications of photography to medicine'.

# Section 28
# Elementary anatomy, physiology and pathology

**Dr A.C. Branfoot**, MA, BM, FRCS, FRCPath
Senior Lecturer in Histopathology
Westminster Medical School

## 28.1 INTRODUCTION

This section of the study guide is not intended to be a comprehensive text on anatomy, physiology and pathology – it serves merely to guide the student as to what to learn (and to what depth) and to introduce the subject generally. In studying anatomy one should always consider the function or physiology at the same time this allows a better appreciation of the reasons for the anatomical appearances and relationships. This in turn makes the study more interesting, often more easy to remember, and paves the way for the study of the abnormal function and anatomical appearances one meets in the study of pathology.

The medical photographer's ability will be assessed not only on his expert knowledge of scientific photography but also on his knowledge of the subjects photographed. He is expected to be fully conversant with the normal structure and functions of the body, the more common pathological changes and the specialist nomenclature of both. He is *not* required to learn in any depth biochemistry, techniques of clinical examination and differential diagnosis, pharmacology, principles of patient management and treatment, or the histological appearance of diseases. Subjects such as anaesthetics, cardiology, community medicine, geriatrics, microbiology and obstetrics need only be touched upon. For obvious reasons the medical photographer will be expected to be fully conversant with visual medicine.

The depth of knowledge required in this area of study varies according to the level of examination, and the numerous examination questions cited at the end of the section will give a clear indication of the type of knowledge required. The student working towards IMBI Primary Certificate or BIPP Basic Medical Photography Certificate should study nursing books such as *Aids to Anatomy and Physiology for Nurses* by Armstrong or *Foundations of Anatomy and Physiology* by Ross and Wilson. The advanced student working towards the Higher Certificates will need to study more comprehensive texts such as *A Textbook of Human Anatomy* by Hamilton or *Gray's Anatomy*, *Medical Embryology* by Langman, *Histology* by Leeson and *Systemic Pathology by St Symmers. An Introduction to the Study of Disease* by Boyd is an invaluable text for first studies in pathology. The student should also have access to a good illustrated atlas such as McMinn and Hutchings, and an illustrated text on surface and radiological anatomy.

Use whatever facilities are available, e.g. anatomical and pathology museums, the library, dissecting and post-mortem room. Each patient and specimen photographed will present the student with a learning opportunity. Try to relate the study of specialist photography to specialist anatomy, e.g. Section 7 to Section 28.13, Section 8 to Section 28.12, etc.

## 28.2 ELEMENTARY HISTOLOGY

The successful photography of normal histological and histopathological material requires a much greater knowledge of histology than is given in these short notes but simple basic knowledge of this subject is essential for a proper appreciation of gross anatomy and physiological processes.

### (1) *The cell*

A basic unit of all tissues and organs. The cytoplasm is dependent upon the nucleus for control of the chemical processes (metabolism) carried on in the cell and for its reproduction. In most animals certain cells perform special kinds of work or make certain chemical substances, and

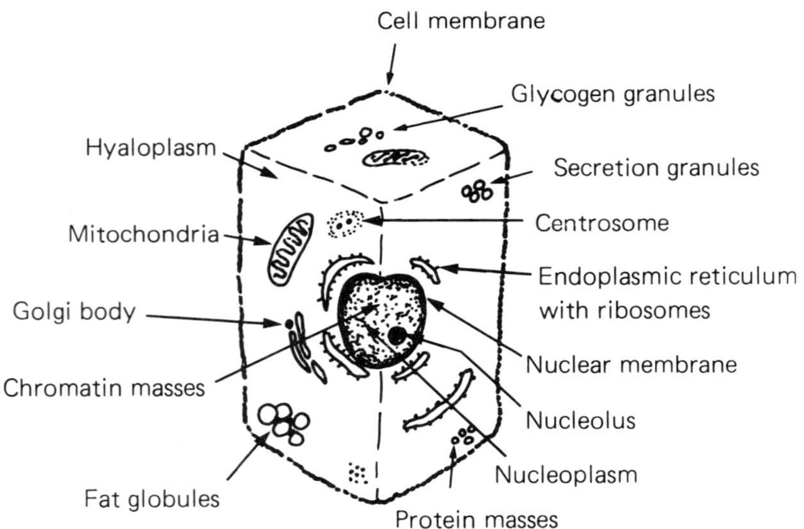


***Figure 28.1*** *A generalized cell*

these cells have, correspondingly, special shapes and compositions. They are differentiated into tissues and organs which carry on particular 'jobs' or functions. They lie in the body in some regions close-packed and in others separate from each other, and all are bathed in the extracellular fluid, from which they derive their nutrition, and which provides a relatively constant environment. The cell membrane is freely permeable to water and selectively permeable to electrolyte ions.

### (2) *Epithelium*

Lines surfaces, e.g. the skin, the interior of the urinary, alimentary and respiratory tracts. Each of these epithelial surfaces shows anatomical features related to its functions. Skin, for example, is multi-layered, the cells firmly attached to each other and the outer surface converted to tough horny material. The respiratory epithelium is a thinner, more simple, surface layer composed of columnar cells, some of which show numerous motile thread-like cilia and some secrete a slimy mucous material.

### (3) *Connective and allied tissues*

In their simplest form these bind together and support other tissues and organs. An intercellular matrix in which fibres and other materials may form, appears more important from a functional point of view than the cells themselves. Fibrous (collagenous) tissue, ligaments, tendons, cartilage and bone belong to this class. They have similar origins in the embryonic mesoderm, and the tumours which develop from these tissues show some similarities of behaviour and differences from the tumours of epithelial origin.

In the processes of repair in these tissues following injury different but allied types of tissue may be found, e.g. bone in fibrous scar tissue, cartilage in fracture callus. This is called metaplasia of tissues.

Massive accumulation of fat in the cytoplasm of some connective tissue cells is seen in adipose tissue which not only acts as a structural padding and insulating material but also is an important storehouse of fatty nutrient material which can be utilized when required.

### (4) *Blood*

Is a specialized fluid 'connective tissue'. An average man has about 6 litres of blood in his body, 60% of this volume being fluid (plasma) and the rest cells. Although there is some variation in the proportions of different blood cells according to age, sex, time of day, state of health, etc., the number of cells is fairly constant.

The red blood cells number about 5 million per cubic millimetre and contain a red pigment, haemoglobin, which is responsible for transporting oxygen efficiently from the lungs to the tissue cells which need it for metabolism. The white blood cells total about 10 000 per cubic millimetre, and are chiefly concerned with combating the effects of infection and other various injuries to the body. The plasma contains chemical substances necessary in the process of clotting or thrombosis, albumin molecules which are necessary to keep up the fluid content of the blood, and globulins which are of special interest in relation to the development of immune antibodies.

The red cells and some of the white cells, the myeloid series, are produced in the connective tissues within bones (bone marrow). Most of the remaining white cells are produced in the lymph nodes and spleen. It is these organs – bone marrow, lymph nodes and spleen, therefore, which are mainly affected in leukaemias and other diseases in which the blood cell production is disorganized.

### (5) *Muscle*

There are three varieties of muscle, striped cardiac, striped voluntary and smooth unstriped muscle which sheaths blood vessels, the alimentary canal, part of the respiratory tree, etc. Voluntary muscle develops in the mesodermal somites in connection with the other mesenchymal tissues, and is closely related with the various connective tissues in the development of the skeletal system.

Enlargement of muscle fibres and increase in bulk of muscle tissue (hypertrophy) occurs when muscles are used excessively, e.g. the heart in hypertension and in valve lesions. The opposite condition (atrophy) occurs in disuse (even with the nerve supply intact), in association with peripheral nerve damage, in old age and in cachexia in patients suffering from some malignant tumours.

The student should also study electron microscope photographs of striated muscle in relation to the physiological processes of contraction of muscle cells.

### (6) *Nervous tissue*

Nervous tissue will be considered in the section on the nervous system.

### (7) *Reproduction of cells*

The student should be completely familiar with the process of cell division (mitosis), and the appearances of cells showing mitotic activity. Great irregularities in the process and increased numbers of cells in mitosis are found in the more malignant tumours.

The importance of the chromosomes and their genetic material has been known for many years, but since 1956 techniques for the counting and photographing of chromosomes in man have been developed and this subject has become of great medical interest. The genetic sex of a patient may be determined by study of the nuclear appearances of cells; some diseases, e.g. mongolism, Turner's syndrome and Klinefelter's syndrome, are associated with abnormal numbers of chromosomes in the patient's cells, and some cases of leukaemia, particularly chronic myeloid leukaemia, have been found to have abnormal chromosomes.

## 28.3 NEOPLASMS (TUMOURS)

Having studied normal tissues and cell division, one must now make a brief acquaintance with neoplasms (tumours), particularly since much of the routine work will consist of photographing patients and specimens affected by this type of disease.

We have noted that muscle tissue may undergo hypertrophy or atrophy according to how much the muscle is utilized. This capacity for increasing the amount of tissue according to the needs of the individual is common in many organs, and such tissue hyperplasia is delicately adjusted to the requirements of the moment. The glands secreting hormones are good examples.

In neoplastic disease, however, tissues grow in an excessive manner and in a way quite unrelated to the physiological needs of the individual. The cause or causes of this are still not fully known but a vital change occurs, in one or more tissue cells, which causes them and their progeny to proliferate in an excessive manner uncoordinated with the surrounding normal cells. As the tumour cells proliferate they usually produce lumps or masses which can be felt and seen, but occasionally the tumour cells are present in small or separate clumps and such tumours are difficult to distinguish with the naked eye and may occasionally be confused with other conditions such as chronic inflammation. Neoplastic tissue may also resemble the normal surrounding tissue very closely and may, therefore, be difficult to separate clearly.

Some tumours grow very slowly and tend to remain limited in one small area, the body tissues try to 'wall them off' with fibrous tissue (a capsule), and many of these growths never spread to more distant parts of the body. They are known as benign or simple tumours.

Others – the malignant tumours – have the capacity to permeate between surrounding normal cells, and these growths often have, therefore, a very irregular and ill-defined edge. Vital structures may be destroyed by such growths and they often penetrate into the capillaries, veins and lymphatics so that tumour cells can spread to distant regions and thus cause many other tumour nodules (metastases).

Although we know only a little about the basic cell abnormality in neoplasms we know a large number of factors which help to initiate them: X-rays, ultraviolet rays, coal tar derivatives, arsenic, chromates, air pollution, etc. Since tumours at any one site, caused by any one of these factors, are apparently indistinguishable from those caused by any other factor we cannot classify tumours according to their cause. The best method is to classify them according to their tissue or organ of origin.

Thus we recognize two big groups of malignant tumours, the carcinomas arising in epithelial tissues, sarcomas which arise in connective and similar tissues and many other smaller groups arising in the various specialized tissues and cells, e.g. gliomas, synoviomas, melanomas, etc.

## 28.4 THE SKELETAL SYSTEM

### 28.4.1 The planes of reference and terms of relative position

The principal planes of reference are shown in Figure 28.2, but note also the terms rotation, proximal and distal, superficial and deep, cranial and caudal, superior and inferior, palmar and dorsal (in the hand) and plantar and dorsal (in the foot).

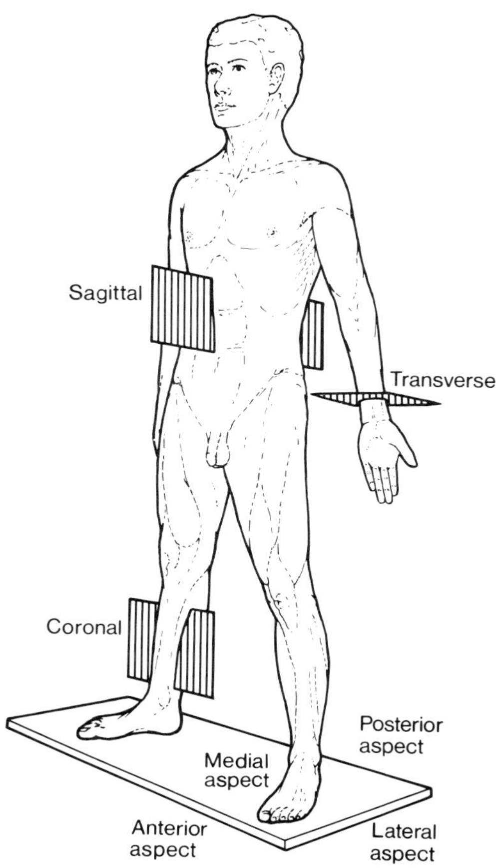


***Figure 28.2*** *The principal planes used in anatomy*

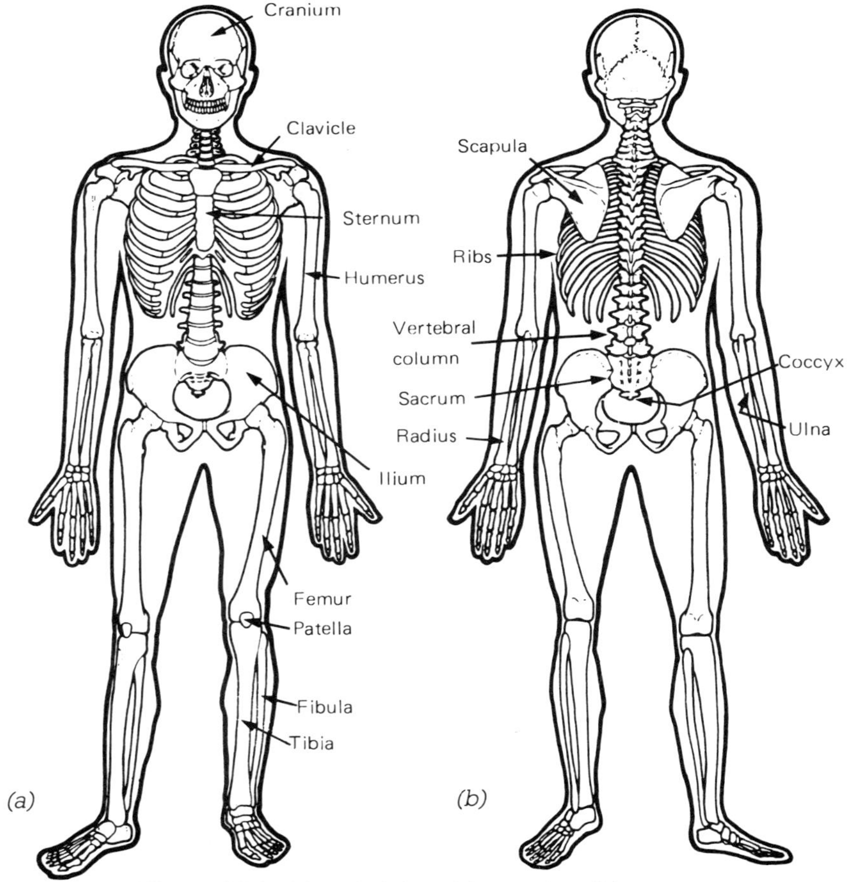

***Figure 28.3*** *The skeleton: (a) anterior, (b) posterior*

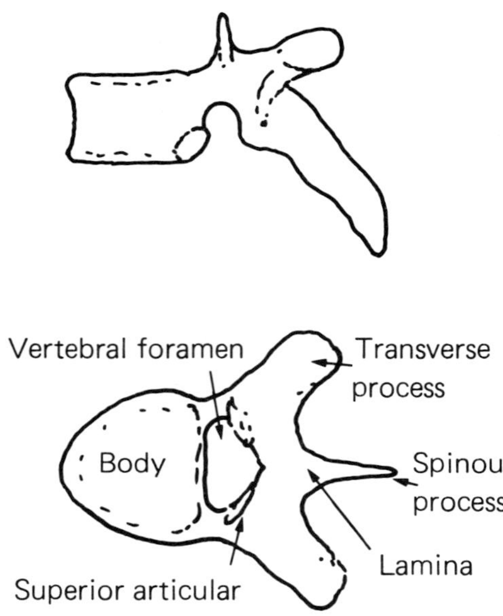


***Figure 28.4*** *A generalized thoracic vertebra. Note the long spinous process – these point downwards and overlap in the thoracic region. Two half-facets are found on each lateral surface of the body and one articular surface on each transverse process; these are used to articulate with the ribs*

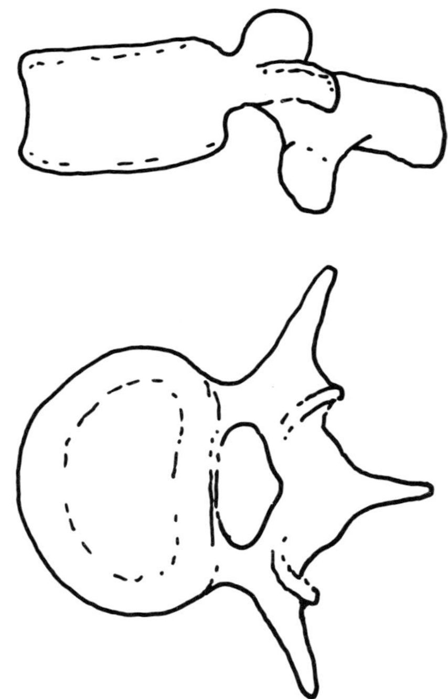

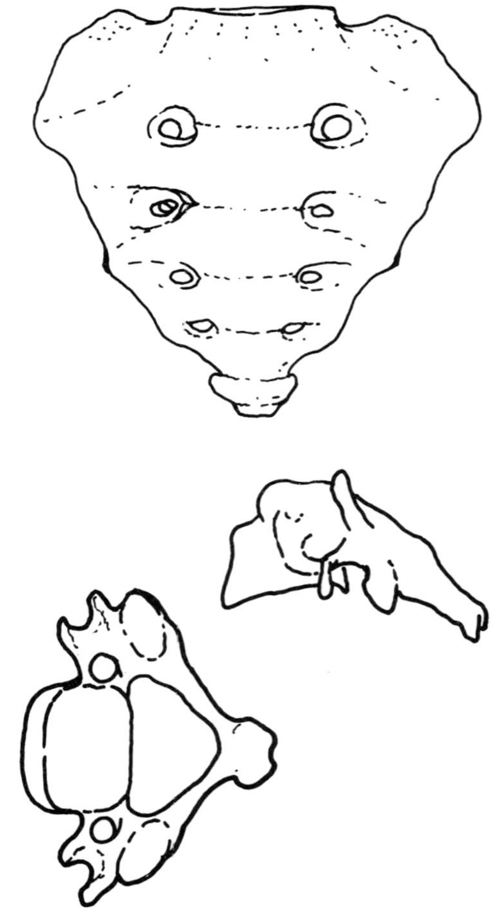

***Figure 28.5*** *(Above) The lumbar vertebra is larger with short, flat spinous processes. (Top right) the sacrum and coccyx are formed from nine rudimentary vertebrae fused together. (Right) the cervical vertebra has a forked spinous process for the attachment of muscles and ligaments and foramina through the transverse processes for arteries*

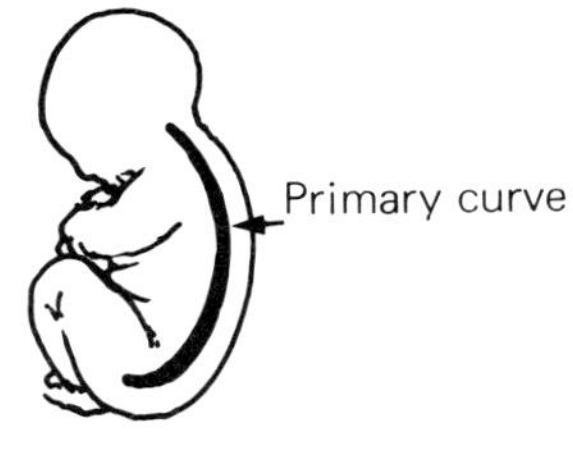


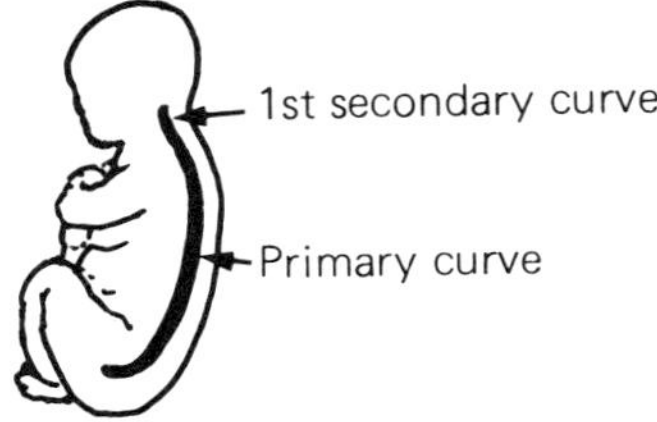


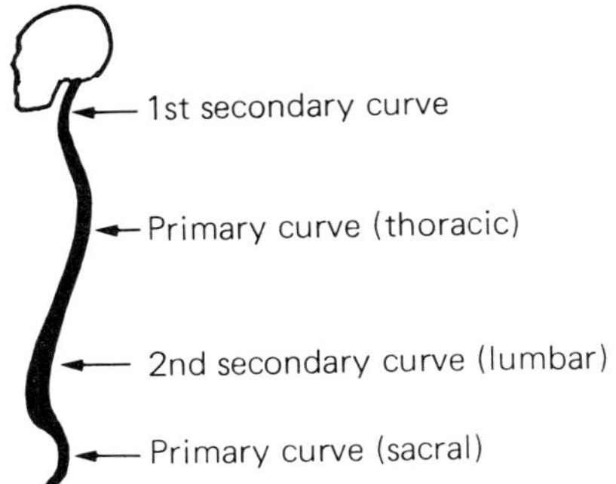


***Figure 28.6*** *The development of the spinal curves*

### 28.4.2 The Skeleton

This is composed of a number of bones which are roughly grouped into:

(1) The axial skeleton – cranium, vertebral column, ribs and sternum, and
(2) The appendages (arms and legs).

The axial skeleton is extremely well-adapted for protection of the brain, spinal cord, lungs and heart. The arms and the 'shoulder girdle' are adapted for tree climbing in our ancestors and for intricate manual operations in modern man.

The spinal cord extends in what is virtually a continuous tube in the centre of the vertebral column and ends at the level of the highest lumbar vertebra.

#### (1) *Vertebral column*

There are five regions:

| | |
|---|---|
| Cervical | 7 vertebrae |
| Thoracic (dorsal) | 12 vertebrae |
| Lumbar | 5 vertebrae |
| Sacral | 5 vertebrae (fused) |
| Coccygeal | 4 vertebrae (fused) |

*Cervical region* – The bodies are small. The first two vertebrae are highly modified, the atlas and the axis. Movements mainly flexion and extension. Rotation is mainly at the joint between axis and atlas. Note the canals for the vertebral arteries which help to supply arterial blood to the brain.

*Thoracic region* – The bodies are more sturdy. Attachments of ribs. Rotation is free but other movements are somewhat limited.

*The ribs* 1–7 join the sternum through intervening cartilages, 8, 9 and 10 are united to the cartilages of the rib above, 11 and 12 are completely free anteriorly. Note that the diaphragm arises mainly from the inner aspects of the lower six ribs.

There are some developmental variations which may occur, e.g., cervical and lumbar ribs, and which may cause symptoms in patients.

*Lumbar region* – the bodies are very bulky and give great support. Sturdy attachment of powerful muscles. Flexion and extension are free, lateral flexion is considerable, rotation fairly limited.

*Sacral region* – note the structures seen in the vertebrae of other regions, e.g. bodies, spinous processes etc., and also that the ribs and intervertebral discs are represented in the sacrum.

*Intervertebral discs* – comprise approximately one-quarter of the length of the vertebral column. Composed of an outer

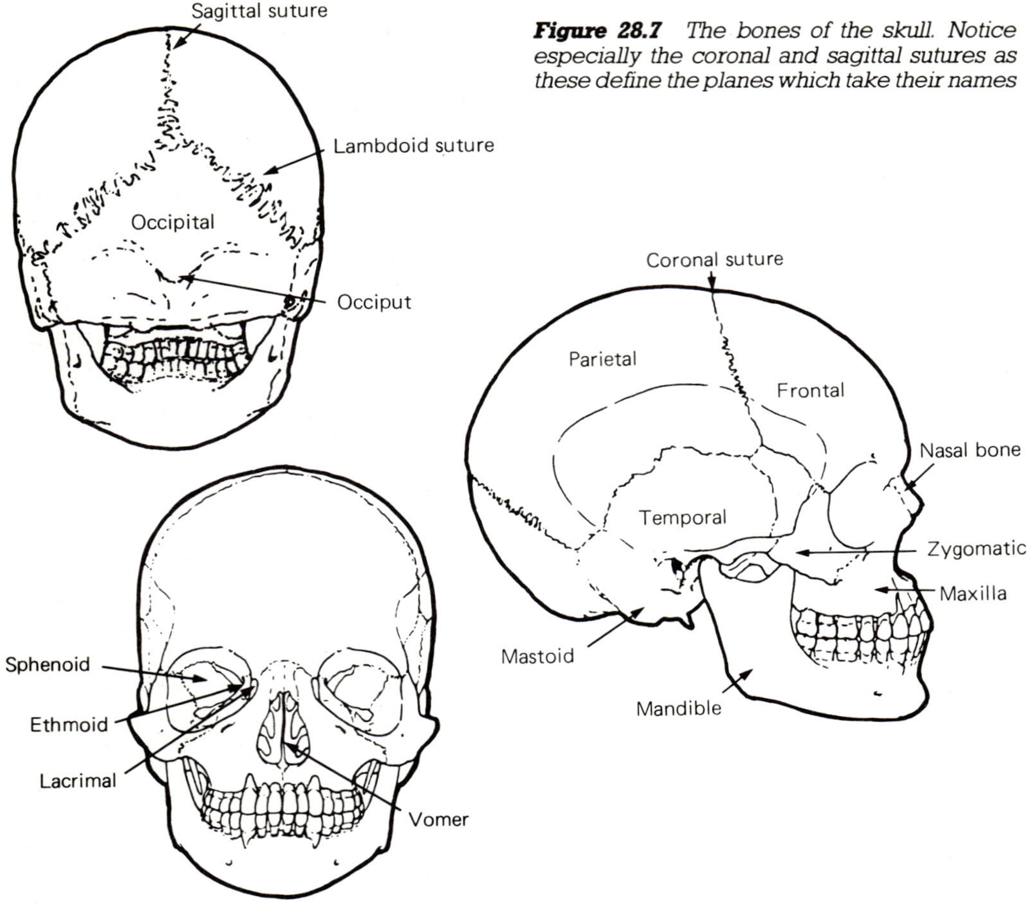


***Figure 28.7*** *The bones of the skull. Notice especially the coronal and sagittal sutures as these define the planes which take their names*

fibrous ring and an inner soft pulp. 'Prolapsed' discs are now recognized quite frequently.

*The primary and secondary curves* of the vertebral column – the primary are present during foetal life, the secondary develop when the child learns to raise the head and to walk.

## (2) *The Skull*

A segmental pattern is actually present in the skull, but it is difficult to see in the adult. The bones may be artificially divided into those which comprise mainly the facial part of the skull and those which serve as a 'brain box' (cranium). Try to get an idea of the arrangement of the individual bones, and the purpose of the various cavities present (nose, sinuses, auditory canal, etc.) and note that several nerves and arteries pass through the skull via holes and gaps which remain owing to incomplete fusion of the individual skull bones. The student must relate the various regions of the cranial cavity to the parts of the brain which occupy them, and remember that the cavity is divided incompletely by partitions (reflections of the dura) extending from the inner aspect of the cranium. Probably the most important of these is the tentorium separating the cerebral hemisphere compartment from the cerebellar compartment below. Note the pocket (sella turcica, pituitary fossa) for the pituitary gland.

### (3) *The teeth*

The shape and functions of these different types of teeth should be noted (see diagrams in Section 5).

| | *Incisor* | *Canine* | *Premolar (bicuspid)* | *Molar (multicuspid)* |
|---|---|---|---|---|
| Permanent, upper | 2 | 1 | 2 | 3 on each side |
| lower | 2 | 1 | 2 | 3 on each side |
| Deciduous, upper | 2 | 1 | | 2 on each side |
| (milk) lower | 2 | 1 | | 2 on each side |

*Approximate times of eruption*

| | | |
|---|---|---|
| Deciduous: | Lower central incisors | 6–9 months |
| | Upper incisors | 8–10 months |
| | Lower lateral incisors and first molars | 15–21 months |
| | Canines | 16–20 months |
| | Second molars | 20–24 months |
| Permanent: | First molars | 6th year |
| | Central incisors | 7th year |
| | Lateral incisors | 8th year |
| | First premolars | 9th year |
| | Second premolars | 10th year |
| | Canines | 11th–12th year |
| | Second molars | 12th–13th year |
| | Third molars | 17th–25th year |

### (4) *The upper limb*

Mobility is the 'key' word; it comprises the following parts:

*The scapula* – is a very mobile bone, anchored only by muscles to the thoracic cage and by ligaments to the clavicle, which is also mobile. The glenoid cavity in dry skeletons is very shallow but, in life, deeper owing to a fibrocartilaginous lip at the margins. Note the smooth surface for the origin of the big muscle masses and how to orientate the bone.

*The clavicle* – is strong, but fairly mobile. Flat in the lateral third. The tuberosity, for the ligament jointing it to the scapula, is on the lower surface. This bone is often fractured in spite of its strength.

*The humerus* – a body and two expanded ends. The upper end (head) articulates with the scapula (glenoid cavity). Note the two tubercles (for tendinous attachments) at the upper end. The lower part of the body becomes flatter anteroposteriorly and shows a slight forward curve. The articular surfaces for the radius and ulna are the trochlea and the capitellum.

*Note* the direction of the trochlear surface to create the 'carrying angle'. The medial projection (epicondyle) is more prominent than the lateral, and the ulnar nerve passes immediately behind it. The olecranon process of the ulna fits into a deep pit (olecranon fossa) in the humerus when the arm is fully extended.

*The radius and ulna* – study these two bones together, noting particularly the shapes of the joint surfaces, both at the upper and lower end of the bones, and between the bones themselves. The upper joints are not very mobile, but the wrist joint is extremely so. Note the very prominent tuberosity for the strong biceps muscle. The interosseous membrane gives a greater surface for the origin of muscles.

*The hand* – note the excellently adapted structures, particularly the thumb, used for gripping objects. Initially it will be easier not to learn all the names of the carpal bones – you will gradually acquire this knowledge.

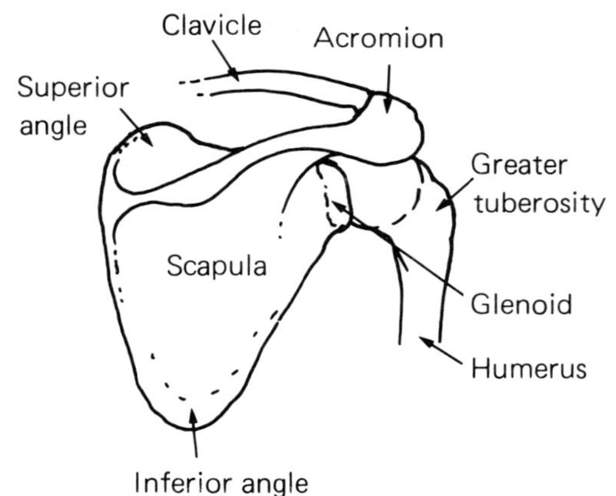


***Figure 28.8*** *(Above) The shoulder joint*

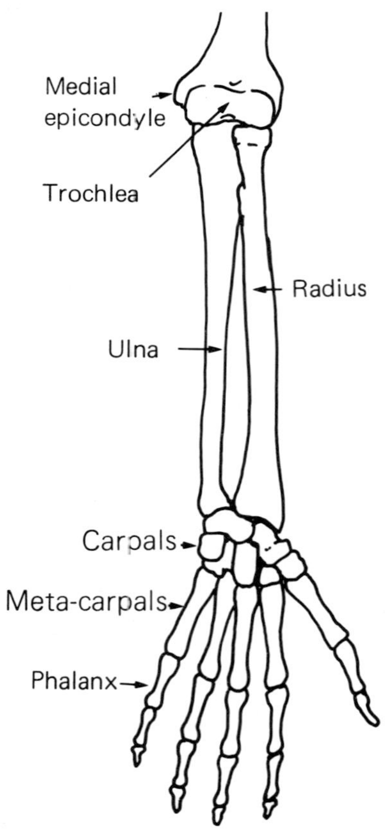


***Figure 28.9*** *(Right) The arm and hand*

### (5) *The lower limb*

Stability is the 'key' word, it comprises the following parts:

*Hip (innominate) bones* – comprising the:

ilium
ischium
and pubis

Together with the sacrum they form the bony pelvis. Note the smooth surfaces where fleshy muscle fibres originate and the strong ridges and processes where ligaments and tendinous muscular attachments occur. The acetabulum is very deep and the joint therefore stable. At the same time a fair degree of mobility is allowed. You should know approximately where the main muscle masses arise. The pubic bones are joined together by a fibro-cartilage, which allows a slight expansion of the bony pelvis. Note how the pelvis is orientated in life.

*The femur* – the longest and strongest bone, it has a cylindrical shaft. The head shows a rough impression for the ligamentum teres and is rather more than a hemisphere. The angle between shaft and neck is about 125°. The neck projects at an angle of about 15° anteriorly to the coronal plane. Note the trochanters and the condyles and the relationship of the patella.

*The tibia and fibula* – the tibia is strong, and firmly joined by ligaments to the fibula. Identify the subcutaneous surface of the tibial shaft and the sharp anterior crest. Note also the attachments of the cruciate ligaments and the semilunar cartilages. An interosseous membrane is also present between the tibia and fibula. The lower joint surface is a very deep, mortice-shaped cavity which articulates with the talus in the foot. The whole arrangement is very stable. Note the point of insertion of the patellar ligament.

*The foot* – do not worry initially about individual names, but note the interlocking of the bones, the strong ligaments and tendons and the arches formed.

## 28.4.3 The ossification of bones

This is best exemplified by the long bones which, in the early foetus, are made entirely of cartilage. Ossification begins typically at the centre of the shaft and later at the ends of the bones (the epiphyses). The newly-formed bone increases gradually, until cartilage only remains at the articular surfaces at the ends (the joint surfaces) and at the junctions between the epiphyses and the shafts. This is the state of affairs during childhood, when active growth by further bone formation occurs at the epiphysial cartilages. During adolescence the epiphysial cartilages disappear one by one, the bone of the shaft fusing with the centres of ossification at the ends of the bones and then further growth is impossible.

Here is a list of the times of fusion in some human bones:

| | | |
|---|---|---|
| Vertebrae | | 20–25 years |
| Humerus | Upper end | 20 years |
| | Lower end | 16–18 years |
| Femur | Upper end | 18 years |
| | Lower end | 20 years |
| Tibia | Lower end | 18 years |
| | Upper end | 20 years |
| Wrist bones | | At varying ages from 1 to 12 years |

Many pathological conditions occur in the region adjacent to the epiphyseal cartilage in young persons. Osteomyelitis (an infection in bone) and osteogenic sarcomas (malignant tumours of bone) are good examples. Since cartilage is avascular, however, the epiphyseal cartilage itself is usually only slowly involved by the disease and, to some extent, acts as a resistant barrier.

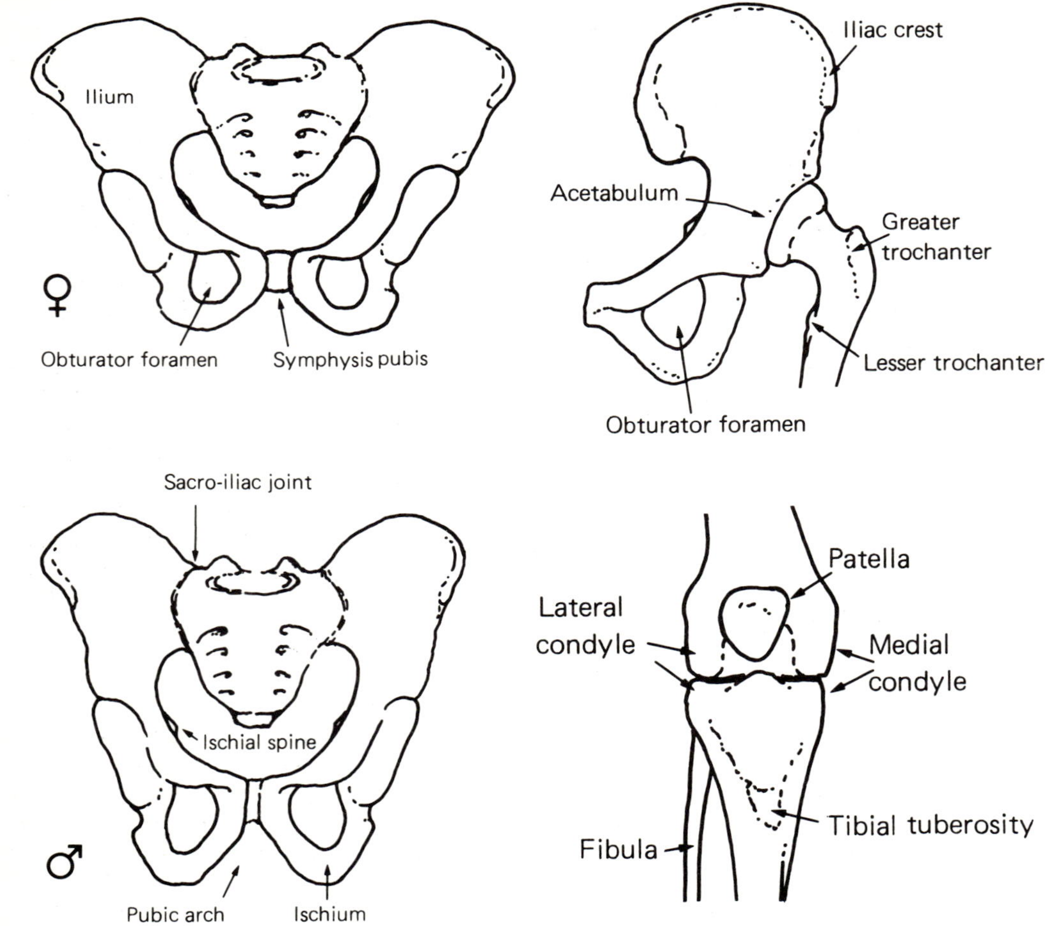

Ilium
♀
Obturator foramen
Symphysis pubis
Iliac crest
Acetabulum
Greater trochanter
Lesser trochanter
Obturator foramen
Sacro-iliac joint
Ischial spine
♂
Pubic arch
Ischium
Lateral condyle
Patella
Medial condyle
Fibula
Tibial tuberosity

Lateral malleolus
Talus
Calcaneum
Tarsals
Metatarsals
Phalanges

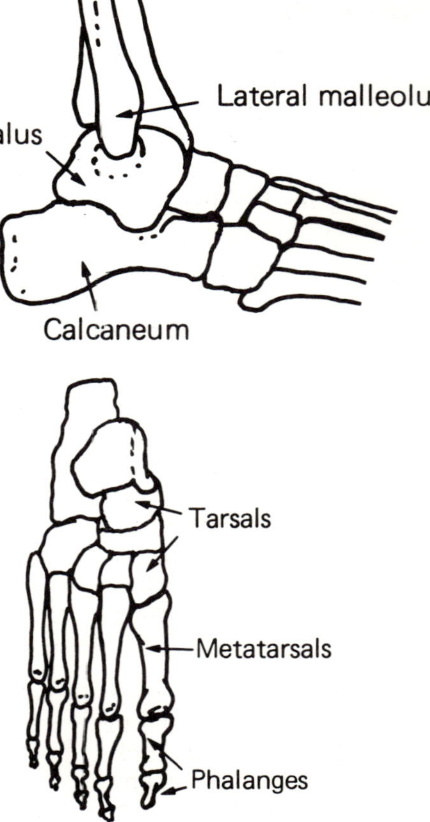

***Figure 28.10*** *The bones and joints of the lower limb. Note the differences between the male and female pelvic girdles*

### 28.4.4 The classification of joints

(1) *Fibrous joints,* e.g. inferior tibio–fibular joint, and skull sutures.
(2) *Cartilaginous joints,* e.g. bone epiphyses and symphysis pubis.
(3) *Synovial joints* are sub-classified into the following types:

   (a) *Plane joint* – gliding movement only, e.g. most carpal and tarsal joints.
   (b) *Hinge joint* – movement in one axis at right-angles to the bones, e.g. interphalangeal joints, elbow and knee joints. Very strong collateral ligaments present.
   (c) *Pivot joint* – movement in one axis parallel to the bones, e.g., the upper radio–ulnar joint and between axis and atlas.
   (d) *Ellipsoid joint* – no axial rotation but all other movements, e.g. wrist joint
   (e) *Saddle joint* – metacarpo–carpal joint of the thumb.
   (f) *Ball and socket joint* – motion around many axes, e.g., shoulder and hip joints.
   (g) *Joint with disc* – allows movement in two axes at right angles to each other, yet still preserves close contact between the joint surfaces, e.g. sterno–clavicular joint.

The student must be familiar with all the joint movements, e.g.

(1) *Gliding*
(2) *Angular* – terms used: Flexion, Abduction, Dorsi-flexion, Extension, Adduction, Plantar-flexion,
(3) *Circumduction*
(4) *Rotation* – terms used: Internal, Medial, External, Lateral,

Anatomical movements utilize the principles of levers, pulleys and other mechanical aids to greater efficiency.

### 28.4.5 Muscles

The student must learn the names of the largest muscles of the body, particularly the large muscle groups and their surface anatomy markings. A knowledge of their points of origin and insertion into the bones usually gives a hint of their physiological action.
Note the following general principles:

(1) Muscles tend to give way to narrow tendons in the region of joints, to keep the latter free for movements.
(2) Synovial sheaths cover many of the tendons to the fingers and toes.
(3) Bands or retinacula often tie down tendons to one point, and thus create a pulley action, e.g. at the ankle.
(4) Muscles are always in a continuous state of partial contraction – muscle 'tone'. In other words, nerve impulses are continually stimulating a small proportion of the fibres in a muscle. When very active contraction is required all the muscle elements are brought into action.
(5) Usually, the muscles acting on a hinge joint are arranged into two main groups, the flexors which bend the 'limb' and the extensors which oppose the action of the flexors and straighten the 'limb'. When both groups are in the state of partial contraction (*see* (4) above) the limb is held rigidly at that joint.

## 28.5 SURFACE ANATOMY

This subject is concerned with those bony points which are palpable through the skin and underlying tissues, and the way in which we can, by utilizing these 'landmarks', chart the positions of deeper organs, blood vessels, nerves etc. There are several specialized books and a chapter in Gray's text-book will give you

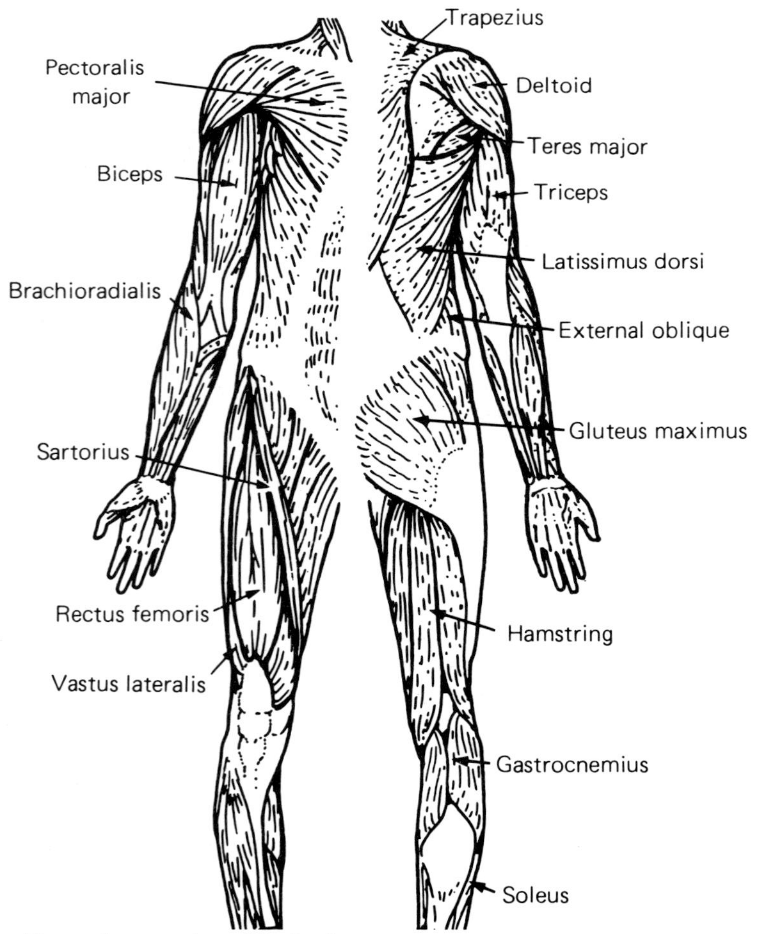


***Figure 28.11*** *The major muscles of the body*

greater detail and these must be studied carefully. The best technique is to explore one's own body for the various palpable bones, correlating these points with the content of the illustrations and making sure one can correctly label the structures indicated.

## 28.6 THE DIGESTIVE SYSTEM

The majority of the digestive apparatus is situated in the abdomen, but certain organs are situated in the mouth region.

### 28.6.1 Food

This may be divided into the following main categories:

| | |
|---|---|
| Carbohydrates<br>Proteins<br>Fats | Broken down before being used. Large molecules disintegrated chemically by enzymes before absorption. Small molecules absorbed, dissolved in water. |
| Salts<br>Water<br>Vitamins | Absorbed and taken up into the body tissues without alteration. |

The student must be aware of the composition of most common foods.

**(1) *Carbohydrates***

The chief source of energy, and essential for muscular contraction, heat and mechanical power. Starch and complex sugars are broken down to simple sugars which are readily soluble in water and are then absorbed. Some of these simple sugars are reconverted to an insoluble carbohydrate (glycogen) and stored in the liver.

**(2) *Proteins***

Proteins are mainly necessary for replacing and building up body tissues, but are usually ingested in greater amounts than strictly necessary. The excess is used for providing more energy. Proteins are very large molecules formed by linking together many amino acid molecules. For digestion these complex molecules have to be split into the constituent amino acids, which are then absorbed in solution from the intestine. Resynthesis of the necessary amino acids into body proteins then occurs.

**(3) *Fats***

Fats have a very high 'calorific' (energy and heat-forming) value. They are easily broken down into glycerol and fatty acids. The glycerol is absorbed as such, but the fatty acids combine with alkali to form soluble 'soaps' before absorption. Resynthesis into fats then occurs, and although some of this may be used immediately by the body some is stored as fat in adipose tissues. In the process of completely burning fats some of the breakdown products need to be combined with products of carbohydrate breakdown and, if the latter is impaired as in starvation and diabetes mellitus, chemical compounds known as ketones may accumulate in the blood stream and cause coma.

### 28.6.2 The digestive apparatus

It consists of several distinct anatomical parts:

**(1) The mouth**

The teeth tear up large masses of food and reduce the small portions to a pulp. Together with the tongue and other muscles they mix up this pulp intimately with the saliva – a secretion derived from the salivary glands and containing mucus and an enzyme (amylase), which starts the splitting up of starch. The salivary glands are: the parotid, submaxillary, sublingual and numerous small scattered glands in the buccal cavity. Note the sites of the glands and the orifices of their ducts. At intervals of time the soft 'bolus' of food is forced by muscular action rapidly into the oesophagus.

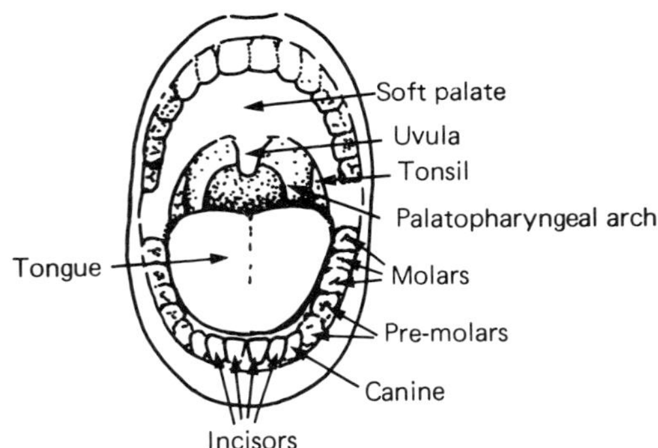


***Figure 28.12*** *The oral cavity*

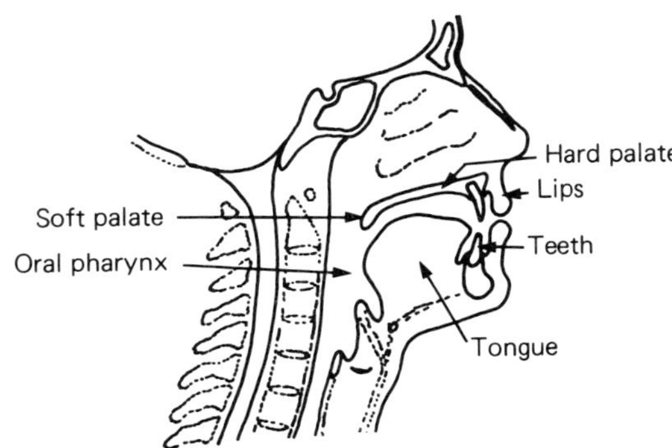


***Figure 28.13*** *The mouth and oral pharynx form the start of the digestive tract*

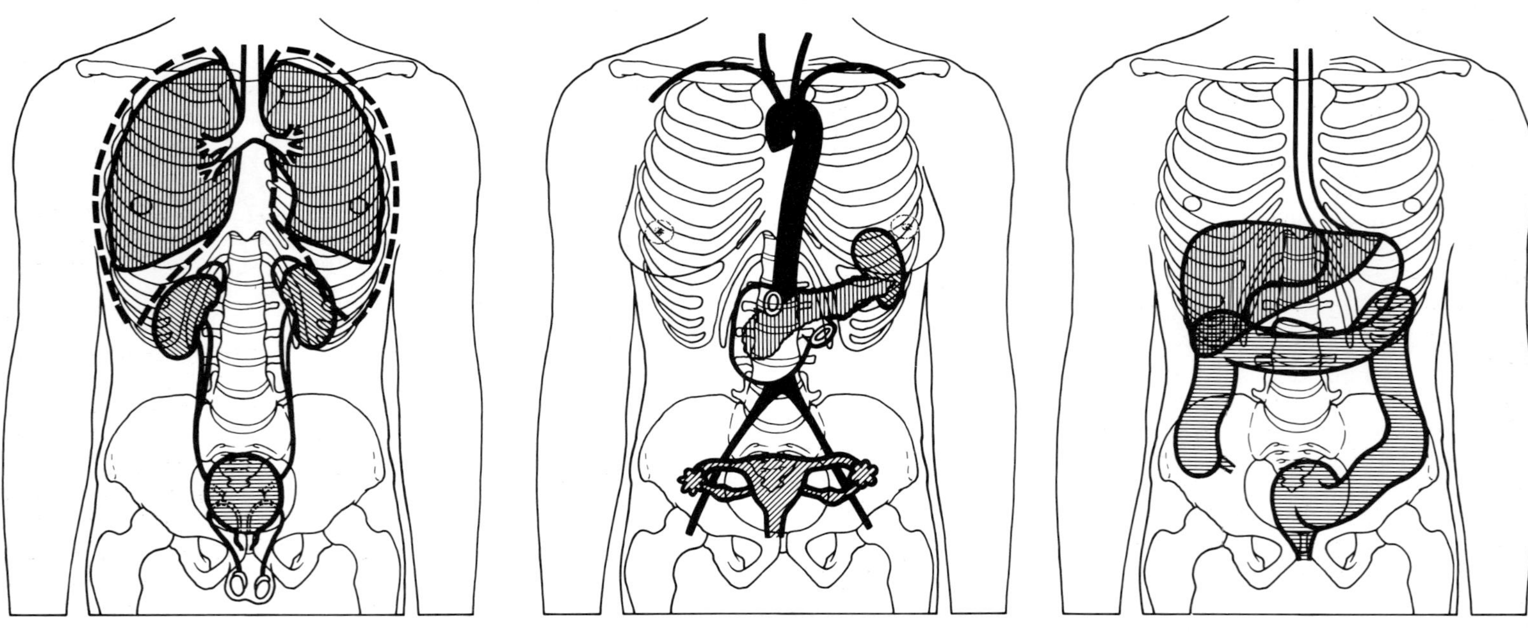

***Figure 28.14*** *The relationships between the thoracic and abdominal organs and the skeleton. It is most important that the student is able to draw these organs onto a skeletal outline*

**(2) *The oesophagus***

A muscular tube about 10 inches long, extending from the level of the 6th cervical vertebra down to the 'cardiac' sphincter at a point just to the left of the midline and at the level of the 11th thoracic vertebra.

At first it is immediately posterior to the trachea and anterior to the thoracic vertebral bodies, but below the level of the 4th thoracic vertebra it gradually inclines to the left, crossing in front of the aorta which lies in the lower part of the thorax and in the abdomen, anterior to the vertebral bodies. The food bolus passes down the oesophagus by *peristalsis*, a rhythmic muscular contraction which passes food down the whole length of the alimentary canal. There may be the opportunity of seeing peristalsis when taking photographs in the operating theatre. Glands in the oesophageal wall secrete mucus which eases the passage of food along the tube. Only residual digestion by the salivary amylase occurs in this part of the alimentary canal. There are three points of slight narrowing at 7 inches, 11 inches and 17 inches from the front teeth. They correspond to:

The sphincter at the upper end of the oesophagus,

The point at which the left bronchus crosses in front, and

The point at which the oesophagus penetrates the diaphragm.

**(3) *The stomach and intestine***

Situated in the peritoneal cavity and largely suspended by peritoneal folds (mesentery, omentum), so that they can remain mobile and undergo free peristalsis. Compare with the pleural and pericardial sacs. Always try to relate the position of abdominal organs to the surface anatomy. The trans-pyloric plane of Addison at the level of the 1st lumbar vertebra is most useful.

(1) *The stomach* – a sac-like dilatation of the alimentary canal where food can be intimately mixed and churned up with the gastric secretion. The cardiac sphincter (valve) at the upper end and the pyloric sphincter at the lower end are fairly fixed anatomical positions, but the shape and position of the rest of the stomach varies enormously with posture, time after food, etc. The mucous membrane contains the secretory glands and produces some 2–3 litres of gastric juice every 24 hours. It contains:

(a) Pepsin, an enzyme which, in acid solution, begins to split up proteins into smaller medium sized molecules (peptones).
(b) Hydrochloric acid to produce the desired acidity and to counteract the saliva, which is alkaline, and
(c) Mucus.

There is also a lipase of no great importance. Peristaltic waves of contraction pass the food through the pylorus into the small intestine.

(2) *Small intestine* – approximately 20 feet long. The first part (duodenum) begins at the pylorus and is closely related to the head of the pancreas. The following parts, the jejunum and the ileum, are attached to the posterior abdominal wall by a mesentery, and otherwise lie free as a coiled tube. The mucous membrane contains glands which secrete enzymes with the following functions:

(a) Medium size protein molecules are split up into small soluble molecules, the amino acids,
(b) Transformation of the pancreatic enzyme trypsinogen (*see* below),
(c) Small amounts of carbohydrates

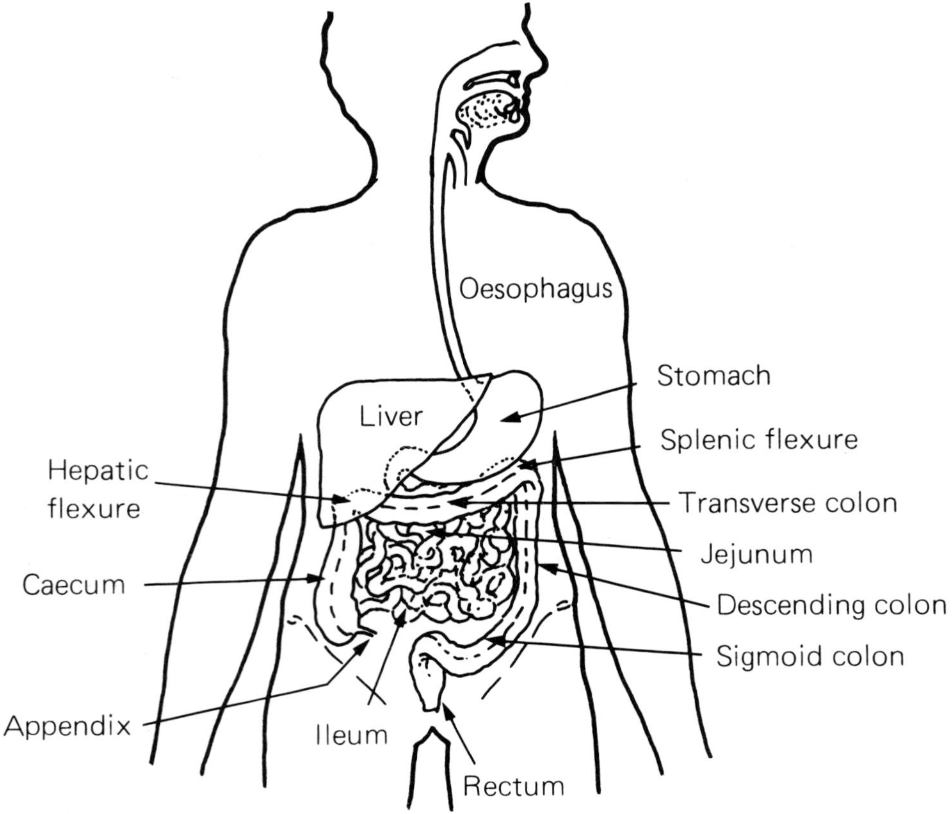

Oesophagus
Stomach
Liver
Splenic flexure
Hepatic flexure
Transverse colon
Jejunum
Caecum
Descending colon
Sigmoid colon
Appendix
Ileum
Rectum

***Figure 28.15*** *The major components of the digestive tract*

Cardiac sphincter
Fundus
Greater curvature
Lesser curvature
Body
Duodenum
Pyloric antrum
Pyloric sphincter

***Figure 28.16*** *The stomach*

R. lobe
L. lobe
Falciform ligament
Gall bladder

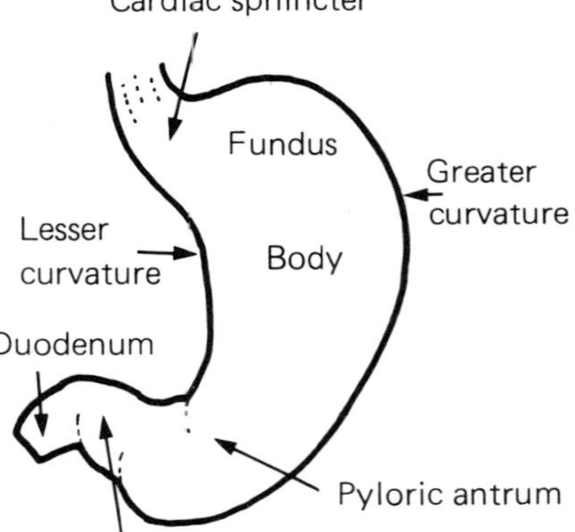

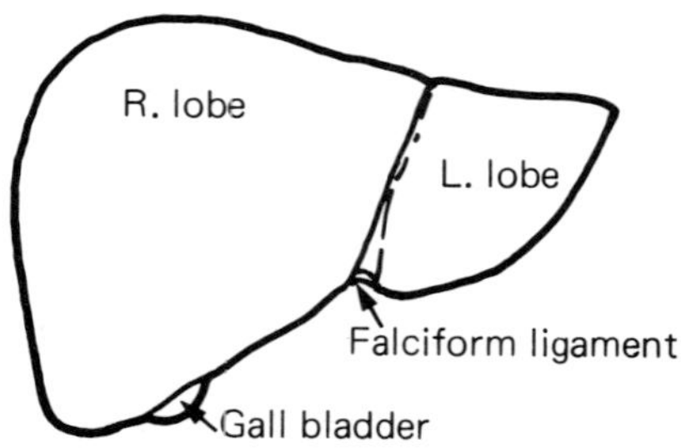

***Figure 28.17*** *The liver*

are broken down into simple sugars.

The duodenum also receives a far more important enzyme secretion from the pancreas and also bile from the liver.

The alkaline pancreatic juice contains:

(a) Trypsinogen, a precursor of the enzyme trypsin, which has the same property as pepsin in splitting proteins into smaller molecules which are in turn further broken down by dipeptidases.
(b) Lipase, an enzyme for splitting fats, and
(c) Carbohydrate – splitting enzymes.

In the small intestine the contents are thoroughly mixed by muscular contraction and gradually passed onwards by peristalsis. The surface of the mucosa lining this part of the bowel shows coarse folds, which are easily seen with the naked eye, and also an enormous number of small projections (villi) which are best seen under a dissecting microscope. Moreover, the electron microscope has revealed that similar but minute folds are present along the borders of the columnar mucosal cells, thus further increasing the absorptive area available in the intestine many times.

(3) *Large Intestine (caecum, colon and rectum)* – the large gut secretes mucus and no digestive enzymes, so that only some residual digestion by the small intestinal and pancreatic enzymes occurs. Absorption of small food molecules occurs, but it is mainly water which is progressively absorbed as the contents pass along the colon to the rectum and anal canal. The faeces – the contents of the rectum and anal canal – are voided at intervals by mass contraction of their muscular walls.

The colon is arbitrarily divided into ascending, transverse, descending and pelvic (sigmoid) sections. Note that the large gut can be recognized by prominent, longitudinal muscle-bands, the taenia coli. These latter help the surgeon (and also the photographer) to differentiate immediately coils of large intestine from the small.

**(4) The liver (weight, 1500g)**

This organ, one of the most vital in the body, is situated in the upper right quadrant of the abdomen below the diaphragm. It has a double vascular supply – arterial blood being brought via the hepatic artery almost directly from the abdominal aorta and venous blood via the portal vein from the intestines and stomach.

The organ is formed of large numbers of closely-packed and ill-defined 'lobules'. Although many cells in the body will immediately utilize some of the simple breakdown products of carbohydrates and proteins absorbed from the gut, some of these materials are stored in the liver as glycogen and fat. Proteins are not stored, as such, in tissues. A good deal of synthesis of proteins, from amino acids, occurs however in the liver, particularly serum proteins.

**(5) The biliary apparatus**

Bile is formed continuously in the cells of the liver at a rate of 500–1000 ml every 24 hours. It is secreted into fine canaliculi running between the columns of liver cells and thence passes into two large hepatic ducts issuing from the lobes of the liver. These ducts join to form one duct which leads to the duodenum and which has an offshoot – the cystic duct and gall bladder – in which bile can be stored. Contraction of gall bladder, with expulsion of bile into the duodenum, which occurs after a fatty meal, can be shown by X-ray techniques (cholecystogram).

Bile contains bile salts, secreted by the liver, which lower the surface tension of fats so that the droplets are divided up into numerous minute globules which afford a better opportunity for the lipases to split them. The bile salts also combine with substances like cholesterol and the fat-soluble vitamins to form water-soluble and therefore absorbable compounds. Note the bile salt cycle whereby 90% of these substances is reabsorbed back into the blood stream and returned to the liver.

### 28.6.3 Some abnormalities and diseases of the alimentary canal

The alimentary canal is a prolific source of clinical and pathological lesions which may need photography. Tumours are without doubt the most common, and are most often seen in the stomach and large intestine, but neoplasms of the oesophagus, pancreas, bile ducts, liver, tongue and buccal cavity are not uncommon.

Other abnormalities and diseases which may be mentioned are:

#### (1) *Peptic ulcers*

These occur almost exclusively in the stomach and duodenum, but occasionally affect the oesophagus or a congenital Meckel's diverticulum in the ileum. The aetiology of these is not fully known, but often excessive secretion of hydrochloric acid plays a large part. Ulcers may be (a) acute, shallow and in these cases often multiple, or (b) chronic and deep, often penetrating through the whole wall of the organ.

#### (2) *Diverticula*

These are localized pouches, or hernias, which seem to 'blow out' from certain sites in the alimentary canal. They are found in the oesophagus, duodenum, small intestine and colon. The causes are several but not all are fully understood.

#### (3) *Congenital megacolon (Hirschprung's disease)*

This is a disorder of the nerve plexus in the 'recto–sigmoid' region of the large intestine. It results in a failure of the normal muscular contractions of the gut, which becomes obstructed and dilated above the site of the lesion.

#### (4) *Portal vein obstruction*

The two main causes are:

Cirrhosis (fibrosis) of the liver.

Thrombosis (clotting) of the portal vein, or obstruction from some other cause.

You should note the results of such venous obstructions as splenomegaly, oesophageal and stomach varices, rectal piles and the opening-up of other collateral vascular channels like the 'caput medusae' seen round the umbilicus.

#### (5) *Cholecystitis and cholelithiasis*

In some individuals the capacity to produce a concentrated bile in the gall bladder without the precipitation of some of its components seems to be impaired. Cholesterol, normally insoluble in water and only held in solution in bile by a complicated process of micelle formation, is the most common constituent of gall stones but bile pigments and calcium salts are usually also present (mixed stones). It is possible to develop stones in the gall bladder and bile ducts without previous infections (pure metabolic stones), but it appears probable that attacks of bacterial inflammation in the gall bladder can predispose to the formation of stones which in turn by their presence can lead to further attacks of infection and inflammation.

#### (6) *Congenital pyloric stenosis*

This is a condition occurring in newborn infants, usually male. It is characterized by spasm and great hypertrophy of the circular muscle fibres of the pyloric sphincter. Obstruction to the passage of stomach contents into the duodenum gives the symptoms of 'projectile vomiting' which usually come on shortly after the first week of life.

## 28.7 CARDIOVASCULAR SYSTEM

The human being has a closed circuit vascular supply, the blood circulating except in the case of the spleen entirely within 'pipes' – the blood vessels – and being pumped by the regularly contracting muscular pump – the heart. This is in contrast with some animals, in which the blood is poured out of the blood vessels, bathing the tissues which are able to take up substances required for metabolism directly from the blood. In man the plasma seeps through the finest blood vessels, and the tissues have been compared with a sponge soaked with this exuded *extracellular fluid*. Only a proportion on this fluid gets directly back into the blood vessels and another system – *the lymphatic system* – is necessary to drain off the excess fluid.

### 28.7.1 The heart (weight 270-360g.)

This organ lies in the pericardial sac in the mediastinum of the thorax. The cardiac muscle has an inherent capacity for rhythmical contraction. For instance,

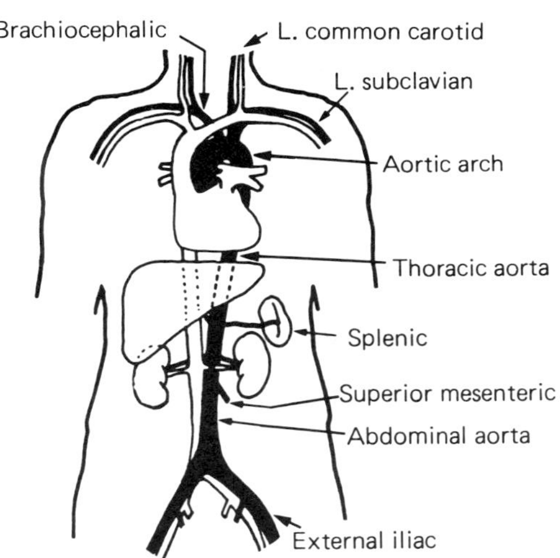


***Figure 28.18*** *The major abdominal arteries*

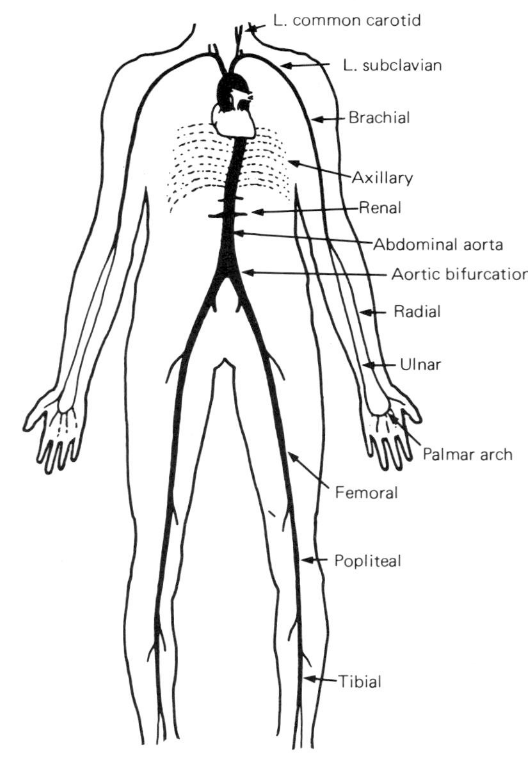


***Figure 28.19*** *The major arterial vessels*

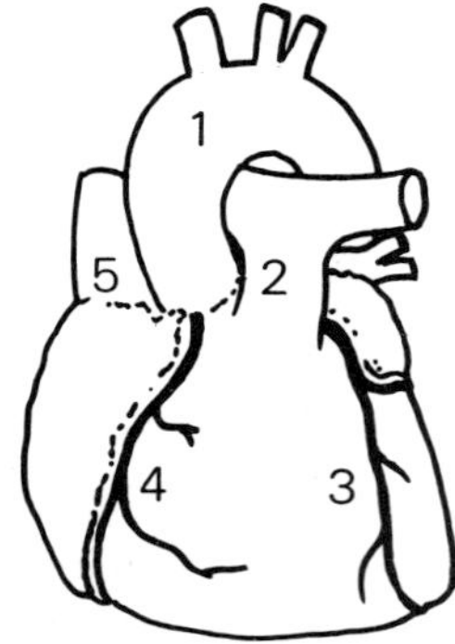


1 Aorta
2 Pulmonary artery
3 L. coronary artery
4 R. coronary artery
5 Superior vena cava

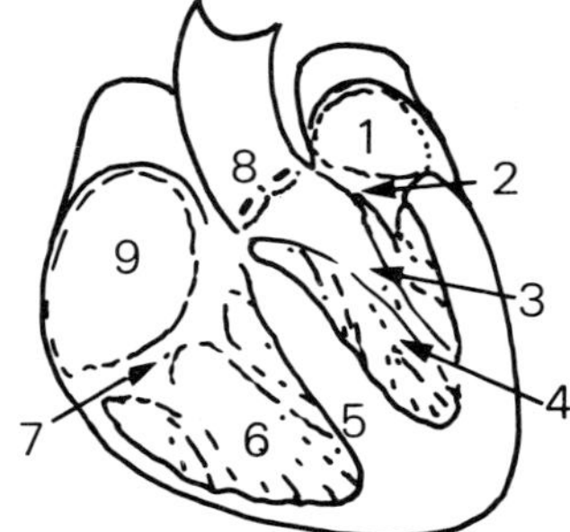


1 L. atrium
2 Mitral valve
3 L.ventricle
4 Papillary muscle with chordae tendinae
5 Septum
6 R. ventricle
7 Tricuspid valve
8 Semilunar valve
9 R.atrium

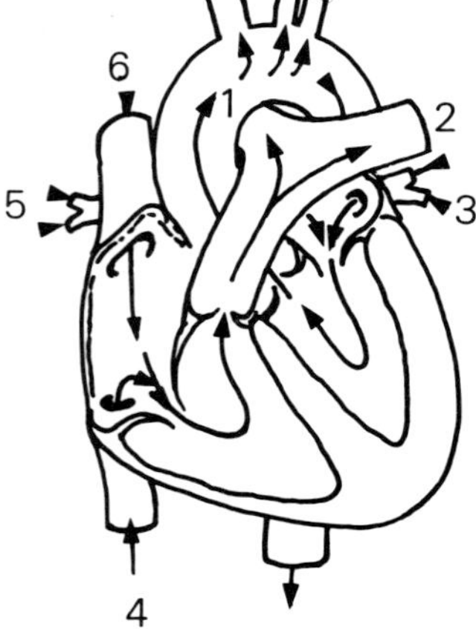


1 Aorta
2 Pulmonary artery
3 Pulmonary veins
4 Inferior vena cava
5 Pulmonary veins
6 Superior vena cava

***Figure 28.20*** *The heart*

myocardial fibre cells cultured from rats' hearts show periodic rhythmic contractions. Some of the fibres have been modified into a conducting type of fibre and into the sino–auricular and atrio–ventricular nodes, which it is believed are largely responsible for the control and conduction of the stimulus which produces a co-ordinated cardiac contraction. The extent of the influence of the nerve plexuses present in the heart is still debated and undetermined. First the auricles (atria) contract, blood passing into the ventricles, and a fraction of a second later the ventricles contract, forcing blood into the arterial 'tree'. The heart is a double pump, the one organ acting for the two circulations, systemic and pulmonary, and normally there is no direct communication between the right side of the heart and the left.

*Note* the position and functions of the cardiac valves.

*Note* that the heart has its own blood supply through the coronary arteries which arise from the aorta just above the aortic valve.

### 28.7.2 The arteries

These are muscular and elastic tubes which gradually decrease in bore as their distance from the heart increases. The aorta is almost entirely composed of elastic tissue to withstand the widely fluctuating pressure. The proportion of muscle fibre increases progressively as the vessels become smaller, so that the small arteries are able to open up or close down the blood supply to different regions of the body as necessary. This function is under the control of the autonomic nervous system.

The photographer must know the names of the *main* arteries and it is useful to know at which points arterial haemorrhage may be controlled.

### 28.7.3 The veins

Their names are important to remember but are often similar to the arteries which they tend to accompany. The special blood supply from the gut to the liver *(portal venous system)* should be studied particularly in regard to portal obstruction and the development of anastomotic channels. *Note* the function of the venous valves in the lower limbs, and the effects of incompetency.

### 28.7.4 Capillaries

The extensive network of these thin-walled structures allows plasma to pass out and come into intimate contact with the tissue cells. Gas exchange between the tissues and the blood can easily occur by diffusion through their walls. *Note* the response in inflammation where the vascular dilatation and increased permeability play a great part in the defence processes and, in repair of tissues, the proliferation of new capillaries is of great importance.

The student should understand the manner in which plasma passes from capillaries by hydrostatic pressure into the tissue spaces, and how much of this fluid is drawn back into the venous circulation by osmotic pressure exerted largely by the serum albumins. Some of the fluid, including cells and particulate matter such as cell debris, bacteria and other organisms, is taken up into the lymphatics.

### 28.7.5 The lymphatic system

This is a network of thin-walled vessels similar to the capillaries and small veins. They tend to follow closely the course of the veins, and, like them, possess valves. The *lymph nodes* (filters) are situated at intervals along the lymphatic chains in well recognized anatomical groups. *Note* the importance of the lymphatics in infections and in the spread of tumours.

### 28.7.6 Cardiovascular abnormalities

Pathological lesions in these organs are legion, but by far the most important, in this ageing population, is *atheromatous* degenerative change which affects predominantly larger and medium sized arteries. You must familiarize yourself with the appearances of the intimal fatty plaques and with their complications – ulceration, thrombosis, stenosis and aneurysm formation. Stenosis and thrombosis cause lack of blood supply *(ischaemia)* and may cause *infarction*. The brain and the myocardium are often so affected. This type of disease is frequently associated with high blood pressure *(hypertension)* which causes the left ventricle to hypertrophy and which may eventually cause myocardial failure.

In the past, lesions due to rheumatic fever, bacterial endocarditis and syphilis were all more common but, with the introduction of antibiotics, have become less frequent.

Look up the various congenital anomalies which may occur in the heart septa, in the valves and the great vessels. One should be able to orientate the heart even if it has been opened and sliced in an unusual manner.

## 28.8 THE RESPIRATORY SYSTEM

Concerned, together with the cardiovascular system, in transporting oxygen to the tissue cells and in removing carbon dioxide from them. The respiratory system comprises:
nose, pharynx, larynx, trachea, bronchi and lungs.
Note the functions of the nose, pharynx, larynx, tonsils and adenoids, including the site of the olfactory nerve endings in the upper part of the nose and the functions of the vocal cords in the larynx.

### 28.8.1 The trachea

This extends from the larynx (level of the 6th cervical vertebra) into the thorax (at the level of the 4th thoracic vertebra), where it divides into right and left main bronchi. Rigidity is given by cartilaginous rings which are deficient posteriorly where the tube is completed by smooth muscle. It is in close relationship throughout its length with the oesophagus behind. *Note* that the distance from the front teeth to the larynx is 15 cm, (6 in) and to the bifurction of the trachea is 27 cm, (11 in).

### 28.8.2 The bronchial tree

The bronchi break up into numerous subdivisions which ultimately supply small ill-defined closely-packed lobules of lung tissue. Cartilaginous plates – less complete than the tracheal rings – and muscle are present in the larger branches, but become progressively less prominent and ultimately absent towards the periphery. Virtually the whole respiratory tract, down to and including the bronchioles, is lined by ciliated columnar epithelium. Some of the columnar cells are modified to mucus-secreting *goblet cells*, and mucous glands in the submucous tissue are also plentiful.

### 28.8.3 Serous sacs in the thorax

The heart and the lungs lie in cavities: the pericardial and pleural sacs. These serous sacs are lined by a smooth shiny membrane which secretes a little fluid. The lubricated surfaces, therefore, glide easily one upon the other, and normally there is only a potential space between them.

Occasionally an inflammatory reaction or some other disease will cause a great increase in the fluid content *(pleurisy with effusion)* or the inflamed serous surfaces may stick and rub together, giving rise to an intense pain (*pleuritic pain*).

### 28.8.4 Lungs (weights: right 500–650g; left, 450–600g)

When the thoracic cage expands owing to the action of the diaphragm, of the intercostal muscles and occasionally of some additional accessory muscles, the lungs themselves are also caused to expand and air is sucked into the respiratory tract and the alveolar spaces. The elastic recoil of the lungs, gravity forces and occasionally some muscle action cause expiration with expulsion of this air from the air passages and lungs.

The pulmonary arteries subdivide side by side with the bronchi and, ultimately, the smallest branches of the respiratory tree (the alveoli) are still closely supplied by blood vessels in the form of a capillary network. The alveoli and atria comprise most of the space in the lungs, and gases can rapidly diffuse from the blood in the capillaries across the thin alveolar walls into the air spaces. These alveolar sacs are about 120 microns in diameter, and it has been estimated that there are 400 million in each lung, giving approximately 121 $m^2$ (1300) of respiratory surface.

Although the *vital capacity* may be about 3500 cc normal respiration may only change about 500 cc of air in the lungs. The *reserve* is, therefore, very great. Oxygenated blood, relatively free from carbon dioxide, is taken back in the pulmonary veins to the left side of the heart and hence to the body tissues. The rate and depth of respiration are controlled by several mechanisms.

A respiratory 'centre', situated in the brain stem, initiates the rhythmic respirations, but this is influenced by the higher centres of the brain, the carbon dioxide content of the blood, and by various nervous stimuli from the lungs and the thoracic cage.

Now consider a number of pathological lesions, which may be encountered during practical work and which will now become more clearly understood. The bronchi and bronchioles can become obstructed by oedematous swelling of their lining mucosa and by a thick mucous secretion in their lumina. These conditions occur in *bronchial asthma* and the patient has great difficulty in forcing air out of the lungs during expiration. Similar airway obstruction can occur as a result of *chronic bronchitis*, a common ailment in Britain and, if obstruction persists for a long period of time, alveolar sacs over-distend and their walls may

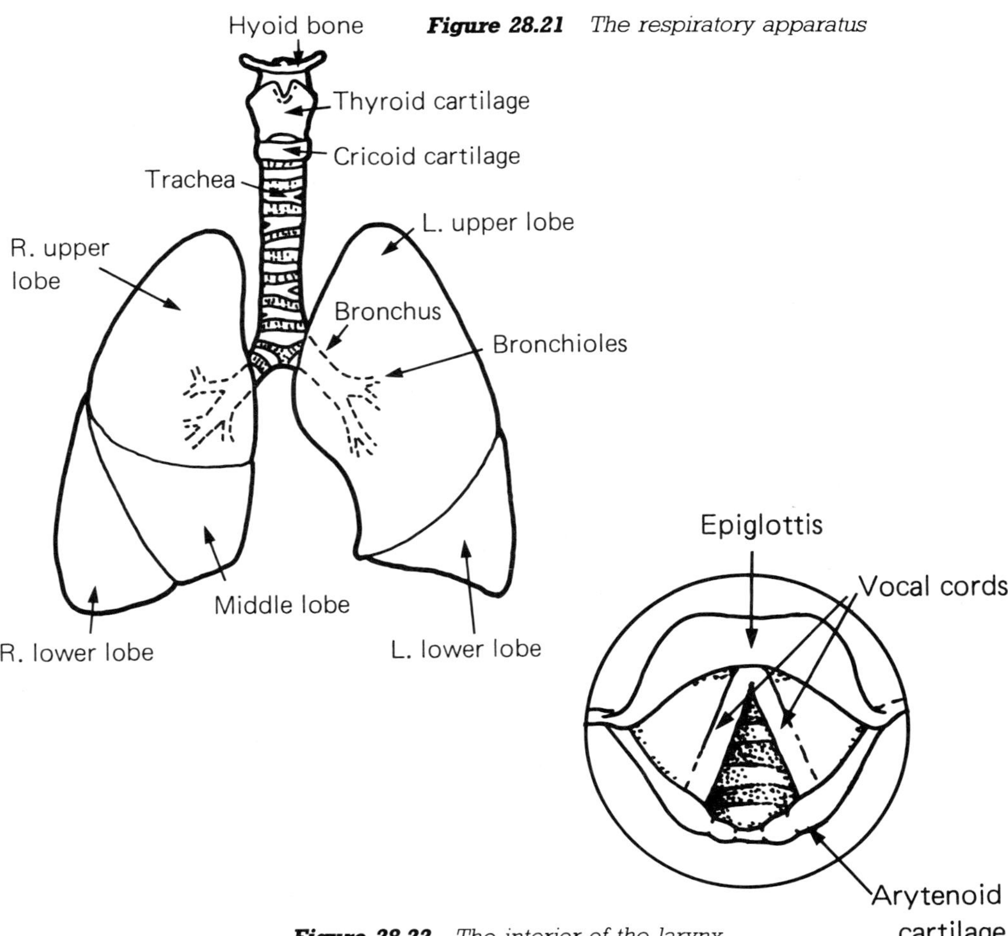


**Figure 28.21** *The respiratory apparatus*

**Figure 28.22** *The interior of the larynx*

rupture with the result that much larger diameter and therefore less efficient air-containing cavities are formed. This condition is known as *emphysema* and quite often the cavities dilate up to *bullae* measuring several centimetres in diameter.

*Bronchiectasis* is an abnormal and permanent dilatation of the bronchi. They usually retain their tubular appearance but occasionally may blow up into saccular or rounded cavities. The lower lobes are most commonly involved and infection in stagnant secretions in these bronchi is usually difficult to cure.

In *pneumonia* an inflammatory fluid *exudate* accumulates in the alveoli, displacing the normal air content and causing the lung tissue to be firm and more rigid than normal. The patient as one might expect is *toxic* (or poisoned by the infection), may be *cyanosed* due to lack of oxygenation of the blood and is short of breath *(dyspnoeic)*.

*Tuberculosis* causes a special type of pneumonic consolidation in which the lung tissue in the centre of the lesions dies and becomes converted into a cheesy (*caseous*) material.

*Neoplastic disease* frequently affects the respiratory tract. The nose, pharynx, tonsils, larynx and bronchi are the most common sites, particularly the bronchi; *bronchial carcinoma* being one of the major causes of death among males in many countries. In this disease the tumour most often grows initially in one of the largest (primary) branches of the bronchial tree, and often spreads to involve the adjacent lymph nodes around the hilum of the lung and the mediastinum. Rather less frequently it may arise in the periphery of the lung in one of the smaller bronchial branches.

## 28.9 THE URINARY SYSTEM

It has already been shown that, in the course of metabolism, numerous waste materials are produced by the body and the majority of these are excreted by the kidneys. The urinary system, therefore, comprises: (1) two complicated filter organs – the kidneys – which retain as much as possible of the essential chemical substances in the blood stream and allow waste substances to pass through, and (2) the duct system – the distal parts of the renal collecting tubules, calyces, pelves, ureters, bladder and urethra – which convey the waste materials out of the body as urine.

### 28.9.1 The kidneys weight about 150g, in the average adult male.)

Note their general and surface anatomy, their blood supply and any features which help to orientate them for photography. The kidney is covered by a fibrous tissue capsule and the cut surface reveals the *cortex, medulla* (pyramids), *calyces* and *pelvis*. Relate each of these anatomical areas to their histological components, and with the aid of the textbooks draw detailed diagrams. The histological structural unit is known as a *nephron* supplied with blood by an afferent arteriole which splits up into numerous capillaries in the filter units known as *glomeruli*. There are about 1.25 million nephrons in the normal kidney each consisting of a filter unit and a complicated twisted tubule which drains the filtrate into the collecting ducts. The tubules also engage in an elaborate active metabolic process by which many chemical ions are secreted from the peri-tubular blood vessels into the urine, and similar ions are also actively reabsorbed back from the urine into the blood stream. This is the basis of an important *homeostatic* mechanism designed to keep the internal environment of the body cells as constant as possible.

*Note* the course of the ureters from the kidney pelves down to the orifices in the bladder. These latter, together with the

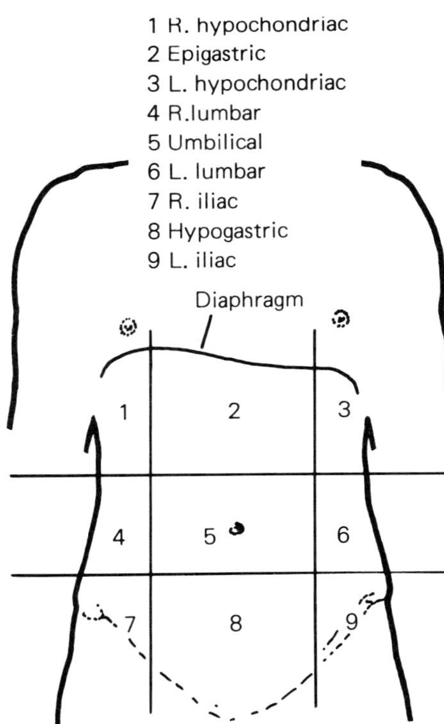


**Figure 28.23** *The regions of the abdomen*

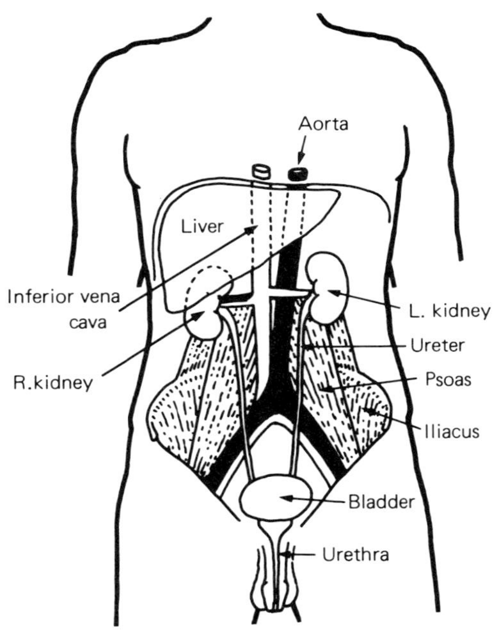


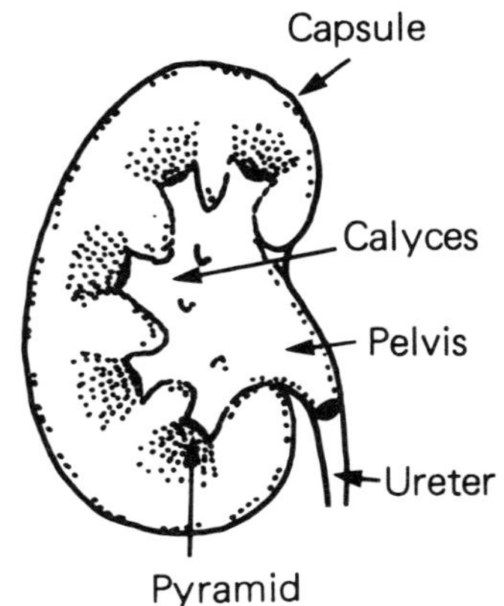


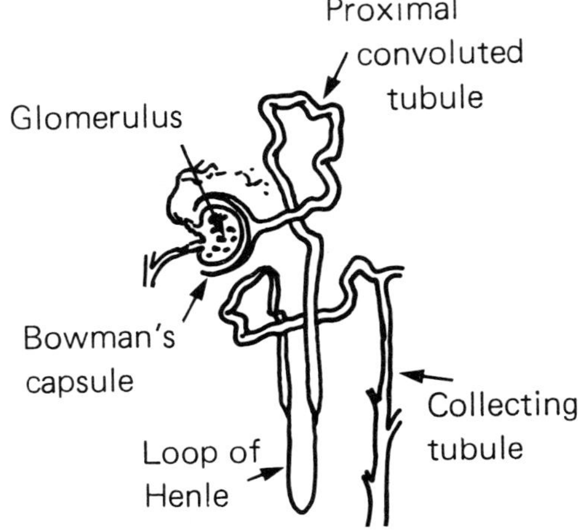


**Figure 28.24** *(Above) The relationship between the urinary organs and the rest of the abdomen. (Top right) The macroscopic appearance of the kidney. (Right) the microscopic structure of a nephron*

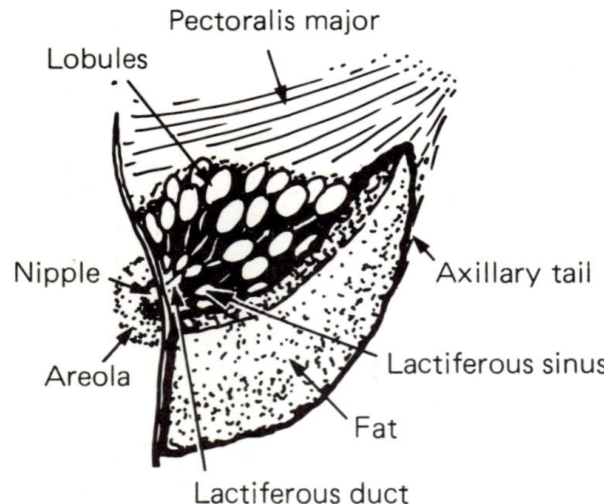


***Figure 28.25*** *The female breast*

internal urethral orifice, form the corners of a smooth, triangular area at the base of the bladder – the *trigone*.

### 28.9.2 Development and anatomical abnormalities of the system

The kidney develops in the embryo from two separate elements, the primitive kidney forms on the posterior wall of the abdominal cavity and develops the glomeruli and the convoluted tubules, and an upgrowth from the primitive bladder forms the ureter, the renal pelvis and, by branching, the calyces and the collecting tubules. Anatomical malformations may be encountered which have been caused by slight variations or defects in this development. For instance, the kidney may completely fail to develop but the ureter may be present. The ureteric bud may branch prematurely, producing two separate pelves, or even two complete ureters on one side. Failure of the two primitive parts to join is thought by some to be the cause of polycystic kidneys.

Specimens which show the results of obstruction to the flow of urine may also be seen. The most common sites of obstruction are in the male urethra, particularly in the region of the prostate. Blocks also frequently occur at the lower end of the ureter, at the pelvi–ureteric junction or within the kidneys. A common cause of blockage is a stone *(calculus)* formed by precipitation of a chemical compound which should normally be held in solution in the urine. Uric acid, oxalates and phosphates are the most common of such chemical substances.

### 28.9.3 The genital system

**(1) *The female mammary glands***

These are considered here although they are modified skin appendages – modified sweat glands. Each consists of about twenty or more units of branched and coiled glands, embedded in adipose and fibrous tissue, and opening by separate ducts on to the surface of the nipple. *Note* the lymphatic drainage of the breast which is of great importance in the spread of breast cancers.

**(2) *The female genital organs***

Note their size, shape, and histological features and how to orientate the pelvic organs for photography. Numerous follicles gradually mature in the ovaries during the life of the female and in these follicles develop the ova. At a certain time during each menstrual cycle a 'ripe' follicle ruptures, discharging the ovum from the surface of the ovary into the Fallopian (uterine) tube. The ovum is carried down this tube by the action of its lining ciliated columnar epithelium and, if fertilized, becomes embedded in the prepared uterus, where it subsequently develops into a foetus. The ovaries sometimes develop cysts and tumours which cause enlargement and malignant tumours may spread to involve adjacent structures.

The uterine muscle very commonly forms simple smooth muscle tumours *(fibroids)* which may cause considerable enlargement, distortion and dysfunction of the organ. Although benign they are responsible for a great deal of pelvic and menstrual symptoms in women and some of their complications can be quite serious. Cancer may develop in the epithelial lining of either the body or the cervix and these two tumours together with those of the ovary and breast constitute the bulk of malignant tumours in the female.

**(3) *The male genital organs***

The germ cells of the male (the spermatozoa) develop in coiled tubules in the testes, normally situated in the scrotal sacs. The sperms, when mature, pass through this coiled duct system through the epididymis to the ductus deferens. This duct passes up from the scrotal sac, along the inguinal canal through the abdominal wall into the pelvis, and ultimately opens into the prostatic part of the urethra. The point where it penetrates the wall of the abdomen is a point of potential weakness and here a *hernia* (rupture) may develop. The seminal vesicles act as a storehouse for spermatozoa, and the volume of seminal fluid is increased by fluid secretions from the seminal vesicles, the prostate gland and the glands of Cowper.

## 28.10 THE RETICULO-ENDOTHELIAL SYSTEM

The reticulo-endothelial system is composed of cells which are widely scattered in the body, but which are found in large numbers in the bone marrow, the spleen, the liver and lymph nodes. The reticulum cells are capable of phagocytic activity and the system was first clearly demonstrated by injecting into the bloodstream finely divided dye particles which were taken up by the reticulo-endothelial cells. They are, of course, also able to ingest other foreign particles like bacteria, and it was soon discovered that this system was also concerned in the formation of specific *antibodies* which help to protect the body against infections. The reticulo-endothelial cells, particularly those in the spleen, are also used in the breakdown of red blood cells.

### 28.10.1 The spleen (weight 160 g.)

It is situated in the abdomen, in the left hypochondrium, and is anatomically related to the left kidney, the tail of the pancreas, the stomach and colon. Apart from its functions as part of the reticulo-endothelial system it can also act in some animals as a reservoir of red cells which can be used quickly in the event of a sudden haemorrhage.

### 28.10.2 Diseases of the reticulo-endothelial system

The medical photographer should at least understand the major groups of these diseases.

*Inflammations* – excess activity is often associated with enlargement of these organs. The large, tender lymph nodes draining a septic focus and the large, soft spleen of *septicaemia* are well known.

*Lipoid storage diseases* – fatty substances may accumulate in the reticulo-endothelial system owing to their faulty metabolism and the organs may become greatly enlarged. *Gaucher's disease* is perhaps the best example.

*Reticuloses or lymphomas* – these diseases generally behave as tumours of the reticulo-endothelial system although

their aetiological background is probably variable. Some may result from virus infection, e.g. *Burkitt's lumphoma*. They usually cause considerable enlargement of one or more organs in this system and several of the lymphomas behave as highly malignant neoplasms.
*Blood diseases* – Leukaemias, Polycythaemia, Splenic anaemia, etc.

## 28.11 THE NERVOUS SYSTEM

The brain and spinal cord show, during development, a basically segmented appearance but while the spinal cord retains this in later life the brain has largely lost its segmented pattern.

The nervous system has many analogies with a telephone system and, indeed, it is known that the nervous impulse, conducted along nerve fibrils, is associated with an electrical change in that fibre. The fibres or 'wires' are the elongated cytoplasmic processes of the cells (neurones) and are known as axons. The energy for working the system is derived from metabolic processes occurring in the nerve cells. The wires are gathered up into bundles or trunks (nerves) and cross connections are made in the central nervous system – the brain and spinal cord which are the main 'telephone exchange'. When an impulse has to 'jump' from one neurone to the next, or from a neurone to a muscle fibre, a chemical substance is formed at the nerve ending (acetylcholine) which acts as the stimulus to the receiving unit.

In the past the axons (axis cylinders) of the nerve cells have been classified as myelinated and non-myelinated, but it is realized now that there are no such inherent differences and that all have at least a fine outer sheath of fatty material (myelin). This is known to be an electrical insulator and is also probably vitally concerned with the propagation of the nerve impulse.

Most of the day-to-day messages controlling the activity of glands, smooth muscle, the heart, etc., are sent without the individual being aware of this activity, and he cannot exercise any conscious control over these messages. A special group of nerves is used for this purpose – the autonomic nerve system. Activity directly under the control of the brain, or which may be controlled at will if necessity arises, is regulated by nerve impulses which pass along the ordinary peripheral nerves. The information passing towards the central nervous system from skin, muscle, joints, etc., travels in afferent (sensory) fibres. Messages passing from the central nervous system to cause muscle contraction pass along efferent (motor) fibres. In each of these types of fibre there is virtually 'one-way traffic' only, but for convenience motor and sensory fibres are usually trunked together into mixed nerves.

Some cranial nerves are mixed but most are purely sensory or motor. Spinal segmental nerves are always mixed – the component fibres separating close to the spinal cord as sensory and motor roots. Be familiar with the anatomical plan of the autonomic nerve system and its two component parts the *sympathetic* and *parasympathetic* systems and note the opposing physiological actions of these two components. Note also the development of miniature relay stations (ganglia) and the close relationship anatomically and physiologically of the sympathetic nerves with the adrenal glands.

The nerve cells in the central nervous system are mainly aggregated into special regions known as the grey matter and the axons of the cells are for most of their course situated in the white matter – white and glistering because of its high myelin content. The neurones and their fibres are supported and maintained by a special type of connective tissue called the neuroglia. Although some degree of correlation between sensation and motor function is undertaken in the spinal cord,

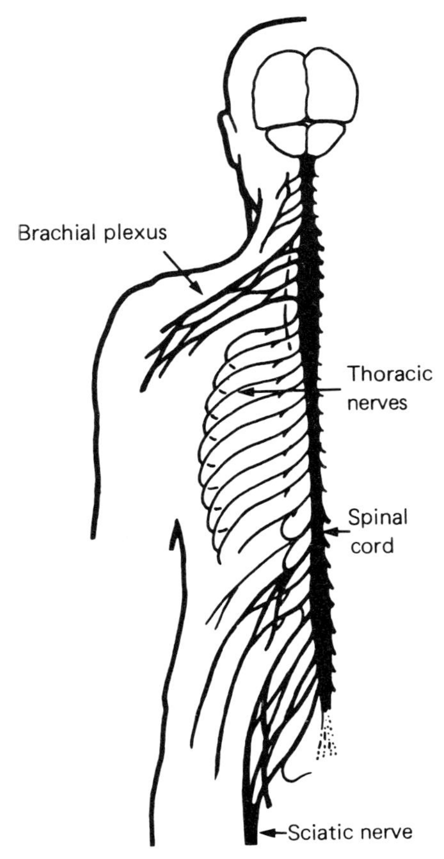


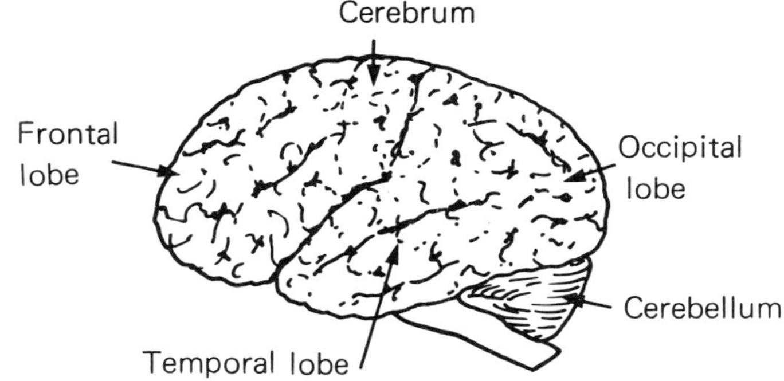


***Figure 28.6*** *(Above) The external appearance of the brain*

***Figure 28.27*** *(Left) The major nerve plexuses and spinal cord*

***Figure 28.28*** *(Below) A mid-sagittal section through the brain*

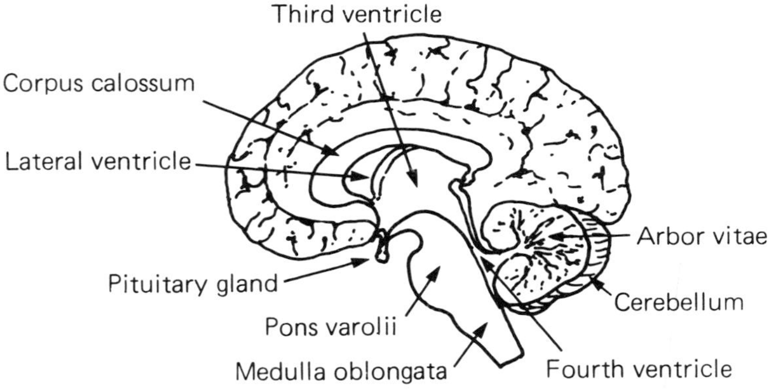

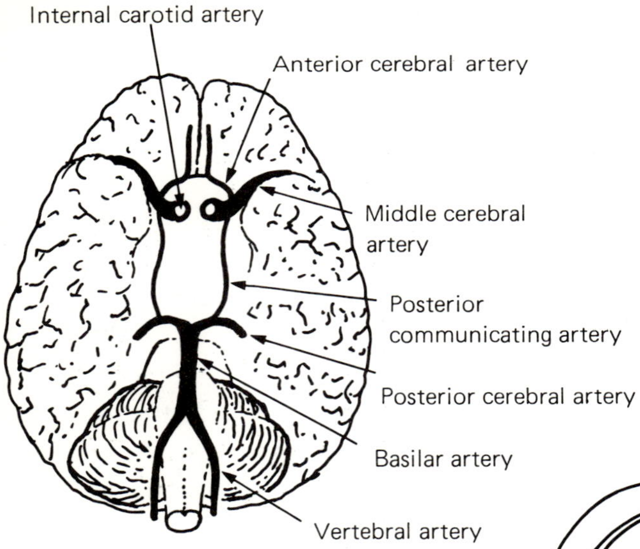

***Figure 28.29*** *(Above) The arterial blood supply to the base of the brain*

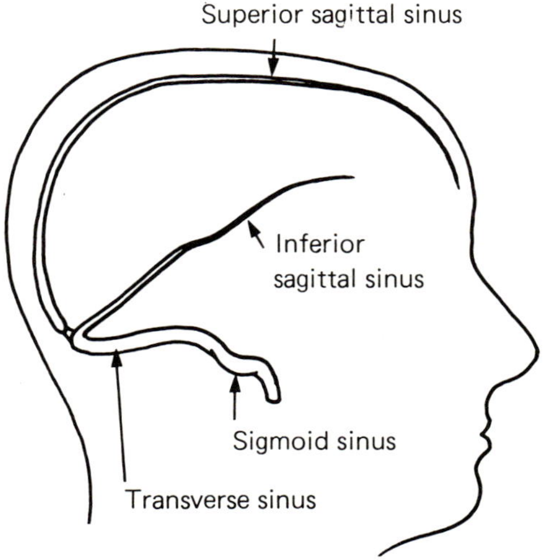

***Figure 28.30*** *(Right) The major venous sinuses of the brain which drain into the internal jugular vein*

the most important and complex correlations and the exercise of 'will' are performed in the cerebral hemispheres of the brain. The *cerebellum* is concerned particularly with the preservation of balance and the many coordinating procedures related to this. A good anatomy or pathology museum or access to post-mortem material would be of great help in learning the various regions of the brain and their relations with the dural folds and the various parts of the bony skull or cranium.

The brain tissue is bathed by a fluid – the *cerebrospinal fluid* (CSF) – which acts in many ways as the lymph does in other organs and tissues, but also forms a fluid cushion between the soft central nervous system tissue and the hard bony skull. It is secreted from the blood in the *choroid plexuses*, which are suspended in cavities – the ventricles – inside the brain. The fluid then circulates through the ventricular system back into the dural venous sinusoids. Make a drawing to ensure you understand this circulation of the CSF. Occasionally this circulation is blocked, and hydrocephalus results, (special photographic techniques exist for recording this - *see Section 10*). The meninges (connective tissue coverings of the brain and spinal cord) are composed of three layers, the outer tough *dura mater* and two delicate inner layers the *pia mater* and the *arachnoid mater*.

The arterial Circle of Willis, situated at the base of the brain, is supplied by the internal carotid arteries and the vertebral arteries. *Berry aneurysms* sometimes develop on this arterial circle or its main branches and these many rupture, giving rise to an often fatal *subarachnoid haemorrhage*. Small branches of these vessels within the brain substances sometimes rupture in hypertensive patients (*cerebral apoplexy*).

Blockage of the cerebral arteries may occur either by a clot *(thrombus)* developing as a result of disease in these vessels or by a portion of thrombus becoming dislodged, circulating in the arterial system *(embolism)* and ultimately impacting in one of the cerebral vessels. Such a block in the vascular supply to the brain often causes death of brain tissue *(infarction)* which may liquefy *(cerebral softening)*.

*Note* the close relationship between the middle ear, in the petrous temporal bone, and the temporal lobe of the cerebral hemisphere above and the cerebellar hemisphere behind. Septic infection in the middle ear cavities may spread into these adjacent regions of the brain.

Tumours of nervous tissues are by no means uncommon. They may occur on peripheral nerves as nerve sheath tumours *neurilommomas* or *neurofibromas* which may be multiple. The dural coat of the meninges generally produces benign tumours – the *meningiomas*, and the central nervous system gives rise to the *gliomas*, which are invariably malignant. While nerve cell tumours *(neuroblastomas)* may occur in the sympathetic nerve plexus and the adrenal glands they are almost unheard of in the central nervous system itself.

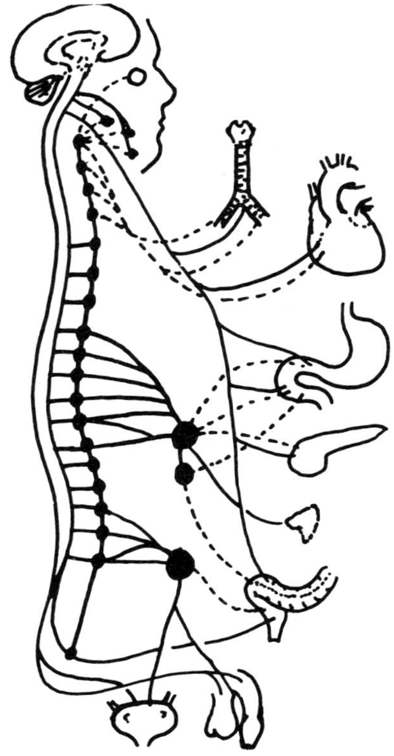

***Figure 28.31*** *A schematic diagram of the sympathetic and parasympathetic nerve pathways*

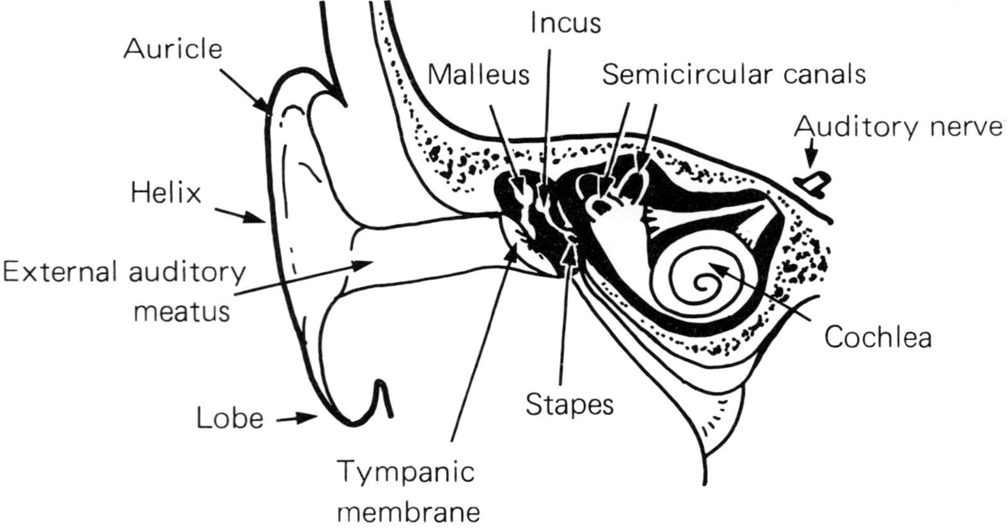


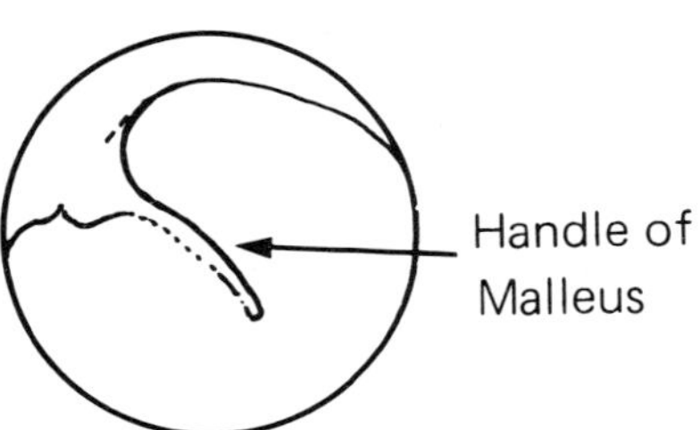


***Figure 28.32*** *The ear in cross-section. The inset (below left) shows the external appearance of the tympanic membrane*

## 28.12 ORGANS OF SPECIAL SENSE

### 28.12.1 The eye

The medical photographer must understand fully the similarities and differences between the eye and the camera. He should also have a clear knowledge of the general anatomy of the eye and its relations in the orbital cavity of the skull. The functions of the ciliary apparatus and the circulation of the aqueous humour in the anterior and posterior chambers should be noted. *Glaucoma* results from abnormal function of this system.

The retina should be viewed through the pupil, using an ophthalmoscope, when it will be possible to see many of the surface blood vessels and the paler *optic disc*, the area where the optic nerve enters – the 'blind spot'. The *macula lutea* is the most sensitive and critical part of the retina, situated in a position where the visual axis strikes the retinal layer. Study of the transverse section of the eye will show that light passes through virtually the whole thickness of the retina before it can influence the *rods* and *cones* – the light-sensitive structures which are situated in the deepest layer of the retina.

The conjunctiva, the iris and the ciliary apparatus may all become involved by various inflammatory reactions. Cysts of the eyelids (*Meibomian cysts*) are quite common and two malignant tumours of the eye, fortunately rather uncommon, are the *malignant melanoma* and the *retinoblastoma*, which occurs in young children. Because of this special knowledge of optics and his involvement in ophthalmic photography the medical photographer will be expected to be *fully* conversant with the structure and functions of the eye and its component parts.

### 28.12.2 The ear

There are two separate anatomical parts:

(1) The apparatus for the reception of sound waves, comprising the *external auditory meatus*, the *tympanic membrane* (drum), the *ossicles (malleus, incus and stapes)* in the middle ear, and the *cochlea*. The mechanism for translating mechanical sound waves into nerve impulses conducted along the cochlear nerve to the brain must be understood.

(2) The apparatus for the preservation of balance, comprising the *semicircular canals* (in three planes at right-angles to each other) and the *utriculus* and *sacculus* (with otoliths). *Note* their bony relations to the petrous temporal bones, their minute anatomical structure and the functions of each part.

Infections may spread up from the nasopharynx via the Eustachian tubes into the middle ear *(otitis media)*, and from there the infection can spread further into the communicating mastoid air cells *(mastoiditis)*, and occasionally even into the adjacent meninges, temporal lobes and cerebellum which are close relations of the petrous temporal bone.

## 28.13 THE ENDOCRINE SYSTEM

The endocrine (ductless) glands are the organs which secrete, into the blood stream, hormones – chemical substances which act, usually for prolonged periods of time, on other tissues and organs. In this way they have a controlling influence on such things as skeletal growth, metabolism, sexual development and behaviour, and the reactions of the body to alarm and various types of stress.

### 28.13.1 The pituitary gland

This has a controlling influence on several other endocrine glands; consists of two lobes – the anterior developed from the pharynx, and the posterior developed from the brain. It lies in the sella turcica in the floor of the cranium.

The anterior lobe is composed of masses of epithelial cells richly supplied by thin-walled blood sinusoids, an arrangement commonly found in endocrine glands, and includes at least three types of cell classified according to their manner of staining as:

The non-granular chromophobes which comprises about 50% of the cells,
Granular eosinophil cells 40%, and
Granular basophil cells 10%.

The chromophobe is a precursor cell, and the granular cells actively secrete the hormones. The eosinophil cells appear definitely related to synthesis of new body proteins and growth of the individual, particularly skeletal growth. Lack of this 'growth hormone' is responsible for some types of *dwarfism* and increased secretion, such as may occur from a tumour (*eosinophil adenoma*), of these cells may cause *gigantism*, in young adults, or *acromegaly* in older persons, in whom most of the epiphyses of the skeleton have united before the adenoma develops.

The basophil granular cells secrete several hormones. The following are well known:

Gonadotrophins luteinizing-hor-

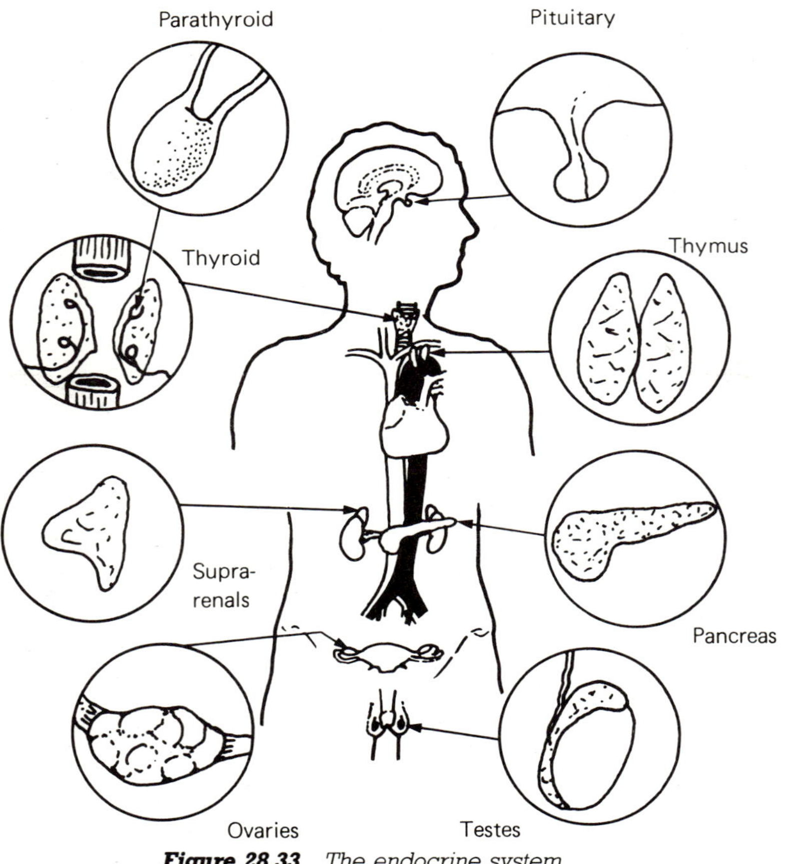


***Figure 28.33*** *The endocrine system*

mone and follicle-stimulating hormones) which have as their target the ovary.

Adrenocorticortrophin which controls some adrenal cortical hormone secretions.

Thyrotrophins which influence the thyroid.

There are several other less well studied hormones secreted by the anterior pituitary cells.

Not only does the pituitary influence these other 'target' organs but a feedback system has been demonstrated, in the case of the adrenal cortex, controlling the secretion of pituitary adrenocorticotrophin. This provides a very delicate balance, maintained according to the body's needs, but on occasion a disturbance of the mechanism may lead to disease. Serious destruction of the pituitary may result from the circulatory collapse associated with a severe post-partum haemorrhage, and death of the patient may occur within a week or two of such a catastrophe. More chronic destruction of the gland occurs by slow compression of the glandular tissue by adjacent tumours or some other expanding pathological lesion. The patient declines gradually with wasting of organs, body tissues and the sexual and other endocrine glands (*Simmonds' cachexia).*

The posterior lobe is intimately related developmentally, anatomically and functionally with the hypothalamic region of the brain above it. There is now evidence that its hormones, the anti-diuretic hormone (vasopressin) and oxytocin, are secreted in the hypothalamus and passed down the pituitary stalk to the posterior part of the gland where they may be stored. These hormones are chemically very similar, and they seem to stimulate smooth muscle to contract, e.g., in arteries, pregnant uterus and breast ducts. The antidiuretic hormone has a powerful effect on the renal convoluted tubules and *diabetes insipidus*, due to damage in the hypothalamic and posterior pituitary tissues, causes the kidneys to secrete a large volume of very low specific gravity urine.

### 28.13.2 Thyroid gland

Situated in the neck below the larynx and fairly firmly adherent to the trachea, it is composed of two lateral lobes and an isthmus. The thyroid, itself controlled by the pituitary, controls the general rate of metabolism (and therefore growth in infancy). It is composed of numerous closely-packed acini of epithelial cells closely related to the blood vessels. The cells secrete a hormone – thyroxine – which may be passed into the blood for immediate use or may be stored in the form of colloid in the lumen of the acini for secretion later. Excessive storage of colloid may occur under various conditions and give rise to a *goitre*. Excessive secretion by a highly overactive epithelium, with little storage, is seen in *thyrotoxicosis* (exophthalmic goitre). Lack of secretion due to deficiency of secretory epithelial cells causes *cretinism* in infants and *myxoedema* in adult life. The clinical pictures of each condition are often striking and photogenic and serial photographs are useful in recording progress.

Another hormone secretion of the thyroid has recently been discovered – *calcitonin,* secreted by a para-follicular cell and having an action physiologically antagonistic to the parathyroid hormone.

### 28.13.3 The parathyroid glands

There are four in all and usually closely apposed to the thyroid capsule posteriorly and often difficult to find. The histological picture is rather similar to the pituitary gland, but only two varieties of cell are described, the chief cell and the oxyphil. The hormone secreted controls the balance of calcification and decalcification of bone and, secondarily, the levels of calcium and phosphorus in the blood. Parathyroid lack causes *tetany* due to a low blood calcium. Increased parathyroid activity causes decalcification, softening and cyst formation in the bones, and the blood calcium rises *(generalized fibrocystic disease of bones).* An adenoma or hyperplasia of the gland can cause this type of disease.

### 28.13.4 The adrenals

These are bilateral organs situated above, and in close contact with, the upper poles of the kidneys. They are composed of:

*Cortex* – epithelial in nature and with abundant yellow lipoid content. *Note* that there is also a brown inner pigmented zone.
*Medulla* – derived from sympathetic nervous tissue, white in colour.

The medulla secretes hormones known as catecholamines, principally noradrenaline and adrenaline, which prepare the body for 'activity', as does the rest of the sympathetic nervous system. The output of the heart rises, blood pressure increases, pulse rate rises and food stores are mobilized.

A tumour of the adrenal medulla

*(phaeochromocytoma)* may cause serious attacks of high blood pressure due to excessive hormone secretion. Another tumour the *neuroblastoma,* occurs mainly in children and usually behaves as a highly malignant neoplasm spreading to the lymph nodes, liver and bones.

In recent years the importance of the adrenal cortex has been established. It secretes hormones which control:

> The correct development of the sex organs,
> The electrolyte (salt) and fluid metabolism, and
> Carbohydrate, protein and fat metabolism.

Severe destruction of adrenal cortical tissue (for instance, by tuberculosis) may cause *Addison's disease*, the patient suffering from low blood pressure, low blood sugar levels, bronzing of the skin and muscle weakness.

The adrenal cortex may undergo hyperplasia or develop simple adenomas or malignant carcinomas. These are often associated with evidence of hypersecretion of the various hormones produced in the cortex. *Conn's syndrome* is due to excessive secretion of aldosterone produced in the outer (zona glomerulosa) region of the gland. The patient develops hypertension, muscle weakness and polyuria. *Cushing's syndrome,* caused by excessive cortisol secretion, produces a well known and highly photogenic condition. The patient has a round 'moon' face, adiposity of the trunk, hirsuties, hypertension, diabetes, etc.

In the *adrenogenital syndromes* one finds a variety of clinical pictures according to the sex of the patient, the severity of the hormone dysfunction and the age at which the disease develops. It may cause *pseudohermaphroditism* if it operates during embryonic life, or an apparent change of sex due to changes in secondary sexual characters if it operates in later life. In some small children both an excessive sexual and muscular development occurs *(infant Hercules type).*

In recent years the damping effects of cortisone (one of the adrenal cortical hormones) upon inflammatory reactions in the body have been noted, and cortisone has been found to be of some therapeutic value in the control of some inflammatory conditions.

### 28.13.5 Pancreas

Apart from the zymogenic tissue, which secretes the enzymes for digestion, the pancreas has 'islet tissue' which secretes insulin into the blood stream. Insulin controls the storage of glycogen in the liver and its breakdown into glucose as required. It is also responsible for the correct utilization of glucose by the muscles and other tissues. If the islet tissue is deficient in cells the supply of insulin is impaired and the patient suffers from *diabetes mellitus.* Hyperglycaemia and glycosuria result and sometimes ketones and similar metabolic products accumulate in the blood stream causing *diabetic coma.* These patients often have to inject themselves with insulin to take over the normal function of the pancreatic islet secretion. Excessive production of insulin sometimes occurs in patients who have *'islet cell tumours',* and in these cases there is an intermittent low blood sugar with all symptoms and signs of an 'insulin overdose'. Recently, it has been recognized that islet cell tumours may in some patients secrete excessive amounts of *gastrin* which causes in turn a greatly increased secretion of gastric acid and the production of *intractable peptic ulcers.*

### 28.13.6 Thymus

This is a lymphoid organ of rather special character situated in the lower neck and superior mediastinum in front of and above the pericardium. It grows in early childhood and then atrophies in adult life gradually becoming replaced by adipose tissue. It appears that certain immunological processes, particularly those concerned with acquired hypersensitivity, e.g. the tuberculin reaction, and with rejection of grafts, are linked with the thymus gland and the circulating lymphocytes in the blood stream, the lymphocytes playing a part in recognizing foreign cells and in destroying them. The thymus gland is included with the endocrine organs since a hormone secretion is suspected but not proven at the present time. There is no doubt that thymectomy in animals impairs these immunological responses, and in human beings there is a connection, which may be on an immunological basis, between the disease known as *myasthenia gravis* and hyperplasias and tumours *(thymomas)* of the thymic gland.

## References

Boyd, W. (1977). *An Introduction to the Study of Disease*. 8th Edn. (USA: Lea and Febiger)

Curran, R. (1972). *Colour Atlas of Histopathology*. (London: Harvey Miller)

England, M. (1983). *A Colour Atlas of Life Before Birth. (Normal Foetal Development*. (London: Wolfe Medical Publications)

Hamilton, W. (1976). *Textbook of Human Anatomy*. (London: Macmillan)

Keogh, B. and Ebbs, S. (1984). *Normal Surface Anatomy and Imaging* (London: Heinemann Medical Books)

Langman, J. (1981). *Medical Embryology*. (Baltimore: Williams and Wilkins)

Leeson, C. (1981). *Histology*. (Philadelphia: W.B. Saunders)

Lockhart, R. (1974). *Living Anatomy*. (London: Faber and Faber)

McMinn, R. and Hutchings, R. (1981). *Colour Atlas of Human Anatomy*. (London: Wolfe Medical Publications)

Miller, A. (1977). *A Summary of Medicine for Nurses and Medical Auxiliaries*. (London: Faber and Faber)

## *Examination questions (basic level)*

Q.1 Describe briefly the Primary function of:
(*a*) Heart,
(*b*) Lungs,
(*c*) Kidneys,
(*d*) Liver.

Q.2 Draw and annotate a cross-sectional diagram of the eye and compare and contrast the mechanism of vision with that of photography.

Q.3 Describe the function of each of the following nerves. Use not more than two sentences in each case.
(*a*) The olfactory nerve,
(*b*) The optic nerve,
(*c*) The oculomotor nerve,
(*d*) The facial nerve,
(*e*) The vagus nerve,
(*f*) The hypoglossal nerve.

Q.4 Describe the circulation of the blood in the heart and lungs naming the parts through which the blood passes. Draw and annotate a diagram and indicate with arrows the direction of blood flow.

Q.5 Explain the relationship between a muscle and its nerve supply and blood supply.

Q.6 State:
(*a*) What are the signs and symptoms of infective disease?
(*b*) What are the access routes of micro-organisms into the body?
(*c*) What is pus?
(*d*) What constitutes a fistula?

Q.7 What is:
(*a*) A disorder of the blood?
(*b*) A disorder of the circulation?
Give examples of each.

Q.8 What is a neurone? What is the difference between motor and sensory nerves? What is the difference between white and grey matter?

Q.9 Draw and annotate a cross-sectional diagram of the skin and briefly explain the function of the parts you have labelled.

Q.10 Draw and annotate a diagram of the main components of the urinary system and briefly explain the function of the kidney.

*Multiple choice (basic level) any of the statements may be true or false.*

Q.11 The following are bones or parts of bones:
(*a*) The olecranon,
(*b*) The ileum,
(*c*) The greater trochanter,
(*d*) The periosteum
(*e*) The hypochondrium.

Q.12 In the normal human adult there is only one of the following:
(*a*) Innominate vein,
(*b*) Cardiac atrium,
(*c*) Portal vein,
(*d*) Thoracic duct,
(*e*) Eustachian tube.

Q.13 The following are all parts of the alimentary canal:
(*a*) Oesophagus
(*b*) Ilium,
(*c*) Thoracic duct,
(*d*) Caecum,
(*e*) Gastrocnemius.

Q.14 The following muscles are all found in the thoracic region:
(*a*) Soleus,
(*b*) External oblique,
(*c*) Intercostal,
(*d*) Buccinator,
(*e*) Vastus medialis.

Q.15 The following arteries are branches of the aorta:
(*a*) Coeliac artery,
(*b*) Renal artery,
(*c*) Mesenteric artery,
(*d*) Popliteal artery,
(*e*) Testicular artery.

## *Examination questions (advanced level)*

Q.1 Describe a reflex arc with full details of how nerve impulses are conducted.

Q.2 Draw an annotated diagram of the female mammary gland, and describe the hormonal control of lactation. List the advantages of breast and bottle feeding.

Q.3 (*a*) Define the following and state their precise location:
(*1*) Pituitary fossa,
(*2*) Suprarenal gland,
(*3*) Lung hilum,
(*4*) Ilium,
(*5*) Aorta.
(*b*) Make a labelled diagram of a transverse section through the mid-thorax.

Q.4 By following the course of a ham sandwich from mouth to anus, describe how the food is digested. Include details of the anatomy of the alimentary canal and the various digestive juices secreted.

Q.5 Name and describe the components of blood, list the functions of the blood and describe briefly a blood dyscrasia with which you are familiar.

Q.6 Draw a sagittal section of the male reproductive system, suitably annotated. Tabulate the differences/similarities of mitosis and meiosis.

Q.7 What and where are the following:
(*a*) The zygomatic arch,
(*b*) The acetabulum,
(*c*) The sinu-atrial node,
(*d*) Wharton's duct,
(*e*) The vomer,
(*f*) The cricoid,

Q.8 Discuss the concept of homeostasis.

Q.9 Describe briefly the following terms:
(*a*) Reticulo-endothelial system
(*b*) Antigen
(*c*) Acquired immunity
(*d*) Autoimmune disease
(*e*) Immunosuppression
(*f*) Antihistamine

Q.10 Draw a detailed and annotated diagram of a kidney nephron. Explain the functions of each component of the nephron.

*Multiple choice (advanced level) any of the statements may be true or false*

Q.11
(*a*) The carpal groove is made into a tunnel by the transverse radial ligament.
(*b*) The shape of the carpus on its palmar aspect from side to side is deeply concave.
(*c*) The muscle which arises from the apex of the glenoid and is inserted into the radial tuberosity, is the glenoid.
(*d*) The clavicle begins to ossify before any other bone.
(*e*) The capitate lies opposite the base of the second metacarpal.

Q.12 The following are all bones in the foot:
(*a*) Navicular,
(*b*) Pisiform,
(*c*) Cuboid,
(*d*) Cuneiform,
(*e*) Scaphoid.

Q.13 The following neoplasms are malignant:
(*a*) Adenoma,
(*b*) Papilloma,
(*c*) Epithelioma,
(*d*) Lipoma,
(*e*) Fibrosarcoma.

Q.14 The trigeminal nerve:
(*a*) Is the third cranial nerve,
(*b*) Supplies the superior oblique muscles,
(*c*) Arises in the cerebellum,
(*d*) Is the smallest cranial nerve,
(*e*) Consists of only sensory nerves.

Q.15 The following structures are to be found in the ear:
(*a*) Canal of Schlemm,
(*b*) Scala vestibuli,
(*c*) Anterior primary rami,
(*d*) Septum lucidum,
(*e*) Basilar membrane.

# Section 29
# Medical terminology

**A.R. Williams**, MPhil, FBIPP, FRPS, FBPA, AIMBI
Head of Medical Illustration and Teaching Services
Charing Cross Hospital and Medical School, London

## 29.1 INTRODUCTION

Student medical photographers are often bemused and bewildered when they first enter the profession by the medical terminology used. It is perhaps easiest to think of it as being another language, the language of hospital practice, with its own vocabulary, syntax, etc., founded in Graeco-Roman roots like any other European language. Like any other language the best way to learn it, to continue the analogy, is to immerse oneself in foreign territory and speak and write the language. Whenever a new term is encountered the student should look it up in a pocket dictionary and make brief notes in a pocket book. Similarly, every time a new diagnosis is met, look it up in the dictionary and make notes on the condition, its cause, what there is to see and photograph. As you gain experience so your vocabulary will grow. The study of anatomy and physiology, and the systematic study of the specialist sections of this book will give a broad foundation on which to build. Three books are invaluable in learning this new language, they are:

*Medical Terms : Their Origin and Construction.* F. Roberts (Heinemann, London)

*Practical Terminology in Hospital Practice.* P.M.Davies (Heinemann, London)

*Dictionary of Abbreviations in Medicine and Related Sciences.* E.Steen (Baillière Tindall, London)

Also a good pocket medical dictionary such as *Livingstone's Pocket Medical Dictionary*, by N. Roper, or Bailliére's *Nurses Pocket Dictionary*, is absolutely essential.

The student will find a certain amount of confusion in medical terminology. Anatomical terms have been changed frequently by various congresses and committees so that some generations of doctors use terms different from those of other generations. Human anatomical terms often also differ from those of comparative anatomy and both will be met in medical photography. Confusion in pathological terms is even worse; mainly arising from the fact that the cause of so many diseases is doubtful or completely unknown. Pathological conditions are sometimes known by the names of people who described them and also by terms which imply an aetiological basis for the disease. Such an example is a particular tumour of the kidney which is variously known as a Grawitz tumour, a hypernephroma and a carcinoma of the renal tubules.

## 29.1 DERIVATION OF THE COMPLEX TERM

The student should not be intimidated by complex terminology – these terms are often derived from simple roots which should be familiar. Take for example the term 'pulmonary hypertrophic osteoarthropathy'. The technique is to split this into simple roots, prefixes and suffixes, as follows:

pulmonary/hyper/trophic/
osteo/arthro/pathy

where pulmonary means relating to the lungs, hyper means excessive, trophic means nutrition/growth, osteo means relating to bones, arthro means relating to joints, pathy means disease. So already we have a disease of the bones and joints with some overgrowth, due to pulmonary influence. One could then logically deduce that there would be pain, swelling and clubbing. It is almost always possible to do this with composite terms but be careful if the parts do not all have a meaning. For example one might be tempted to split 'gastrocnemius' into 'gastro' meaning pertaining to the stomach, and 'cnemius' of unknown definition – thus guessing it to be a disease of the stomach. Whereas in actuality, of course, it is a muscle in the leg.

## 29.3 PREFIXES, SUFFIXES, AND ABBREVIATIONS

Medicine, like any speciality, has a large number of abbreviations in common usage and the student must consult the texts quoted above for a complete glossary. A short list of the more commonly used prefixes, suffixes and abbreviations, is recorded here for the convenience of the student.

### Prefixes and suffixes

a– – absence of
ab– – away from
acro– – extremity
actino– – ray
ad– – towards
adamant– – hard
aden– – gland(s)
adip– – fat
–aemia – blood
–aesthesia – sensation
algi– – pain
amb– – both
an– – without
andr– – male
angio– – vessel(s)
ankylo– – bent, adhesion
ante– – before
anti– – opposed to
arthr– – joints
–ase – enzyme
astheno– – weak
atelo– – incomplete
aur– – ear(s)
auto– – self

bi– – two
bil– – bile
bio– – life
blepharo– – eyelid
brachio– – arm
brachy– – short
brady– – slow

calc– – calcium
cardi– – heart–orifice to stomach
caud– – tail–lower part of the body
–cele– – swelling containing fluid
–centesis – perforate
cephal– – head
cervico– – neck
cholangi– – bile ducts
chole– – biliary system
cholecyst– – gall bladder
choledoch– – common bile duct
chondr– – cartilage
chromo– – colour
–cide – destroy
circum– – around
cleido– – clavicle
–coele – swelling containing fluid
col– – colon
con– – together, with
cranio– – skull
cryo– – cold
crypto– – concealed
cyano– – blue
cyst– – bladder
cyto– – cell

dactyl– – fingers or toes
dent– – tooth
derm– – skin
–desis – binding
dextro– – right
di– – two
dia– – through
diplo– – double
dorso– – back
dys– – difficult

e– – out
–ectasis – dilate
ecto– – outside
–ectomy – cutting out, removal
ectra– – outside
–emesis – vomit
en– – in or into
encephal– – brain
end– – inside, inner
enter– – intestine
epi– – upon
epiphysi– – epiphysis
erythro– – red

| | |
|---|---|
| eu– | – well, easy |
| ex– | – out |
| extra– | – on the outside |
| fibro– | – fibrous connective tissue |
| –fugal | – move away from |
| gastr– | – stomach |
| gen– | – referring to production |
| –genic | – producing |
| genu– | – knee |
| gloss– | – tongue |
| –graphy | – recording |
| gyn– | – female |
| haem– | – blood |
| hemi– | – half |
| hepat– | – liver |
| hetero– | – dissimilar |
| hidro– | – sweat |
| homo– | – similar |
| hydro– | – fluid |
| hyper– | – above – in excess |
| hypo– | – beneath, less than normal |
| hyster– | – uterus |
| iatro– | – medicine |
| idio– | – self |
| in– | – in |
| infra– | – below |
| inter– | – between |
| intra– | – within |
| isch– | – deficiency |
| iso– | – same |
| –itis | – inflammation |
| juxta– | – near |
| karyo– | – nucleus |
| kato– | – down, against |
| kera– | – horny |
| kinesi– | – movement |
| koilo– | – hollow |
| labio– | – lips |
| laparo– | – abdomen |
| leuko– | – white |
| lien– | – spleen |
| linguo– | – tongue |
| lipo– | – fat or lipids |
| lith– | – stone |
| –logy | – science |
| lymph– | – lymphatic system |
| lymphangi– | – lymph vessels |
| -lysis | – dissolve |
| macro– | – enlarged |
| mal– | – bad |
| –malacia | – softening |
| mamm–<br>mast– } | – breast |
| mega– | – big |
| men– | – month |
| meso– | – middle |
| meta– | – change |
| myel– | – bone marrow or spinal cord |
| myo– | – muscles |
| nano– | – small |
| necro– | – death |
| neo– | – new |
| nephr– | – kidneys |
| neuro– | – nerve |
| ob– | – in front of |
| ocul– | – eye(s) |
| odont– | – tooth |
| –odynia | – pain |
| –oid | – form |
| oligo– | – few |
| –ology | – study of (loosely) |
| –oma | – tumour |
| onycho– | – nail |
| ophthalm– | – eye(s) |
| or– | – mouth |
| orchi– | – testis(es) |
| ortho– | – straight |
| os– | – bone(s) |
| –ostomy | – making a hole in |
| ot– | – ear(s) |
| pachy– | – thick |
| palin– | – again |
| pan– | – all |
| para– | – change or near |
| –pathy | – abnormality |
| ped– | – child |
| –penia | – deficiency |
| per– | – through |

peri– – around
phago– – devour
–phila – affinity for
phleb– – vein(s)
–plasia – form
–plasty – moulding
–plegia – paralysis
pneum– – lung(s)
–pnoea – breath
poly– – many
port– – portal vein
post– – after
pre–, pro– – before
proct– – rectum
proto– – first
pseudo– – false
psyche– – of the mind
–ptosis – falling
pyel– – kidney(s)
pyo– – pus

retro– – behind
–rhagia – excessive flow
–rhea – flow
rhin– – nose
–rrhaphy – suturing

salping– – uterine tube
sangui– – blood
sapro– – decay
sarco– – flesh
schisto– – divide, cleft
sclero– – hard
scolio– – twisted
sial– – salivary gland(s)
soma– – body
spondyl– – vertebra(ae)
–stasis – standing still
stetho – chest
stomato– – mouth
sub– – under
super–, supra– – above
syn– – together
syringo– – tube

terato– – monster
thrombo– – clot
tomo– – section
–tomy – cutting or cutting into
toxic– – poison
trachelo– – neck
trans– – through, across
–trophy – nourish
–uria – urine

vaso– – blood vessel
vesic– – urinary bladder

xantho– – yellow
xero– – dry

## Abbreviations

### A

ACH – adrenal cortical hormone
ACTH – adrenocortico trophic hormone
AE – after evacuation
AEG – air encephalogram
AF – atrial fibrillation
AFB – acid fast bacilli
AFM – after fatty meal
AI – aortic incompetence
AI(D) – artificial insemination (donor)
AM – after micturition
AOD – arterial occlusive disease
AP – anteroposterior
– artificial pneumothorax
APC – aspirin-phenacetin-cafein
APM – anterior poliomyelitis
ARD – acute respiratory disease
AS – aortic stenosis
ASD – atrial septal defect
AV – arterio-venous

### B

Ba – barium
BBS – battered baby syndrome
BCC – basal cell carcinoma
BCG – Bacille Calmette–Guérin TB test
BD – twice a day

BI – bony injury
BID – brought in dead
BMR – basal metabolic rate
BP – blood pressure
BS – breath sounds
BSR – blood sedimentation rate

## C

Ca – carcinoma
CBD – common bile duct
CCF – congestive cardiac failure
CDH – congenital dislocation of hip
CH – crown heel foetal
CR – crown rump measurement
CHD – coronary heart disease
CNS – central nervous system
CSF – cerebrospinal fluid
CT – coronary thrombosis
CVA – cerebrovascular accident
CVD – cerebrovascular disease
CXR – chest X-ray

## D

D&C – dilatation and curettage
DD – differential diagnosis
DJD – degenerative joint disease
DLE – disseminated lupus erythematosus
DNA – did not attend
DOA – dead on arrival
DR – diagnostic radiology
DS – disseminated sclerosis
DU – duodenal ulcer

## E

ECF – extracellular fluid
ECG – electrocardiogram
ECT – electroconvulsive therapy
EDC – expected date of confinement
EDD – expected date of delivery
EEG – electro encephalogram
EKG – ECG
EM – electron microscopy
EMG – electromyogram
ENT – ear, nose and throat
EOA – examination, opinion and advice
ESR – erythrocyte sedimentation rate
EUA – examination under anaesthetic

## F

# – fracture
FB – foreign body
Fe – iron
FF – fat-free
FFI – free from infection
FH – family history
FHS – foetal heart sounds
fl – flexion
FMD – foot and mouth disease
FTT – failure to thrive
FUO – fever of undetermined origin

## G

GB – gall bladder
GC – gas chromatography
GE – gastro enterology
GI – gastro intestinal
GIT – gastro intestinal tract
GM – grand mal
GSW – gun shot wound
GU – gastric ulcer
– genito urinary

## H

Hb – haemoglobin
HD – Hansen's disease -
– leprosy
H&E – haematoxylin and eosin
Hg – mercury
HH – hard of hearing
HID – headache, insomnia and depression
HPI – history of present illness
HS – herpes simplex
H&T – hospitalization and treatment

HVD – hypertensive vascular disease

***I***

ICU – intensive care unit
IDK – internal derangement of knee
IF – immuno fluorescence
IH – inguinal hernia
IO – intra ocular
IR – infrared
ISQ – *in statu quo* - as before
ITT – insulin tolerance test
IU(C)D – intra uterine (contraceptive) device
IUD – intrauterine death
IV – intra venous
IVC – inferior vena cava
IVP – intra venous pyelogram
IVT – intra venous transfusion

***K***

KUB – kidneys, ureter, bladder
KS – ketosteroid

***L***

L – left
– lateral
LAO – left anterior oblique
LB – loose body
LBP – low back pain
– low blood pressure
LCM – left costal margin
LE – lupus erythematosus
LIF – left iliac fossa
LKS – liver, kidney, spleen
LL – left lateral
– lower lobe
LMP – last menstrual period
LOM – limitation of movement
LP – lumbar puncture
LV – left ventrical
LVF – left ventricular failure
LZ – lower zone

***M***

MC(J) – metacarpal (joint)
MCP – metacarpo-phalangeal
MD – mentally deficient
– mitral disease
MI – mitral incompetence
– myocardial infarction
MLS – medial/longitudinal section
MM – mucous membrane
MPB – male pattern baldness
MR – mentally retarded
MS – multiple sclerosis
– mitral stenosis
MSU – midstream urine specimen
MT – metatarsal

***N***

NAD – no abnormality detected
NAI – non-accidental injury
NBI – no bone injury
NG – new growth
NOS – not otherwise specified
NSU – non-specific urethritis
NTP – normal temperature and pressure
NYD – not yet diagnosed

***O***

OA – osteo arthritis
O&C – onset and cause
OHD – organic heart disease
OPD – out patient department
OR – operating room

***P***

PA – posterior anterior
PAN – polyarteritis nodosa or
– periarteritis nodosa
Pb – lead
PH – past history
PIC – pain in chest
PID – prolapsed intervertebral disc
PIP – proximal interphalangeal
POP – plaster of paris
PM – post mortem
– petit mal

PMH – past medical history
PP – pustular psoriasis
PPH – post partum haemorrhage
PR – per rectum
PS – pulmonary stenosis
PTB – pulmonary tuberculosis
PTA – prior to admission
PU – peptic ulcer
pass urine
PUO pyrexia of unknown origin
PV – per vaginam
PVD – peripheral vascular disease

***R***

R – right
RA – rheumatoid
Ra – radium
RAO – right anterior oblique
RBC – red blood cells
Rep – repeat
RHD – rheumatic heart disease
RIF – right iliac fossa
RP – retrograde pyelogram
RT – radiotherapy
RTA – road traffic accident
RV – right ventricle
Rx – prescription

***S***

SBE – sub-acute bacterial endocarditis
SBP – systolic blood pressure
SCB – strictly confined to bed
SCL – scleroderma
SI(J) – sacral iliac (joint)
SI(Unit) – international system of units
SIW – self inflicted wound
SLE – systemic lupus erythematosus
SNS – sympathetic nervous system
SOB – short of breath
STS – soft tissue swelling
– serological test for syphilis
SVC – superior vena cava
SVT – supra ventricular tachycardia

***T***

T&A – tonsils and adenoids
TB – tuberculosis
TDS – three times a day
TLC – tender loving care
TMJ – temporo-mandibular joint
TNM – tumour, node, metastases
TP – terminal phalanx
TPR – temperature pulse and respiration

***U***

UCHD – usual childhood disease
UVF – ultraviolet fluorescence
UVL – ultraviolet light

***V***

VC – venereal disease
VDH – valvular disease of the heart
VH – ventricular failure
VM – vasomotor
VOD – venous occlusive disease
VSD – ventricular tachycardia
VV – vulva and vagina

***W***

WBC – white blood cells
WNL – within normal limits
WR – Wassermann reaction

## 29.4 EPONYMS AND FAMOUS NAMES

Very many diseases are named after the men who discovered the disease, or who first reported it. A favourite examination question in the past has been 'name ten famous men in medicine and give a brief description of the disease for which they are chiefly remembered.'

The advanced student should certainly consult texts on medical biography and history to obtain brief biographical detail of the commonly occurring names in medical photography, i.e. those diseases which are often photographed.

A 'model' answer might read as follows:

*Dupuytren's contracture* – a thickening and drawing together of the skin and then underlying tissues in the palm of the hand causing gradual and permanent bending of the fingers. Cured by surgery.

Born into a poor family in 1777 Dupuytren was educated in Paris at the cost of an army officer who took a fancy to him. He had an incredible struggle as a medical student; living for 6 weeks on bread and cheese and using the fat of dissected subjects to make oil for his lamp. He was a very determined man and in 1814 became a surgeon-in-chief, at Hotel Dieu. He was a great teacher and lecturer. He saw 10 000 patients a year and was regarded as a brilliant surgeon. He was cold, overbearing and miserly and tolerated no rivals – but all were forced to admit his abilities. He became a multi-millionaire.

His most famous works were excision of the lower jaw, amputation of the cervix, establishment of an artificial anus, ligation of the subclavian artery and the classification system for burns. He died at the age of 57 in 1835 as a result of a stroke two years earlier.

The same answer at a basic level would not include all the biographical detail. The following is a list of the names which commonly occur in medical photographic practice:

Addison, Albright, Apert, Basedow, Bazin, Behcet, Bell, Bowen, Buerger, Colles, Collins, Crohn, Crouzon, Cushing, Down, Dupuytren, Ehlers, Erb, Fallot, Fröhlich, Gull, Gun, Hashimoto, Heberden, Henoch, Hirschsprung, Hodgkin, Horner, Huntington, Hurler, Hutchinson, Kaposi, Klinefelter, Klippel, Koplick, Ludwig, Marfan, Meibom, Munchausen, Osler, Paget, Parkinson, Peutz, Plummer, Pott, Raynaud, Recklinghausen, Reiter, Robertson, Robin, Sezary, Sjogren, Sprengel, Stevens, Sydenham, Trendelenburg, Turner.

The student must familiarize himself with the diseases or syndromes named after these men. (A syndrome is a set of signs and symptoms that appear together with reasonable consistency.)

## References

Dox, I., Melloni, B. and Eisner, G. (1979). *Melloni's Illustrated Medical Dictionary*. (Baltimore: Williams and Wilkins)

Jablonski, S. (1969). *Illustrated Dictionary of Eponymic Syndromes and Diseases*. (Philadelphia: W.B. Saunders)

Rickards, R. (1980). *Understanding Medical Terms*. (Edinburgh: Churchill Livingstone)

Steen, E. (1971). *Dictionary of Abbreviations in Medicine and Related Sciences*. (London: Baillière Tindall and Cassell)

# Index